Natural Cancer Handbook

Alternative Cancer Treatments

ISBN-13: 9781482368222
ISBN-10: 1482368226

Front cover photograph: Source Image and description:
Dr. Raowf Guirguis. National Cancer Institute Author:
Susan Arnold (photographer)

TABLE OF CONTENTS

Legal Disclaimer:

The information and reference materials contained here are intended solely for the general information of the reader. It is not to be used for treatment purposes, but rather for discussion with the reader's own physician.

The information presented here is not intended to diagnose health problems or to take the place of professional medical care. The information contained herein is neither intended to dictate what constitutes reasonable, appropriate or best care for any given health issue, nor is it intended to be used as a substitute for the independent judgment of a physician for any given health issue.

All content, including text, graphics, images and information, contained in this book is for general information purposes only. If you have persistent health problems or if you have further questions, please consult your health care provider.

1. Introduction

Why You Should Consider Alternative Cancer Treatments

Those who question orthodox medical treatment are often harassed. To specify "orthodox", we mean surgical treatment, chemotherapy and radiation therapy as approved by health authorities and supplied broadly by medical experts.

The alternatives to orthodox treatments are just that - alternate options.

There are a number of questions that may arise about orthodox treatments, but they usually boil down to just one question: which of the orthodox remedies are you going to receive? There are a number of different options among the orthodox treatment options.

The number and type of treatments depends upon exactly where your cancer is situated, the stage at which it has been identified, if it has spread to other locations, your age, and general health status.

In most cases, orthodox cancer treatments will have a powerful effect on a patient's wellbeing. Generally, a patient who is young, fit and healthy (apart from the cancer), is going to be much more able to endure the rigors of conventional cancer therapy than the frail, aged patients who make up the bulk of the cancer statistics.

Virtually all orthodox treatments have unwanted side effects, and in the case of most common cancers, are ineffective as well. They create misery and expense for cancer patients, and do not prolong their lives.

Even though the decision may be made not to use any alternative treatment options, that doesn't mean there is no variation within the types of orthodox treatment. There are multiple combinations of surgery, radiation and chemotherapy.

You are responsible for making the ultimate decision on which treatments you'll receive. You'll base your final decision on knowledge of all of the facts. What are the side effects of a particular kind of treatment? How much will it improve survival from the cancer? You'll need to know the pros and cons of each therapy prior to making your decision.

Keep in mind that professionals may not be correct on their prediction of your prognosis – whether your cancer is curable or incurable, if the advised treatment is going to do exactly what is anticipated, and whether the side effects of treatment will be mild or severe. Even today, medicine is an inexact science.

In the event you accept only orthodox treatment, you will join a group of many millions of cancer patients who have complied previously. Many people have beaten cancer utilizing orthodox treatment. Due to social pressure, it requires courage to decline any type of orthodox treatment, even though a number of patients do so. Many alternative treatments can be used alongside conventional treatments. It is not an all-or-nothing situation.

It is your body and your decision.

Are Inexpensive, Natural Cancer Treatments Widely Available?

Yes.

The problem is that patients will not normally try natural cancer treatments until they find out that the traditional cancer treatments such as chemo, radiation and surgery don't work for them. At that point, they panic and will try anything, often the first alternative treatment they run across, which may or may not be the best for their particular situation.

Cancer is a debilitating and eventually lethal disease, and it is imperative to use reliable and effective cures.

For orthodox physicians, cancers cannot ever be completely cured, and must be managed using radiation, anti-neoplastic drugs or surgery. Patients are never said to be "cured", only to have survived for 5 or 10 year periods before the cancer returns to take their lives. However, practitioners of alternative medicine are claiming that cancers can be cured permanently using purely natural substances such as fruits, vegetables, oils and minerals.

For practitioners of alternative healthcare and therapy, there are many ways to cure cancers. But, how affordable and available are the natural cancer treatments?

In terms of costs, you will always find natural alternatives for cancer irrespective of the depth of your pockets. There are some alternative health clinics which are extremely expensive, while others are close to charitable organizations. Thus, you can be sure of getting something 'natural' to cure cancer – it can be ridiculously cheap or very expensive.

In terms of availability, there are countless outlets through which patients can get access to information about natural cancer treatments. If you read the newspapers and magazines regularly, you would have come across one or two. However, the best source of information is the Internet. While online, the only issue you will have to deal with is that of choice. In fact, there are so many treatments offered online, that consumers often become confused when trying to evaluate which one is best.

Although it has been mentioned that natural cancer treatments can be affordable and are widely availabe, it is important to point out some pitfalls. Some of the so-called alternative health practitioners on the Internet are nothing but scammers and fraudsters. Their only intention is to take advantage of cancer patients desperate for a cure and rip them off. Therefore, one has to be very cautious and wary when dealing with such people online.

A product that claims to eradicate deep-rooted cancer in a matter of days is most likely a fraud. If the claim sounds too good to be true, it probably is. We have tried to include only treatments for which there are numerous anecdotal accounts, or at least some scientific studies.

2. What To Do When You Find Out You Have Cancer

If you have any doubts at all, get retested first to make absolutely sure you have cancer. Considering the cost and trauma of cancer treatment, it is absolutely imperative to be sure of the diagnosis.

The *Journal of Clinical Oncology* has reported that misdiagnosis of some forms of cancer (especially breast cancer, which seems particularly prone to error) is as high as **44 percent.**[1]

There are many non-invasive diagnostic aids to confirm whether you actually have cancer, as opposed to some benign condition. Many tumors produce biochemical tumor markers such as HCG, which can be detected by blood tests. Another example is CA125, an antigen present on 80% of nonmucinous ovarian carcinomas.

The majority of patients will try conventional methods first. After their cancer returns, they begin looking for alternative treatments.

References

(1) Singh H et al, "Errors in cancer diagnosis: current understanding and future directions." J Clin Oncol 25:5009, 2007

3. How To Use This Book

The book is divided into chapters and individual numbered pages.

1. After you have been told you have cancer, get a second opinion.

2. Go to Chapter 8 and remove the most common dietary and environmental causes of cancer. Clean up your internal environment as much as possible.

3. Read the chapter on Vitamin D. Up to 70 % of cancer can be prevented by upgrading your Vitamin D levels, and it also increases the survival rate in cancer patients. Most people have inadequate Vitamin D levels. Take a Vitamin D blood test, which you can do yourself, and send it in by mail. You can buy an accurate Vitamin D test on the web for $75 from ZRT Laboratories.

http://www.zrt.lab.com

4. Start taking coffee enemas, if necessary have a clinic perform them.

5. Make your internal environment slightly alkaline by changing your diet to an alkaline diet. Eat very little meat, no dairy products, and no white flour or white sugar, because these foods have a very acidifying effect on the body's pH level. Eat lots of fruit and vegetables.

6. Read chapter 10 and start following the Johanna Budwig diet. This concise summary spells out exactly what foods to drink and eat and how to modify your body's pH. Remember, cancer cannot live in a well-oxygenated, alkaline environment.

A 90% success rate is quoted by some alternative practitioners in curing cancer with this diet, which can happen in as little as 90 days. Disadvantages are that you will have to continue the diet for the rest of your life, and it has to be followed meticulously.

7. If you have had several courses of chemo and now have multi-drug-resistant cancer, start taking Paw Paw. This plant seems to be an effective alternate treatment against MDR tumors. WARNING: if you do not take Paw Paw at the exact same time every day, it may not work successfully. Take it with food, or you may have severe stomach upset.

8. Take as many of the following anti cancer fighting substances in chapter 10 as you can. None of these have any negative side effects:

Budwig Diet
Beta 1,3D Glucan
Green Food Supplements (Barley Grass, Chlorella, Spirulina)
Melatonin
Noni
Resveratrol
Canadian Resonant light generator
Baking Soda
The Hulda Clark generator

9. Try the secondary anti-cancer substances found in Chapter 11, and consider the treatments listed in Chapters 12-15.

Specific Treatment For Types Of Cancers

The most common cancers worldwide are cancers of the lung, breast, prostate and colon. In America, the most deadly cancers are, in decreasing order: lung, colon and rectal, breast, pancreatic, prostate, leukemia, non-hodgkin lymphoma, liver and intrahepatic bile duct, ovarian, and esophageal.

Several types of cancer are listed below, along with any specialized alternative treatments reputed to be especially effective for that specific cancer.

Adenocarcinoma

ASA

Bone

Artemisinin
Tetracycline

Brain

Note: while many substances test effective against brain cancer cells in-vitro, in-vivo the blood-brain barrier excludes many of them. The following, especially the psychoactive or opiate-related agents, are known to cross the blood-brain barrier.

Cantron/Protocell
Curcumin (optimized bio-available form)
DCA
Low-dose naltrexone
Marijuana (hash oil)
Noscapine
Oleander
Paw paw

Breast

AVOID ALL DAIRY PRODUCTS
Cranberry Juice
Chaparral
Ginger root
Green Tea (ECGC)
Iodine
DCA
Garlic
Tocotrienol

Colon

Black raspberries
Cimetidine
Curcumin
Ginger root
Fucoidan

Gastric

Curcumin

Leukemia

Artemisia
Capsaicin
Fucoidan
Green Tea (ECGC)

Liver

Agaricus blazei
Tocotrienols

Lung

Graviola
Capsaicin

Lymphoma

Artemisia
Curcumin

Oral

Curcumin
Spirulina

Ovarian

Dark red grape juice (resveratrol)
Cranberry Juice
Ginger root
Crinum

Green Tea
Noscapine

Pancreatic

Curcumin

Prostate

Stop ingesting any dairy products
Capsaicin
Cranberry Juice
Crinum
Graviola
Modified Citrus Pectin
Tocotrienols

Skin

Non-Melanoma
BEC 5

Melanoma

tocotrienol

Read all other chapters at your convenience

4. Commonly Used Terms In Cancer Research

In drawing conclusions about the effectiveness of a given cancer cure, scientists use a variety of experimental methods and studies.

Apoptosis

This refers to the self-destruction of cancer cells. This process includes changes which include cell shrinkage, fragmentation of the cell nucleus, chromosomal and nuclear fragmentation. Unlike **necrosis** (death of tissues due to trauma), apoptosis produces cell fragments called apoptotic bodies which are quickly removed by macrophages before the cell contents can spill out onto surrounding tissue and cause inflammatory damage.

Normal cells have a finite lifespan governed by the length of telomeres in the cell. Cancer cells, because of their altered biochemistry, are no longer subject to this control, and reproduce endlessly. Various drugs can restore the normal regulatory function in the cancer cell, at which point the cancer cell dies.

Caspases (the name is derived from **c**ysteine **asp**aspartic prote**ases** or **c**ysteine-dependent **asp**artate-directed prote**ases)** are a family of cysteine proteases, a group of enzymes that break down the amino acid cysteine. These enzymes play an essential role in apoptosis, necrosis, and inflammation. They also regulate maturation in a wide variety of cells. Researchers performing studies of cancer cells frequently mention Caspase activation as a mechanism for apotosis. Twelve caspases have been indentified in humans as of 2009.

It is preferable to induce apoptosis in cancer cells, rather than just poisoning them with toxic chemicals and causing necrosis, because it is a self-contained process that results in the natural death of cancer cells without damage or inflammation affecting normal tissue.

Hormesis

More is not always better, and the paradoxical phenomenon of hormesis is an example of this. Hormesis refers to a protective effect of a substance at low doses, and a completely opposite effect at higher exposures. In cancer research, this produces a U-shaped curve in a graph of exposure vs. tumor incidence.

Studies

Whenever possible, scientific studies have been quoted about the various cures described. There are several methods of study, some producing more reliable results than others. Studies should not be considered as infallible evidence, as irreproducable results can occur due to error, fraud and simple natural variation. For any given substance, the greater the number of independent studies and the larger the sample size, the more accurate the results.

In-Vitro

This literally means "in glass", and it refers to experiments done on cell cultures, either human or animal, grown in a test tube or petri dish. Just because a drug kills cancer cells in a petri dish does not mean it will be effective when given to a human being. The drug may absorb poorly from the intestinal tract if it is given orally, or it may fail to cross the blood-brain barrier in the case of brain tumors, or it may be prohibitively toxic to tissues other than cancer. However, it is a sign that the drug has potential.

In-Vivo

Literally, "in a living organism". These experiments are done on whole animals, usually rats or mice.

Human Studies

These are more difficult, expensive and time-consuming than studies on animals. Ethically, it is important to test all substances on animals first to insure safety before administering them to humans. Because of this, there are often hundreds of animal studies done for every human study.

Retrospective Studies

These studies examine groups of test subjects (in this case, cancer patients) to find something in their histories that differentiates them from people who do not develop cancer. This sort of study is handicapped by the fact that many people do not accurately remember habits and environmental exposures of many years' duration; also, correlation is not the same as causation.

Prospective Studies

These studies, which tend to be the most accurate, start by randomly separating a group of identical patients into two or more subgroups, exposing them to different drugs or environmental factors, and following them to see whether their outcomes differ. If neither the subject nor the researcher knows in which group a given subject is placed, the study is said to be "double-blind". This avoids the researcher or patient being able to manipulate the outcome through their expectations.
Often, one group of patients is administered the drug to be tested, while a second group (the control group) is given a placebo. This accounts for the "placebo effect," which causes patients to feel better even when administered an inert substance.

Testimonials/Anecdotal Reports

Statements from, or stories about, individuals who have experienced cancer treatments. These accounts lack any control group or scientific oversight, and fail to take into account the fact that tumors occasionally undergo spontaneous remission.

A lot of the evidence on the products and methods mentioned in this book is anecdotal; that is, no large multi-million-dollar scientific studies have been done on them. These substances are inexpensive, unpatentable and unprofitable for large pharmaceutical firms, who therefore have no profit motive to fund such studies.

However, lots of people have tried them (usually thousands of people), and found that they worked. Any cure with thousands of positive patient testimonials cannot be dismissed easily.

Unlike chemo, surgery or radiation, almost all of these products are harmless at any dose, and quite inexpensive. That's good enough reason to give them a try.

Tumor Regression/Remission/Cure

Oncologists hesitate to use the word "cure" when speaking of cancer, probably because they rarely offer one. Instead, they speak of 1-year, 5-year, and 10-year survival. Often, tumors return a few years after initial treatment, and treatment of these "drug resistant" tumors is often unsuccessful.

There is no other disease on the planet that is even associated with this sort of terminology, and it is a true admission of failure on the part of the medical establishment. Imagine if doctors started speaking in terms of "1-year survival" when dealing with pneumonia, or strep throat. Patients would laugh at these quacks and never patronize their clinics again. However, it is standard practice in dealing with cancer, and the public is used to it and takes it for granted. A true cure is not even thought to be possible.

Spontaneous Regression

It is commonly believed that without treatment, all cancer progresses from a single mutated cell to a large tumor mass, a process which finally ends with the death of the cancer patient. However, this progression is not inevitable.

Dr. Barnett Kramer of the National Institute of Health states that it is becoming increasingly obvious that tumors require more than just genetic mutations to progress. They require the cooperation of surrounding tissues, a lack of immune responses, and hormones to fuel their growth. Kramer describes cancer as an interactive process, whereas it was once seen as "an arrow that moved in one direction" (that is, from bad to worse). This has implications for cancer prognosis and treatment.[1]

The disappearance of cancer without any treatment at all is not as uncommon as was once believed. Thousands of cases have been documented by various researchers throughout medical history.

The rate of spontaneous remission was once estimated at about 1 in 100,000 cancers.[2] In fact, one carefully designed mammography study from 2008 found that 22% of all diagnosed breast cancers disappeared spontaneously.[3] According to breast surgeon Susan Love of UCLA, at least 30% of tumors found on mammograms will go away without any treatment.

In the case of breast cancer, one may wonder if the lesions detected were true cancers to begin with, as mammography often picks up benign conditions such as DCIS and misdiagnoses them as invasive tumors. However, the 2008 study deliberately left out cases of DCIS, following only cases of invasive carcinoma.

Melanomas, lymphomas and neuroblastomas are also prone to disappear without treatment. For instance, melanomas sometimes regress completely, along with their metastases; there are more than 30 well-documented cases of this on record.[4] Dr. Ross Barnetson, at the Royal Prince Alfred Hospital at the University of Sydney, Australia, estimates that the rate may be as high as 10-20 %, based on histological studies showing that 25% of melanomas display evidence of partial regression, usually associated with lymphocyte infiltration. According to Dr. Alan Houghton, chief of immunology at Memorial Sloan-Kettering Cancer Center, New York, the phenomenon may not be more frequent in the case of melanoma, just more likely to be noticed than with internal cancers such as those of the lung.

A study of precancerous cervical cells (discovered on PAP tests) found that 60 percent of these abnormalities revert to normal within a year, up to 90 percent within three years.[5]

The "overdiagnosis" of lesions which would regress by themselves, or never progress, leads to inappropriate medical intervention that is in itself dangerous. After a review of numerous randomized trials, they found an overdiagnosis rate of approximately 25% of mammographically detected breast cancers, 50% of chest x-ray and/or sputum-detected lung cancers, and 60% of prostate cancers detected by elevated PSA levels.

Observational studies and population-based cancer statistics also suggest overdiagnosis in CAT scan detection of lung, kidney and thyroid cancers, melanoma, and neuroblastoma. The researchers concluded, "patients must be adequately informed of the nature and the magnitude of the trade-off involved with early cancer detection."[6]

Historically, spontaneous cancer remissions occur most often after a febrile illness, as tumors do not tolerate high temperatures as well as normal tissues; also, infection activates the immune system, which eradicates cancer cells along with infectious agents.[7] In this case, the tumor has not gone away of its own accord, but rather has been subjected to an internally generated course of hyperthermia and immunostimulation.

Malfunctioning cells are constantly generated, and removed naturally, by our bodies. We are arbitrarily said to be suffering from cancer when the growths get so large that they can be detected by diagnostic tools. Because of this basic fact, we should not underestimate our own natural capacity for healing.

References

(1) Gina Kolata, "Cancers Can Vanish Without Treatment, but How?", The New York Times, October 27, 2009: Gina Kolata

(2) Hobohm, U., "Fever and cancer in perspective." Cancer Immunol Immunother, 2001, 50: 391-396.

(3) Per-Henrik Zahl; Jan Mæhlen; H. Gilbert Welch, "The Natural History of Invasive Breast Cancers Detected by Screening Mammography." Arch. Intern Med., 2008;168(21):2311-2316.

(4) High WA et al., "Completely regressed primary cutaneous malignant melanoma with nodal and/or visceral metastases: a report of 5 cases and assessment of the literature and diagnostic criteria." J Am Acad Dermatol. 2005 Jul;53(1):89-100

(5) Anna-Barbara Moscicki, M.D., et al., "Regression of Low-grade Squamous Intra-epithelial Lesions in Young Women." The Lancet, November 6, 2004: 364(9446); 1678-1683.

(6) H. Gilbert Welch, William C. Black, "Overdiagnosis in Cancer." J Natl Cancer Inst (2010) 102 (9): 605-613.

(7) Hobohm, U.,"Fever therapy revisited." British Journal of Cancer, 2005; 92, 421 – 425.

5. What Is Cancer?

The basic cause of uncontrolled cell division (cancer) is thought to be a metabolic disorder, anaerobic metabolism, due to the cumulative effects of cytotoxic agents such as pollutants (such as tobacco smoke), inherited or acquired genetic defects (BRCA1 or BRCA2 breast cancer genes; radiation-induced DNA damage), infectious agents (such as the Human Papilloma Virus linked to cervical cancer), and radiation.

Cancer Is Man Made

The cancer epidemic is a modern phenomenon. After careful studies of Egyptian mummies, professional research teams have reported that out of hundreds of examinations, only one case of cancer was found to exist.

When compared to the fact that one out of every four deaths in today's world is said to be the result of some form of cancer, this leads us to wonder why there is such an amazing difference. What are we doing in today's world that our long ago ancestors did not do? Or perhaps we should also ask what they did in their time that we are not doing today?

Since there are different forms of cancer, we should think carefully about the differences between early and modern times in more than one category.

Environmental pollution is a major factor causing the modern cancer epidemic. In today's world, we pollute the air with our automobiles, lawn mowers and other forms of fuel operated machinery.

We might want to consider the fact that these earlier ancestors used a much different form of transportation, one that was fueled by food stuffs and whose excretion or "pollution" could be recycled naturally as manure.

There is also the matter of food. In today's world we often use various pesticides and herbicides on our crops in order to protect them from weeds and from insects that would decrease our yield. These chemicals were not invented until the 1940s.

We also use artificial preservatives in our foods. Formerly, preservation methods were limited to drying, salting and fermentation.

We also might want to consider what our ancestors included in their diets and compare this to what we tend to eat on a regular basis. We do know that they didn't have what we refer to as fast food joints. This isn't to say that cancer is necessarily a byproduct of McDonald's or Burger King, but perhaps we should give careful thought to just how much "junk food" we are consuming daily.

What about other facets of our life style? We take advantage of our modern appliances and cars to avoid even minimal amounts of exercise. Perhaps today's world tends to produce more couch potatoes than it does those of the vegetable variety.

Few people would be happy to revert to the hard life of our ancient ancestors, but perhaps we should examine our current lifestyle so that we may, as the old song says, eliminate the negative and accentuate the positive.

Cancer Is A Symptom Of A Metabolic Disorder

Otto Warburg received the Nobel Prize in 1931 for showing that cancer cells have anaerobic, as opposed to normal aerobic metabolism.

Cancer is the end-product of metabolic dysfunction, and develops when cells are so poorly oxygenated that they must use alternate metabolic pathways to survive. Aerobic, or oxygen-based metabolism, occurs in the mitochondria, organelles within the cell used to produce energy. When the cell switches to anaerobic, or non-oxygen-using metabolism, it bypasses the mitochondria.

Unfortunately, the mitochondria also control the process of apoptosis, so this function is lost at the same time, and the cell becomes immortal. The altered metabolism of a cancer cell is not an all-or-nothing proposition; often, some residual mitochondrial function remains. If aerobic metabolism can be restored, the mitochondria are reactivated, and the cancer cell reverts to normal.

Relationship Between Infection & Cancer

For more than a century, alternative cancer researchers such as Hulda Clark and Virginia Livingstone have suspected infectious agents of causing cancer. These scientists blamed a single microbe, a mycoplasma species, for initiating tumors. However, until recently, mainstream medicine refused to accept this hypothesis, and stated that only a small minority of cancers were caused by any infectious agent.

This idea has been gradually changing over the past 2 decades, and currently it is acknowledged that infection causes approximately 1/6, or 16%, of all cancers worldwide, with a rate 3 times higher in the developing world than in first-world societies. Using information from a number of sources including a cancer-incidence database covering 27 cancers from 184 countries, researchers found that of the 12.7 million new cancer cases diagnosed in 2008, approximately 2 million (16%) were attributable to infections.

There was no single microbe found to be responsible, but rather a variety of infectious agents. The main culprits were human papillomavirus (HPV) which causes cervical and oropharyngeal cancer, the gastric bacteria Helicobacter pylori which causes stomach cancer, and the hepatitis B (HBV) and C viruses which cause liver cancer.

Study authors Dr. Catherine de Martel and Dr. Martyn Plummer, from the International Agency for Research on Cancer in Lyon, France concluded, "Infections with certain viruses, bacteria, and parasites are one of the biggest and preventable causes of cancer worldwide ... Application of existing public-health methods for infection prevention, such as vaccination, safer injection practice, or antimicrobial treatments, could have a substantial effect on future burdens of cancer worldwide."[1]

Some carcinogenic infections can be treated with antibiotics, but many are viruses that respond poorly to conventional drugs.

In some cases bacterial infections may lead to cancer, especially if the infection is recurring or chronic. Bacteria may cause cancer in a variety of ways.

Chronic inflammation disrupts regular cell functions causing inflammation and promoting cancerous growth.

Bacteria can damage DNA, causing mutations which alter control of the cell division and maturation process.

Chronic infection may weaken and suppress the immune system, which would otherwise keep cancer in check.

Also, keep in mind that if you have had a certain infection linked to cancer and have successfully treated it, there still may be a residual risk of subsequent cancer.

References

(1) Dr Catherine de Martel, et al., "Global burden of cancers attributable to infections in 2008: a review and synthetic analysis." The Lancet Oncology, Early Online Publication, 9 May 2012 doi:10.1016/S1470-2045(12)70137-7

Cancer Stem Cells

More than 100 years ago, a British doctor, John Beard, noted that cancer cells behaved much like human trophoblasts (embryonic cells), which are referred to today as stem cells. In 1911, he published a book called, "The Enzyme Treatment of Cancer and Its Scientific Basis," in which he expounded on his theory that cancer was caused by these primitive precursor cells, and that enzymes could be used to treat the disease.

Dr. Beard noticed that the placenta (which forms from part of the fertilized egg) had many similarities to a tumor, in that it exhibits uncontrolled and invasive growth. Some tumors, like placental cells, even secrete the hormone HCG. Placental cells multiply unchecked until the fetal pancreas begins secreting enzymes, at which point the placenta stops growing. This led Dr. Beard to the conclusion that enzymes might also inhibit the growth of tumor cells. Tests on mice implanted with tumors showed that injections of pancreatic enzymes caused their tumors to shrink. Dr. Beard then tested enzymes on human patients, with positive results.

However, Dr. Beard's theory never caught on with the scientific establishment, and he died in obscurity in 1924.

However, it appears that Dr. Beard was correct all along. New research shows that tumors do in fact originate from stem cells, which form the basis for the recurrence of tumors, and also for the development of chemotherapy resistance. Most forms of chemotherapy and radiotherapy kill only the quickly-dividing progeny of cancer stem cells, temporarily destroying the bulk of the tumor. However, if even one stem cell survives, it will soon recreate the original tumor. Breast cancer patients found to have an increased number of cancer stem cells after cancer treatment have a poorer prognosis.[1] Finding a way to wipe out the cancer stem cells is a growing concern for cancer researchers seeking a permanent cure.[2,3]

A number of natural cancer therapies have been shown to affect cancer stem cells. These include andrographalide (Andrographis), curcumin (turmeric), genistein (soy and coffee), piperine (black pepper), quercetin (onion), resveratrol (grape skins and japanese knotweed) and sulforaphane (broccoli sprouts).

References

(1) Lee, Kim, Choi, Kang, Chung, Ryu and Park, "An increase in cancer stem cell population after primary systemic therapy is a poor prognostic factor in breast cancer." British Journal of Cancer (2011) 104, 1730-1738.

(2) Bonnet D, Dick JE., "Human acute myeloid leukemia is organized as a hierarchy that originates from a primitive hematopoietic cell." Nat Med. 1997 Jul ;3(7):730-7.

(3) Germann M, et al., "Stem-Like Cells with Luminal Progenitor Phenotype Survive Castration in Human Prostate Cancer." Stem Cells. 2012 Mar 21. Epub 2012 Mar 21.

Inflammation & Cancer

Chronic inflammation is responsible for the development of at least 20% of human cancer.[1]

One ubiquitous protein involved in the development of cancer is NF-kappaB, a signalling molecule which has a pivotal role in activating genes controlling pro-inflammatory biochemical pathways. These include pro-inflammatory cytokines, such as IL-1, IL-2, IL-6, and TNF-alpha; chemokines such as IL-8, MIP-1alpha, MCP1, RANTES, and eotaxin; adhesion molecules such as ICAM, VCAM, and E-selectin; inducible enzymes such as COX-2 and iNOS; growth factors; some of the acute phase proteins; and immune receptors. All these factors play critical roles governing the inflammatory process. Low-level activation of NF-kappaB has been implicated in multiple degenerative diseases.

Many natural substances inhibit the NF-kappaB pathway, including lignans, sesquiterpenes, diterpenes, triterpenes, and polyphenols such as resveratrol and quercetin.[2]

Well-known natural health products which are known to be NF kappaB inhibitors are allicin (garlic), vitamin D, curcumin (turmeric), ECGC (green tea), eugenol (cloves), gingerol (ginger), IP6 (rice bran), quercitin (apple skins, onions), resveratrol (grape skin and knotweed), tocotrienols (palm oil), sulphoraphane (broccoli), and thymoquinone (black cumin).

References

(1) Pikarskey E, et al., "NF-kappaB functions as a tumour promoter in inflammation-associated cancer." Nature, 2004 Sep 23;431(7007):461-6.

(2) Nam NH, "Naturally occurring NF-kappaB inhibitors." Min Rev Med Chem,2006 Aug;6(8):945-51.)

Cancer Is A Failure Of The Immune System

We each have a certain number of cancerous cells in our bodies, which is not a problem with a correctly operating immune system to keep them in check.

Ironically, damage to the immune system by chemotherapy drugs and radiation is one of the reasons for cancer recurrence after conventional treatment.

6. Traditional Cancer Treatments

A Huge, Lucrative, Self-Protective Industry

In 2011, the average oncologist earned a mean income of $295,000. Roughly 65% of this income was derived from the sale of chemotherapy drugs.[1] Insurance companies are becoming increasingly aware of a profit motive behind the use of chemotherapy, and at least one American insurer, UnitedHealthCare, has decided to offer oncologists a flat rate fee for the total care of cancer patients, and will only compensate oncologists for drugs at the manufacturer's wholesale cost.[2]

According to one study, between 1983 and 1999, American spending on cancer treatment increased by 49% (in 2010 dollars). By comparison, spending in 10 European countries surveyed increased by only 16 percent.

The average cancer patient in America spends $61,000 for cancer care. For patients diagnosed with cancer between 1995 and 1999, the average survival from time of diagnosis in the U.S. was 11.1 years, compared to 9.3 years in Europe.[3]

The cancer care industry in the United States is now a behemoth that rakes in billions of dollars per annum. The management rather than the cure of cancer is one huge money machine. As Dr. Bob Beck, a well-known alternative practitioner, used to say,"a patient cured is a customer lost." Perhaps this explains why the conventional cancer care industry is so vehemently opposed to inexpensive, self-administered alternative treatments.

References

(1) Lee N Newcomber, "Trying Something New: Episode Payments for Cancer Therapy." JOP May 2011 vol. 7 no. 3S 60s-61s

(2) Lynne Taylor, "US cancer care plan "splits doctors' income from drug sales." Pharmatimes, Oct 26, 2010

(3) Tomas Philipson, et al.,"An Analysis Of Whether Higher Health Care Spending In The United States Versus Europe Is 'Worth It' In The Case Of Cancer. Health Aff April 2012 vol. 31 no. 4 667-675

Over Time, Little Improvement In Survival Rates

In America, the overall 5-year relative survival rate for all cancer sites combined was approximately 50% in 1970, and it may be up to approximately 60% today.

Some of the lengthening in survival rates is due to better treatment, but it is also due to statistical manipulation. Because of screening programs such as PSA tests, colonoscopies and mammograms, tumors are caught earlier. Even if this has no impact at all on the effectiveness of treatment, a patient caught earlier in the natural course of an illness will live longer from the time of discovery than one found only at a later stage of the disease. The inclusion of non-cancerous lesions with naturally low mortality rates, such as DCIS (ductal carcinoma in situ of the breast), also skews the survival figures. One must view the official claims of improvement with some skepticism.

Breast cancer survival rates are a good example of this. According to the Komen Foundation, the 5-year survival rate for breast cancer in America has improved from 63% in the early 1960s to 90% today, a 27% improvement. However, when adjusted for stage at diagnosis, the difference shrinks to only approximately 15%.

For patients in the Netherlands (a Western nation that uses conventional treatment comparable to, or perhaps slightly worse, than that used in America) diagnosed with breast cancer from 1955-

1959[1], compared to Americans diagnosed today and treated with the best that modern medicine has to offer, improvement in survival is as follows (current survival statistics from the American Cancer Society):

Localized Disease (Stage I-II)
Dutch Patients Diagnosed 1955-1960 **65%** 5-yr (50% 10-yr)
American Current 5-yr **74%-81%** (10-yr statistics unavailable)

Regional Spread (Stage III)

Dutch Patients Diagnosed 1955-1960 **37%** 5-yr, (25% 10-yr)
American Current 5-yr **49%-67%** (10-yr stats unavailable)

Distant Metastasis (Stage IV)

Dutch Patients Diagnosed 1955-1960 **12%** 5-yr (0% 10-yr)
American Current 5-yr **15%** (10-yr stats unavailable)

Drug trials tend to overstate the actual amount of improvement produced. Often, expensive new pharmaceutical drugs extend the life expectency of patients by only a few months. If the standard survival time for a given tumor is 1 month, a treatment that extends it to 2 months will be hailed as a "100% improvement!"

References

(1) Nab H.W., "Trends in incidence and prognosis in female breast cancer since 1955 : registry-based studies in south-east Netherlands." Doctoral Thesis, 1995, University of Erasmus Medical Center, Rotterdam, Netherlands

Iatrogenic Illness

"Iatros" is the Greek word for healer. Iatrogenic illness refers to disease caused by medical practitioners. Statistics suggest that the medical industry itself is the third leading cause of death in America, behind heart disease and cancer.

Iatrogenesis caused between 225,000 – 284,00 deaths per year in the United States, depending on which statistics are used. These deaths were mainly caused by negative effects of medications not caused by errors in dosage or administration (106,000), hospital-acquired infections (80,000), in-hospital errors not related to medications (20,000), unnecessary surgeries (12,000), and in-hospital medication errors (7,000).[1,2,3,4]

Dealing with the medical-industrial complex is not without risk, as every prescription, invasive procedure, or hospital admission has a small but significant chance of producing undesirable results. Also, procedures such as chemotherapy, radiotherapy and surgery are absolutely guaranteed to have harmful side effects; however, patients are advised to undergo them anyway, since the medical establishment claims they are the only cures available.

References

(1) Starfield B, "Is US health really the best in the world?" (PDF), JAMA 284 (4): 483–5. (July 2000).

(2) Leape L, "Unnecessary Surgery." Annual Review of Public Health 13: 363-383 (May 1992).

(3) Phillips DP, Christenfeld N, Glynn LM, "Increase in US medication-error deaths between 1983 and 1993." Lancet 351 (9103): 643–4. (February 1998).

(4) Lazarou J, Pomeranz BH, Corey PN, "Incidence of adverse drug reactions in hospitalized patients: a meta-analysis of prospective studies." JAMA 279 (15): 1200–5. (April 1998).

"Doctors Refuse Chemotherapy For Themselves!"

There is a widespread internet rumor that doctors refuse chemotherapy for themselves and their families, while foisting it on hapless patients, presumably entirely due to a profit motive. There are two problems with this meme. The first is that it is factually inaccurate. Secondly, it misses the non-financial factors that also encourage physicians to perpetrate the cancer industry.

The Facts Behind The Rumor

In multiple surveys, oncologists themselves were less than universally enthusiastic about chemotherapy, and displayed no widespread consensus on exactly what circumstances warranted the use of these drugs.

A 1985 survey of 118 doctors by McGill Hospital in Montreal asked whether they would personally accept treatment by six then-experimental drugs including cis-platinum. Of the 79 doctors responding to the survey, 64 out of 79 would refuse to use cis-platinum, and 58 out of 79 would refuse all the experimental treatments.[1]

One 1991 Harvard Medical School study was tellingly entitled "Oncologists vary in their willingness to take anti-cancer therapy." While most would accept chemotherapy under some circumstances, there was little general agreement on exactly when it was justified. In only 37% (or 30 hypothetical cases) was there agreement over 85% on what should be the appropriate treatment. Doctors were also more likely to approve of the use of one particular experimental drug for spouses or siblings than for themselves.[2]

A 1997 study of 126 health professionals was entitled, "Would oncologists want chemotherapy if they had non-small-cell lung cancer?" It found that 65.5% of hematologists/oncologists, 33% of other specialists (radiation oncologists and other physicians), 67% of nurses, and 0% of two hospital administrators would take chemotherapy if they had metastatic non-small-cell lung cancer.[3]

Over time, the studies showed an increasing willingness by medical staff to undergo chemotherapy, perhaps because of improvements in drugs and methods to limit toxicity. However, there is no universal consensus on the appropriateness of chemotherapy. Overall, not exactly a ringing endorsement of chemotherapy, but no outright rejection of it, either.

References

(1) Mackillop WJ, O'Sullivan B, Ward GK, "Non-small-cell lung cancer: How oncologists want to be treated." Int J Radiat Oncol Biol Phys 13:929-934, 1987

(2) Lind SE, et al., "Oncologists vary in their willingness to undertake anti-cancer therapies." Br J Cancer 1991 Aug;64(2):391-5

(3) Thomas J. Smith, MD, "Would Oncologists Want Chemotherapy If They Had Non-Small-Cell Lung Cancer?" ONCOLOGY, Results of a 1997 Survey Vol. 12 No. 3

(4) Steel K, Gertman PM, Crescenzi C, Anderson J (1981). "Iatrogenic illness on a general medical service at a university hospital." N. Engl. J. Med. 304 (11): 638–42.

(5) Starfield B (July 2000). "Is US health really the best in the world?" (PDF). JAMA 284 (4): 483–5.

(6) Leape L (May 1992). "Unnecessary Surgery." Annual Review of Public Health 13: 363-383.

(7) Phillips DP, Christenfeld N, Glynn LM (February 1998). "Increase in US medication-error deaths between 1983 and 1993." Lancet 351 (9103): 643–4.

Motives For The Continued Use Of Ineffective Therapies

Financial

Due to the large amount of personal income generated for oncologists through the sale of chemotherapy drugs, there is considerable conflict of interest. It is hard to escape a suspicion that financial gain may be one driving force encouraging the use of these toxic drugs. Obviously, elaborate, drawn-out treatments performed in high-tech hospital settings generate more income than cheap natural substances which can be prepared and consumed at home.

When doctors are threatened with loss of income and livelihood, expect a tenacious defense of the "status quo."

Lack Of Knowledge Of Alternatives

Medical schools do not teach anything about alternative medicine for any disease, except to dismiss these approaches as quackery. These institutions function in lock-step with the pharmaceutical industry.

Only straight-A students, used to spending all their waking hours memorizing and regurgitating information approved by educational authorities, are admitted to these highly competitive professional degree programs. This tends to select for ambitious, conformist and authoritarian personalities.

Once enrolled, these students are subjected to exhausting work hours, with 36-hour shifts being common in internship and residency, a workaholic lifestyle that continues in private practice. Doctors do not have the time to research therapies that are out of the mainstream; in fact, many of them do not even have time to read all the mainstream peer-reviewed medical journals that are published. Annual conferences, which the majority of physicians do not have the time to attend, are one means to share new discoveries; but since these meetings are open only to the initiated, they often function merely as echo chambers.

To a great extent, the skill set that doctors have upon graduation from medical school is the one they utilize for the rest of their careers. It is hard for doctors to prescribe alternative therapies if they do not know about them. They genuinely believe there is nothing but toxic chemotherapy available to treat cancer.

Psychological

In addition, there is an emotional component involved: professionals are loathe to think that their investment of several years of university, plus the rigors of internship and residency, has imparted in them only faulty, harmful beliefs that are detrimental to the public welfare. To make a bad pun, this is a very bitter pill for most doctors to swallow.

Due to the long work hours, doctors do not have extensive personal lives; their professional identity often consumes them to the point where it becomes their entire identity. Other professionals do not have this specific quirk: openly ignore or contradict the professional advice of a lawyer or an engineer, and it will not be taken personally. A doctor, however, may take it as a personal offence.

Doctors are held in high esteem in society, and doctors have absorbed that opinion. There is an old joke, "What is the difference between a doctor and God? God doesn't believe he's a doctor." Unfortunately, there is more than a little bit of truth to this humor. Doctors have extremely high opinions of themselves and their profession, and bristle if it is so much as hinted that they may be less than infallible. The fact that iatrogenic death (often from drug side effects) is currently the 3rd-leading cause of mortality in America[4,5,6,7] has had little obvious effect on the high regard given to the medical profession by the public and medical practitioners themselves, and the idea that Americans are grossly overmedicated and overtreated is considered heresy.

Between vested interest and overinflated self-esteem, expect an irrational and extreme level of defensiveness from any physician whose advice is challenged.

Legal "Standard of Care" & Incompetence

It is difficult to sue a physician successfully for incompetence if the doctor can prove that the medical care provided was up to established norms. Even if a patient is being blatantly harmed or killed by a useless medical treatment, this will be forgiven by the courts if the doctor can prove the regimen was in accordance with medical precedent.

Who and what sets the precedent? The fossilized medical establishment itself, of course. While there is something to be said for discouraging the immediate adoption of unproven new techniques, blind adherence to tradition wears itself into a deep rut very quickly.

On the other hand, a doctor who saves patients through means not sanctioned by the establishment will be told by professional licensing bodies to conform to established methods, or else face loss of license to practice.

The courts not only defend medical tradition, but under some circumstances even enforce it. A parent seeking alternative cancer remedies for a child may face legal loss of custody, and the child will be forced to undergo conventional treatment by an oncologist.

The FDA also acts as an enforcer for the pharmaceutical industry. No health claims may be made for any supplement not approved by this regulatory authority.

Summary

Considering all the above factors, it is not surprising that so few doctors use alternative methods; in fact, it is surprising that any do so at all.

This is also why vital conversations between patients and doctors in regards to alternative therapy may be strained (at best), or may not ever occur at all. If tentative probing of a doctor's views on alternative therapy yields only a dismissive attitude, further argument is unlikely to produce agreement. A cancer patient is probably best advised to take a polite leave of an uncooperative doctor's practice, and find a practitioner who is already more open-minded.

Some University Hospitals Beginning To Test Natural Cures

For millennia, cancer has been one most intractable of human diseases, with a correspondingly long search for the ideal and ultimate cure. Long before modern "conventional" cancer treatments such as chemo and radiotherapy ever existed, various folk medicines were used, some with good effect. Only in this century has a medical monopoly pushed these cures to the margins. Rather than being the norm, this narrow limitation of cures is a historical anomaly.

However, there are signs that natural cures are returning to the mainstream of cancer treatment. Even though the conventional medical establishment is sluggish in embracing the use of natural methods for treating cancers, these cures are becoming more prevalent, largely due to the insistence of patients dissatified with the failure of conventional treatments.

Today, there are numerous university (also called teaching) hospitals carrying out tests on the use of natural substances as therapeutic agents. Some of these institutions are large, well known, and modern, such as the Johns Hopkins Hospital. Through its Johns Hopkins Center for Complementary and Alternative Medicine (CAM) in Cancer, the institution is pursuing studies aimed at testing the feasibility of using natural substances in the battle against cancers –especially those of the breast and prostate. The Center is funded by the NIH National Center for Complementary & Alternative Medicine. A sum of $7.8 million has already been released for research over a period of years.

In one of the research studies carried out, a combination of eight Chinese herbs called PC-SPES was analysed and evaluated for its property in reducing DNA damage in prostate cancer patients.

The use of soya beans and sour cherries in alleviating cancer pain was also investigated. Researchers from St. George's Hospital (London), University of California and Harvard University have also conducted studies into how vitamin D derived from sunlight could be of benefit in preventing breast cancer.

For those that have observed the fierce antagonism between the practitioners of orthodox medicine and holistic medicine, the fact that university hospitals are now teaching medical students and physicians some aspects of alternative medicine is surely good news. It leads us to believe that beneficial discoveries will improve the integration of the healthcare industry in the near future.

In a situation in which a patient would have access to both effective orthodox treatment and sound natural alternatives from a single source, the treatment of cancers would have entered another phase. However, on a deeper analysis, this should not come as a surprise, as medicine is simply going back to its roots –the use of herbs, plants, oils, fruits and vegetables in curing diseases.

Ironically, 62% of cancer drugs approved by the FDA between 1981 and 2002 were of natural origin.[1]

References

(1) Gonzales G.F, "Medicinal plants from Peru: a review of plants as potential agents against cancer." Anticancer Agents Med Chem, 2006 Sep;6(5):429-44.

Costs Of Traditional Versus Alternative Cancer Treatments

Traditional cancer treatments will bankrupt the average American without health insurance. In fact, medical bills (for all diseases) are the leading cause of personal bankruptcy in America. In the majority of cases, the patient had some form of health insurance.

Chemo alone can cost $4000 per injection, and monthly oral drugs can easily reach $1600. Total traditional cancer treatment often costs between $100,000 and $350,000.

Alternative cancer treatments are much more affordable. 5 lbs of Chlorella, which can be purchased for less than $100, will last a year. The Budwig diet costs less than $2 per day.

7. Forms Of Conventional Cancer Treatments

Conventional cancer treatment usually takes the form of chemotherapy, radiation therapy, and surgery; and in specific cases, therapy with miscellaneous targeted anti-cancer drugs such as hormone blockers for hormone-sensitive tumors, or anti-tumor antibodies.

Before you consent to any of these therapies, exercise informed consent and be aware of the problems these procedures can cause. In some cases, mitigating treatments are available.

Chemotherapy

Disadvantages Of Chemotherapy

Low Effectiveness

According to the National Program of Cancer Registries (NPCR) of the Centers for Disease Control and Prevention, the commonest cancers in America are prostate, breast, lung, colon, and skin cancer, leukemia, and non-Hodgkin's lymphoma. This means that the great majority of cancer patients have tumors for which chemotherapy is ineffective.

A 2004 study found that the addition of chemotherapy to cancer treatment increases average survival time of cancer patients by a factor of only 2% (2.1% in America, 2.3% in Australian cases). Survival times were only extended significantly for cancer of the cervix (by 12%), ovarian cancer (8.7%), and a few rarer cancers, such as cancer of the testis (41.8%), Hodgkin's disease (35.8%), non-Hodgkins lymphoma (10.5%). In cancers of the head and neck, lung, stomach, and pancreas, improvement in survival time was less than 5%.[1]

Roughly 75% of cancer patients take chemotherapy, even those with types of tumors proven unresponsive to this mode of treatment, because they are told by medical authorities that this is is the best that conventional medicine has to offer.

Temporary Results

With the exception of some rarer cancers such as seminomas and some types of leukemias and lymphomas, chemotherapy is rarely curative. It buys time for the patient, but survival is measured in 1-year, 5-year, and 10-year intervals. Permanent cure is highly unlikely. This is true for the most common cancers such as breast, prostate, lung, stomach and pancreatic.

Chemotherapy and radiotherapy are most effective against rapidly-dividing cells, and do not discriminate between tumor cells and fast-growing normal cells, such as hair follicles, the gastrointestinal epithelium, and the bone marrow.

Due to systemic toxicity of chemotherapy, patients may experience hair loss, difficulties in chewing and swallowing, constipation or diarrhea, fatigue, nausea, and anemia. These side effects are almost universal, and oncologists warn their patients about them before commencing treatment.

Most of the side effects are temporary, but some can linger long after the therapy is completed. Some chemotherapy drugs cause irreversible damage to major organs, such as the liver, kidneys, heart, brain and reproductive organs.

Many patients complain of "chemo brain", dementia caused by brain damage from chemotherapy. This alarming side effect may be permanent in some cases.[2]

Some chemotherapy drugs can cause infertility, which may also be permanent.

Chemotherapy suppresses the immune system, leaving any remaining cancer cells free to proliferate and create recurrent disease.

Due to the mutagenic nature of chemotherapy drugs, years after completion of treatment, a patient may acquire another kind of cancer. Once patients have a history of cancer, their susceptibility to other kinds of cancer is greatly increased.

Chemotherapy damages normal tissue, and causes secretion of proteins that actually increase tumor growth, leading to faster-growing, treatment-resistant cancer.

Initially, tumours often respond well to chemotherapy, unfortunately followed by rapid regrowth and resistance to further chemotherapy. Rates of tumour cell reproduction have been shown to accelerate between chemotherapy treatments. A recent study of prostate cancer has found a biochemical reason for this phenomenon, aside from the survival of cancer stem cells, which is a separate issue.

Researchers discovered that chemotherapy agents caused genetic damage to primary prostate fibroblasts (non-cancerous cells in the prostate), leading to the secretion of tumor-promoting proteins, including one particularly potent substance called WNT16B. Genotoxic stress increases the secretion of WNT16B through NF-κB , β-catenin and other biochemical pathways known to be involved in tumor growth. WNT16B promotes both the growth and invasiveness of prostate carcinoma, and it also increases the resistance of prostate cancer cells to further chemotherapy. Researchers found they could attenuate the chemotherapy resistance by blocking WNT16B, β-catenin or NF-κB signaling.

Researchers commented, "Our results indicate that damage responses in benign cells... may directly contribute to enhanced tumour growth kinetics."
The researchers reproduced their findings with breast and ovarian cancer tumours. An antibody to block WNT16B, if it could be developed, might improve the response to chemotherapy, and allow smaller doses to chemotherapy to be effective.[3]

Extreme Cytotoxicity Of Chemotherapy Drugs

The toxicity of cytotoxic chemotherapeutic drugs cannot be overstated. It is not an exaggeration to call these drugs poisons at almost any level of exposure.

These types of drugs can be lethal to the patient receiving them and also cause serious health damage or injuries to the experts administering the chemicals. Protocols for medical staff include wearing double gloves and treating an inadvertent spill as a hazmat area. Chemotherapeutic agents are described as hazardous drugs by the National Institute for Occupational Safety and Health (NIOSH), the American Society of Health-System Pharmacists (ASHP), and the Oncology Nursing Society (ONS).

Professionals engaged in managing these types of drugs risk toxicity due to exposure to them. Because of the adverse health defects brought on by all these toxic agents, healthcare units are focusing more on finding out efficient solutions for reducing the potential risks of exposures.[4]

Cytotoxic drugs cause chromosomal modifications, abnormalities associated with the reproductive system and respiratory systems and in many cases cancer. These have generally a high potential to generate significant side effects in the patients who are treated with these types of noxious drugs.

In chemotherapy techniques, the cytotoxic agents are transmitted from the vial to the syringe and eventually injected from the syringe into the infusion bag. Along the way of exchange, there exists a possibility of inequality in the vial's pressurization which can lead to direct exposure of cytotoxic contaminants in the operating atmosphere.

Therefore, any kind of negligence in handling, administering and preparing these types of medications can result in health risks which may be moderate as well as temporary including skin ailments and allergies, or serious and also long-term such as infertility and cancer. An increase in leukemia[5] as well as reproductive problems[6,7] has been noted in staff dispensing cytotoxic agents, and mutagenic agents have been found excreted in the urine of these workers.[8] However, other studies have found no health problems, probably because of improved safety measures such as laminar airflow in laboratories where the chemo drugs are prepared.[9]

If exposure to trace amounts of these chemicals causes such deleterious affects in healthy individuals, it is obvious the results will be much worse in patients who are actually administered the bulk of the medication. Patients are literally being poisoned with the hope that their tumors will succumb before the rest of their cells are killed.

54

References

(1) Morgan G, et al., "The contribution of cytotoxic chemotherapy to 5-year survival in adult malignancies." Clin Oncol, 2004 Dec;16(8):549-60)

(2) Kopplemans V et al., "Neuropsychological performance in survivors of breast cancer more than 20 years after adjuvant chemotherapy." J Clin Oncol 2012 Apr 1;30(10):1080-6. Epub 2012 Feb 27.

(3) Yu Sun, Judith Campisi, Celestia Higano, Tomasz M Beer, Peggy Porter, Ilsa Coleman, Lawrence True, Peter Nelson, "Treatment-induced damage to the tumor microenvironment promotes prostate cancer therapy resistance through WNT16B." Nature Medicine (2012) Published Online 05 Aug 2012

(4) "OCCUPATIONAL EXPOSURE TO ANTINEOPLASTIC AGENTS." National Institute for Occupational Safety and Health

(5) Skov T, Maarup B, Olsen J, Rørth M, Winthereik H and Lynge E. "Leukaemia and reproductive outcome among nurses handling antineoplastic drugs." Brit J Ind Med. 1992; 49:855-861.

(6) Selevan SG, et al., "A study of occupational exposure to antineoplastic drugs and fetal loss in nurses." N Eng J Med,1985 Nov 7;313(19):1173-8.

(7) Stucker I., Caillard J-F., Collin R., Gout M., Poyen D., Hemon D. "Risk of spontaneous abortion among nurses handling antineoplastic drugs." Scand J Work Environ Health 1990; 16: 102-107.

(8) Bos RP, Leenaars AO, rheuws JLG, Henderson PT. "Mutagenicity of urine from nurses handling cytostatic drugs, influence of smoking." Int Arch Occup Environ Health 1982; 50:359-69.

(9) Nguyen TV, Theiss JC, Matney TS. "Exposure of pharmacy personnel to mutagenic antineoplastic drugs". Cancer Res 1982;42:4792-6.

Minimizing Chemotherapy-Induced Illness

Some disadvantages of chemo, especially the temporary ones, can be alleviated. It is vital for a patient to drink plenty of fluids while undergoing chemotherapy, and it is also advisable to eat more than three meals – preferably five to six small meals – a day. Herbal therapies, nutritional supplements and antioxidants prevent toxicity to normal tissues and support the immune system.

Careful selection of chemotherapy drugs prevents useless treatment cycles, and it may be possible to lower the dosage by combining chemotherapy with insulin.

Pinpoint Your Chemotherapy

If you decide, regardless of all these warnings, that you must have chemotherapy, you may as well pick the drug to which your cancer is most susceptible, so you can have the most effective chemotherapy possible.

Precision Therapeutics has developed an assay called ChemoFx to test several different chemotherapeutics on tumor cells in vitro (in the laboratory) to see which chemical is the most efficient in killing specific cancer cells.

By testing multiple chemotherapies on a patient's cancer cells before treating a cancer patient, ChemoFx helps determine the therapy most likely to be effective, while avoiding needless toxicity of treatment with ineffective drugs.

Patients who received a treatment determined by ChemoFx to lead to the best tumor response had an overall survival 1.4 times longer than those receiving a treatment shown by ChemoFx to be ineffective.

Progression-Free Interval was 14 months for ovarian cancer patients treated with drug found by Chemo Fx to be of intermediate effectiveness, compared to 9 months for patients treated with drugs found by ChemoFx to have the lowest effect. The PFI for patients treated with the drug shown to produce the greatest sensitivity was unavailable at the time the study was published.[1]

Another study followed 206 patients with stage II-IV primary epithelial ovarian who were tested by ChemoFx between 1997 and 2003. Patients had already undergone at least one round of chemotherapy. The study evaluated differences in Overall Survival (OS) between patients who were given chemotherapy that produced responsive, intermediate-responsive or non-responsive results according to ChemoFx cell testing.

Of the 206 patients followed:
• Median OS of Assay non-responsive patients was 39.2 months
• Median OS of Assay intermediate-responsive patients was 62.5 months
• Median OS of Assay responsive patients was 80.4 months

Despite the fact that all patients had the same form of cancer, 88% of patients exhibited varying degrees of response to different chemotherapy drugs in the in-vitro test. The analysis also found that nearly 2/3 of patients' tumors were more responsive to a treatment identified by ChemoFx, than to the treatment they had been given.

In a statistical model predicting overall survival if patients were treated with a therapy that caused a greater tumor response, the median OS of patients treated with an Assay non-responsive drug could be improved from 39.2 to 62.5 months. Median OS of patients treated with an Assay intermediate-responsive drug could be improved from 62.5 to 101.3 months. The analysis found that the median OS could be extended as much as 23 to 38 months.[2]
"These overall survival data demonstrate that the responsiveness to treatment established by this sensitivity assay in the laboratory setting, may in fact translate into meaningful clinical outcomes for patients," said Thomas J. Herzog, MD, director of gynecologic oncology at the Columbia University Medical Center and lead investigator of the study. "If these results are confirmed in current ongoing trials, this will be a significant step towards establishing individualized treatment strategies for patients who will require chemotherapy."

The assay requires a live sample of tumor tissue, derived from a biopsy, aspiration or surgical procedure. It can be used in primary, recurrent, and metastatic tumors.

ChemoFx can be used for all solid tumor types, with ovarian and breast tumors being most frequently tested.

http://www.chemofx.com

References

(1) Gallion H, et al., "Progression-free interval in ovarian cancer and predictive value of an ex vivo chemoresponse assay." Int J Gynecol Cancer 2006 Jan-Feb;16(1):194-201.

(2) T. J. Herzog, "A chemoresponse assay and survival in primary ovarian cancer." J Clin Oncol 26: 2008 May 20 suppl; abstr 16522

Insulin Potentiation Therapy (IPT)

Insulin Potentiation Therapy was developed in Mexico City in 1932 by Dr. Donato Perez Garcia, Sr. He treated patients with a wide variety of tumors, and taught the method to his son and grandson, also medical practitioners. IPT is currently being promoted by Dr. Stephen Ayre, who studied under Dr. Perez.

In 2000, the NCI's Cancer Advisory Panel on Complementary and Alternative Medicine (CAPCAM) asked Drs. Perez Garcia and Ayre to give a presentation on IPT as part of the NCI's Best Case Series program. However, since then, CAPCAM has performed no more further into IPT.[1,2]

How It Works

IPT is based on the theory that metabolic differences between normal and cancerous cells can be manipulated to enhance the effects of chemotherapy. Cancer cells have abnormally rapid growth, and any glucose present in the bloodstream is rapidly absorbed, feeding the tumor and starving the patient.

Because they are so dependent on a continuous supply of glucose, cancer cells have many more insulin receptors per cell than normal cells in order to facilitate glucose absorption. Insulin is a substance secreted by the pancreas which instructs cells to take in glucose circulating in the blood.

For example, breast cancer cells have 7 times as many insulin receptors, and 10 times as many igf receptors.[3,4,5]

The overexpression of insulin and growth factor receptors has also been noted in other tumor cell lines. In addition to their hypersensitivity to circulating insulin, cancer cells themselves have developed the ability to produce insulin and insulin-like growth factor (IGF), thus becoming autonomous from the body's own secretion of these substances.[6-16]

When treated with insulin, cancer cells respond with a higher than normal intake of glucose, and theoretically, any other substances present in the bloodstream, such as chemotherapy drugs. In addition, the intake of glucose fuels a growth spurt in the tumor, pushing more tumor cells into division, the part of the cell cycle when they are most susceptible to chemotherapy (non-dividing cells are much less affected by these drugs). By using insulin in conjunction with chemotherapy drugs, significantly lower doses of chemotherapy (only 10-15 % of the standard dose) can be used, thus minimizing side effects and damage to normal cells.

Studies

In-vitro studies of breast cancer cells found that substances which increase the rate of proliferation of tumor cells, such as 17 beta-estradiol, epidermal growth factor, hydrocortisone, and insulin, make the cells much more sensitive to the chemotherapy drug doxorubicin. The effect was seen in 20/25 cells cultures tested, with the most pronounced effect in hormone-responsive cells. A growth-inhibitory breast cancer drug, tamoxifen, had the opposite effect, causing a decrease in sensitivity. In contrast, the sensitivity of normal bone marrow stem cells was affected to a much lesser degree. Researchers concluded, "tumor tissue-specific growth-stimulatory hormones can improve the in vitro efficacy of cell cycle-active anticancer drugs."[17]

Another in-vitro study of MCF-1 human breast cancer cells found that insulin increased the cytotoxicity of methotrexate up to 10,000-fold. The effect was not due to increased intracellular levels of methotrexate, increased cell growth rate, or greater number of cells in the S-phase of cell division (which is specifically targeted by methotrexate), but rather seemed to involve biochemical pathways controlling cell growth, even in cells not performing DNA synthesis.[18]

Human Studies

A 2004 clinical trial of IPT in the treatment of breast cancer was done in Uruguay, and researchers stated, "The group treated with insulin + methotrexate responded most frequently with stable disease" compared to patients treated with either methotrexate or insulin by it self.[19]

In 2009, a 3-year Bulgarian study was published on the use of IPT combined with low-dose chemotherapy (1/10 the conventional dose). The study included 196 patients with various cancers, 143 of them with advanced metastasic disease, and some who had become unresponsive to conventional chemotherapy. Patients exhibited few side effects and had improved quality of life, and some showed complete remission of their disease over the course of the study. [20,21]

Caution

High doses of insulin can cause coma and can be potentially fatal. This treatment should only be used in a medical clinic by a doctor.

Clinics Offering IPT

A large website offering detailed information about IPT and multiple doctor listings:

http://iptq.com/

References

(1) "Minutes of the Third Meeting". Cancer Advisory Panel for Complementary and Alternative Medicine (CAPCAM). September 18, 2000. Archived from on October 29, 2007

(2) NCI Office of Complementary and Alternative Medicine. Spring 2009 "These collaborations are particularly relevant to CAM practices that have been identified through the NCI Best Case Series Program and warrant NCI-initiated research but have not ascertained enough data for a larger project. Examples of such therapeutic regimens include ... insulin potentiation therapy...""

(3) Ayre SG, Garcia y Bellon DP, Garcia DP Jr, "Insulin, chemotherapy, and the mechanisms of malignancy: the design and the demise of cancer." Med Hypothesis 2000 Oct;55(4):330-4.

(4) Vincenzo Papa, Vincenzo Pezzino, Angela Costantino, Antonio Belfiore, Dario Giuffnda, Lucia Fnttitta, Gabriella B. Vannelli, Richard Brand, Ira D. Goldfine, and Riccardo Vigneri "Elevated Insulin Receptor Content in Human Breast Cancer." J Clin Invest 1990 Nov;86(5):1503-10.

(5) Cullen KJ, Yee D, Sly WS, Perdue J, Hampton B, Lippman ME, Rosen N, "Insulin-like growth factor receptor expression and function in human breast cancer." Cancer Res 1990 Jan 1;50(1):48-53.

(6) Hilf R. "The actions of insulin as a hormonal factor in breast cancer." In: Pike M.C., Siiteri P.K., Welsh C.W.,eds. Hormones and Breast Cancer, Cold Spring Harbor Laboratory. pp. 317–337 1981.

(7) Gross G.E., Boldt D.H., Osborne C.K. "Pertubation by insulin of human breast cancer cell kinetics". Cancer Research 1984 44 (8): 3570–3575.

(8) Zapf J., Froesch E.R., "Insulin-like growth factors/somatomedins: structure, secretion, biological actions and physiological role". Hormone Research 1986 24 (2–3): 121–130.

(9) Goustin A.S., Leof E.B., Shipley G.D., Moses H.L. "Growth Factors and Cancer". Cancer Research 1986 46 (3): 1015–1029.

(10) Goustin A.S., Leof E.B., Shipley G.D., Moses H.L. "Growth Factors and Cancer". Cancer Research 1986 46 (3): 1015–1029.

(11) Cullen J.K, Yee, Sly W.S, et al. "Insulin-like growth factor receptor expression and function in human breast cancer". Cancer Research 1990 50 (1): 48–53.

(12) Raile K, et al., "Human osteosarcoma (U-2 OS) cells express both insulin-like growth factor-I (IGF-I) receptors and insulin-like growth factor-II/mannose-6-phosphate (IGF-II/M6P) receptors and synthesize IGF-II: autocrine growth stimulation by IGF-II via the IGF-I receptor." J Cell Physiol 1994 Jun;159(3):531-41.

(13) Quinn K.A., Treston A.M., Unsworth E.J. et al. "Insulin-like growth factor expression in human cancer cell lines". J Biol Chem 1996 271 (19): 11477–83.

(14) Holdaway I.M., Freisen H.G. "Hormone binding by human mammary carcinoma". Cancer Research 1997 37 (7 Pt 1): 1946–1952.

(15) Rasmussen A.A., Cullen K.J. "Paracrine/autocrine regulation of breast cancer by the insulin-like growth factors". Breast Cancer Res Treat 1998 47 (47(3)): 219–33

(16) Yee D. "The insulin-like growth factors and breast cancer - revisited". Breast Cancer Res Treat 1998 47 (47(3)): 197–199

(17) Hug V, Johnston D, Finders M, Hortobagyi G. "Use of growth-stimulatory hormones to improve the in vitro therapeutic index of doxorubicin for human breast tumors". Cancer Res 1986 46 (1): 147–52.

(18) Alabaster O, Vonderhaar B, Shafie S., "Metabolic modification by insulin enhances methotrexate cytotoxicity in MCF-7 human breast cancer cells". Eur J Cancer Clin Oncol 1981 17 (11): 1223–8.

(19) Lasalvia-Prisco E, Cucchi S, Vázquez J, Lasalvia-Galante E, Golomar W, Gordon W. "Insulin-induced enhancement of antitumoral response to methotrexate in breast cancer patients". Cancer Chemother Pharmacol 2004 53 (3): 220–4.

(20) Damyanov, C., Gerisimova, D., Dyukmedzhieva, D., Stoeva, D., "Insulin Potentiation Therapy in the treatment of malignant neoplastic diseases: a

three-year study." Medical Center "Integrative Medicine", Sofia, Bulgaria, 2009.

(21) Damyanov, C., Radoslavova, M., Gavrilov, V., Stoeva, D. "Low dose chemotherapy in combination with insulin for the treatment of advanced metastatic tumors." Journal of BUON. 14: 711-715, 2009.

Avoid Hair Loss Due To Chemo

Hair loss can be prevented through the use of a hypothermia cap applied to the scalp while chemo is being given, especially when anthracyclines or taxanes are used (but not if the two are used together). Many oncologists and hospitals do not know about this hair-sparing technology.
Cold temperature causes blood vessels around hair follicles to constrict, limiting flow of blood carrying chemotherapy drugs. Also, cold temperature inhibits cell metabolism and division, making the cells less suscepible to chemotherapy.

The two most common cap systems are the DigniCap Scalp Cooling System and the Penguin Cold Cap. Both systems are used in Europe, but currently only the Penguin caps are available in America. FDA evaluation is ongoing.

The DigniCap uses a coolant circulated by a compressor, with temperature sensors to maintain the proper cooling. It is a complete miniature refrigeration unit.

The Penguin Cold Cap is a less consumer-friendly product. These caps are filled with crylon gel refrigerated down to -22 degrees Fahrenheit. The caps are changed every half hour during the chemotherapy infusion process, and must be chilled in a separate freezer. Unfortunately, many hospitals do not have a freezer in the facility that can maintain the required temperature, so patients must supply their own freezing unit.

Studies

Success rates vary across different studies, they are currently from 73% to 100%. Differences in cooling time and temperature as well as the specific chemotherapy drug used all affect the outcome.[1,2,3]

Scalp cooling cannot be used if the patient has widespread blood-borne metastases, or cancer such as leukemia, but it is useful for solid tumors. Fears that sparing the scalp from chemotherapy will lead to scalp metastasis are unfounded. A 2009 study of 553 breast cancer patients found a 1.1% incidence of scalp metastasis in women who used the cold caps, compared to a 1.2% incidence among women who did not use them.[4]

Suppliers

The Rapunzel Project, founded by two breast cancer patients, Shirley Billigmeier and Nancy Marshall, donates freezers to cancer patients around the country who wish to use this treatment. Their website offers updated information about hypothermia caps.

http://www.rapunzelproject.org/

References

(1) Grevelman EG, "Prevention of chemotherapy-induced hair loss by scalp cooling.". Annals of oncology: official journal of the European Society for Medical Oncology / ESMO March 2005 16 (3): 352–8.

(2) Weiss, Stefanie, "Breast cancer patient uses super-chilled headgear to try to retain her hair". Washington Post Jan 11, 2011

(3) Braff, Danielle, "Cold caps show promise in keeping hair through chemo". Chicago Tribune Jan 4, 2012

(4) Lemieux J, Amireault C, Provencher L, Maunsell E, "Incidence of scalp metastases in breast cancer: a retrospective cohort study in women who were offered scalp cooling". Breast Cancer Research and Treatment 2009 Dec;118(3):547-52. Epub 2009 Feb 25.

Huang Qin Tang Heals Gastrointestinal Damage

Huang Qin Tang is a traditional Chinese medicine, a mix of plant extracts, roots and fruit that has been used for hundreds of years to gastrointestinal problems. Researchers have found that it not only protects patients from the intestinal toxicity of chemotherapy, it also boosts the effectiveness of the drugs.[1]

A start-up pharmaceutical company called PhytoCeutica has developed a standardized version of the traditional product which they have named PHY906. The formula consists of four herbs, extract of peony and skullcap flower, liquorice and buckthorn fruit.

Researchers treated mice with implanted colon and rectal cancer with chemotherapy, which caused massive destruction of the animals' intestinal lining. The mice were given the herbal extract along with the chemotherapy.

PHY906 did not protect the animals' intestines from the initial DNA damage and apoptosis caused by chemotherapy, but by 4 days after CPT-11 treatment, PHY906 caused the regeneration of the intestinal epithelium by promotion of stem cells and several biochemical signaling components. It also exhibited anti-inflammatory effects by decreasing the infiltration of macrophages and neutrophils, tumor necrosis factor–α expression, and plasma levels of proinflammatory cytokines. PHY906 also inhibited nuclear factor κB, cyclooxygenase-2, and inducible nitric oxide synthase. Compared to a control group of mice, the intestinal lining of the treated mice contained more dividing and fewer dying cells.[2]

In mice implanted with pancreatic cancer, PHY906 was found to potentiate the effects of chemotherapy.[3]

Researchers have also conducted Phase I/II human trials. The patients lost less weight and experienced greater therapeutic effectiveness of chemotherapy drugs.[4]

"Chemotherapy causes great distress for millions of patients, but PHY-906 has multiple biologically active compounds, which act on multiple sources of discomfort," said Professor Yung-Chi Cheng, lead author of the study published in Science Translational Medicine.

"This combination of chemotherapy and herbs represents a marriage of Western and Eastern approaches to the treatment of cancer. We will continue to refine these processes to better study and understand the sophisticated nature of herbal medicines. Revisiting history may lead us to discovering future medicines."

Instructions

The researchers used PHY906 800mg twice daily on days 1-4 of chemotherapy.

Suppliers

200 capsules for $40 at

http://eagleherbs.com

Beta-Glucan

Beta-glucan, mentioned in its own chapter as an immune system booster, reduces the chromosomal damage to normal cells caused by common chemotherapy drugs adriamycin, cisplatin and cyclophosphamide by 41-57%. The mouse study which discovered this used a pre-treatment beta-glucan dose of 100mg/kg weight.[5]

References

(1) Ewen Callaway, "How an 1,800-year-old herbal mix heals the gut." Scientific American, Aug 18 2004

(2) W. Lam, S. Bussom, F. Guan, Z. Jiang, W. Zhang, E. A. Gullen, S.H. Liu, Y.C. Cheng, "The Four-Herb Chinese Medicine PHY906 Reduces Chemotherapy-Induced Gastrointestinal Toxicity." Sci Transl Med 18 August 2010: Vol. 2, Issue 45, p. 45-59

(3) M. W. Saif, S. Liu, A. Elfiky, Z. Jiang and Y. Cheng, "Synergistic activity of PHY906 with capecitabine in pancreatic carcinoma." Journal of Clinical Oncology, 2007 ASCO Annual Meeting Proceedings (Post-Meeting Edition)Vol 25, No 18S (June 20 Supplement), 2007: 15116

(4) Yen Y et al., "Phase I/II study of PHY906/capecitabine in advanced hepatocellular carcinoma." Anticancer Res, 2009 Oct;29(10):4083-92.

(5) Tohamy A.A., "Beta-glucan inhibits the genotoxicity of cyclophosphamide, adriamycin and cisplatin." Mutat Res 2003 Nov 10;541(1-2):45-53

Radiotherapy

Roughly fifty percent of all cancer patients are subjected to some form of radiation therapy during their course of treatment, often as adjunct therapy. If used by itself, as it often is in inoperable head and neck cancers, it is usually only palliative.

Disadvantages Of X-Rays & Radiotherapy

Radiation destroys surrounding tissue as well as cancer cells.

Radiation has immediate local side effects. Like chemotherapy, it is selectively toxic to rapidly-dividing cells, but damages normal tissue to some extent as well. If radiation is specifically targeted toward the head or neck area, side effects may include difficulty swallowing, soreness, dry mouth, earaches and even changes in the way food tastes. If radiation is being used in the chest area, side effects may include coughing, shortness of breath, and swallowing difficulties.

Irradiation of the abdomen and pelvis areas may cause vomiting, diarrhea, frequent urination and bladder irritation. These symptoms usually subside as the tissues heal.

Radiation directed at the brain can cause symptoms similar to dementia such as memory loss and confusion, which can be permanent. Other long-term, permanent side effects can include scarring or fibrosis of tissues, infertility after pelvic radiotherapy, as well as the induction of secondary tumors. Also, while hair loss due to chemotherapy is usually temporary, radiotherapy of the head causes permanent hair loss.

Ironically, radiotherapy itself causes cancer by producing breakage and damage to cellular DNA, either directly by the emissions of the radiographic method, used or by the creation of charged particles called free radicals within the cell.

All radiation is carcinogenic, with a straight-line relationship between radiation exposure and cancer. According to a 2005 report by the National Academies of Sciences, there is no true "safe threshold" of radiation exposure.

Patients subjected to multiple X-rays, CAT scans or radiotherapy have an increased risk of secondary cancers, sometimes years later.

The most common cancer caused by radiation is a sarcoma, usually a tumor of muscle, bone, or blood vessel tissue; however, other types of cancers have also been noted. Medical literature documenting secondary cancers dates back at least 60 years. In a 1948 report entitled "Sarcoma Arising in Irradiated Bone," Dr. Cahan and his colleagues set forth three characteristics associated with cancers caused by radiation therapy: different histologic features of first cancer and secondary cancer; location of the secondary cancer within the region previously treated with radiation; and development of the secondary cancer at least 5 years after the first tumor.[1] These are not ironclad rules, but they are a good general reference when trying to decide whether cancer was likely to have been caused by radiotherapy.

A 2004 study, which compared breast cancer patients who had received radiotherapy with those who had not, found increased risks of various tumors years after treatment:

Myeloid leukemia was increased 199% at 1-5 years.
Lung cancer was increased by 62% 10-14 years post-treatment, and 49% 15+ years later.

Secondary breast cancer was increased by 34% 10-14 years post-treatment, and 26% 15+ years later.

Esophageal cancer at 15+ years was increased by 119%.[2]

References

(1) Cahan G, Woodward Q, Higinbotham NL, et al, "Sarcoma arising in irradiated bone: Report of eleven cases." Cancer 1:3-29, 1948

(2) Roychoudhuri R., et al, "Radiation-induced malignancies following radiotherapy for breast cancer." Br J Cancer 2004 Aug 31;91(5):868-72.

Targeted Radiotherapy - Stereotactic Radiation Therapy

Due to "collateral damage" to surrounding tissues, single-beam therapy can only be used to a limited extent. The amount of radiation that can be given must not be too high, particularly if the cancer is located close to the bowel or to the spinal cord.

Stereotactic radiation treatment provides greater accuracy than ordinary radiotherapy, and limits exposure to high levels of radiation to a much more confined area. It is external beam radiation that takes just one to five days to complete rather than several weeks in standard radiation therapy.

Stereotactic radiotherapy involves several radiation beams directed at a tumor from different angles. The convergence of the beams provides a high dose of radiation to a cancerous region while sparing surrounding tissue. With this method, tumors can be subjected to much higher doses of radiation than they could be with single-beam radiotherapy.

Stereotactic radiotherapy can focus radiation on even the smallest cancers and is the preferred method of treatment for small, well-defined tumors.

It relies on computerized 3-D treatment planning and very precise set-up prior to the procedure in order to provide an accurate radiation dose to the right place. Doctors first do careful measurements of where the tumor is located within the body. This can be done using an ultrasound, a CT scan or an MRI examination. The radiotherapist then makes specific semi-permanent markings on the body to indicate where the beams of radiation should be aimed.

The doctors must be very careful to direct each of the beams directly at the site of the tumor. Placement must be very precise so the tumor will not be missed by any of the external beams used. An immobilization device or technique is used to make sure the patient cannot move even a centimeter during the procedure. Some more expensive machines can track the slight movements of the patient and adjust the beams accordingly.

There are at least two types of stereotactic radiotherapy. The first is stereotactic radiosurgery and involves one or more treatments with radiation to the brain or the spine. This treatment is particularly useful for brain tumors located in inoperable areas. A neurosurgeon and a radiation oncologist almost always collaborate on this form of radiation therapy. Another type of surgery is stereotactic body radiation therapy. This involves using stereotactic surgery in any part of the body, exclusive of the spine or the brain.

All stereotactic radiotherapy equipment uses multiple narrow radiation beams that target very small areas precisely. All provide for high dose radiation and most need only one to five sessions to be effective. Some of the devices only treat brain tumors, while others are specifically designed for head and neck tumors.

Radiofrequency Ablation

Radiofrequency ablation (RF ablation) can be used in the treatment of numerous types of cancer, as well as for metastasis.

It is a viable medical technique that is used in the top medical hospitals in the world. It has been approved by the US FDA as a minimally invasive, alternative approach to cancer treatment when other options, such as surgical therapy, have been unsuccessful or cannot be used due to tumor location or other factors. It requires the cooperation of a team of surgeons, oncologists, and radiologists.

RF ablation uses localized heat and radiation to destroy cancer cells within a small area. The doctor uses a thin needle and guides it into the tumor using a CT scan or an ultrasound.

Once the needle is properly positioned, electricity is applied through the needle, causing heat to build up in the tip of the needle. The heat kills a portion of the tumor, and the dead cells are removed by the body or form scar tissue over time. In a short ablation procedure, general anesthesia is used to keep the patient comfortable.

It may take only one session in order to treat the cancer sufficiently. Each procedure takes about an hour to perform. Some patients require multiple treatments spaced over time. For each treatment, the patient stays overnight and is released the next day. It works extremely well for small tumors, which are often treated in a single session.

There are many advantages of radiofrequency ablation compared to standard radiotherapy or surgery. For one, it is a much less invasive procedure than surgery and can be easily used on multiple metastasis—something not usually done with surgical approaches.

While all procedures do carry some risk, this is a relatively safe procedure. There is no skin incision involved and the pain is also minimal. Since patients are anaesthetized, they feel no pain during the procedure, and often very little thereafter due to minimal damage to tissues surrounding the tumor.

The hospital stay is less than with surgeries, often an outpatient procedure or a one-day hospital stay. The procedure can be repeated again if more cancer occurs in the same location, or if tumors show up in other body areas.

There are very few contraindications to RF ablation. Doctors must not use the procedure for any tumor close to or attached to an abdominal viscus (stomach or intestines) or a major blood vessel. There can be bleeding from loss of integrity of the blood vessel, and there can be perforation of the abdominal organ, resulting in peritonitis and possible sepsis.

It is primarily used for tumors such as liver cancer or metastasis to the liver, which are very difficult to treat surgically due to high risk of severe bleeding. Kidney cancers of some types can also be treated with ablation rather than surgery. Lung cancer, primary or metastatic, can be treated easily with ablation therapy. Ablation therapy can be used for bone metastasis to control pain and to debulk the tumor.

8. Causes Of Cancer

Just because you already have cancer does not mean it is too late to clean up your environment. The same toxic influences which cause cancer also encourage its growth.

Tobacco Smoking

Top on the list of environmental carcinogens is tobacco smoke. A whiff of tobacco smoke is said to contain thousands of chemicals, many of which are carcinogenic.

According to the World Health Organization, tobacco smoke is the single most important factor in cancer development. Roughly one-third of all the deaths from cancer are directly linked to cigarette smoke. Beyond the obvious link to lung cancer, it is also associated with cancers of the esophagus and larynx, bladder, kidneys and colon. Cigarette smoking is associated with greater than 85% of all lung cancers and greater than 75% of all oral, pharyngeal, and laryngeal cancers.

Smoking has even been implicated in the development of breast cancer, a connection not as widely publicized as the link with lung cancer. A survey of studies done by the Public Health Agency of Ottawa, Canada, showed that even exposure to secondhand smoke by teenagers increased the rate of premenopausal breast cancer by 14%-119%, depending on exposure levels. Premenopausal female smokers increase their chances of developing breast cancer by 30%-40%.

It's Never Too Late To Quit!

Cancer patients who continue to smoke have lower survival rates than non-smokers. Patients with early lung cancer who stop smoking double their chances of survival. According to a British study, lung cancer patients who continued smoking had a 29 to 33% chance of surviving 5 years, compared to 63-70% of those who quit after being diagnosed.[1]

It's true that old habits die hard, but when it comes down to habits that both kill you and hurt your wallet, cigarette smoking offers an unparalleled proposition. If you were asked to pay for a daily addiction known to increase exponentially your risk of developing all major forms of cancer and cardiovascular disease, you'd probably chuckle and disregard the salesman.

Unfortunately, there are approximately 1 billion tobacco smokers on this planet, and many of them are unaware of the health impacts of tobacco use. Fortunately, new pharmaceutical advances have now enhanced the ability of individuals to quit smoking. What are you waiting for?

How To Quit

Conventional medical practitioners will recommend antidepressant drugs which block nicotine receptors in the brain, and/or nicotine patches and gums.

Another extremely effective method is hypnosis, which can be done by a hypnotist, or by smokers themselves. The book "Easy Way to Quit Smoking," written by British accountant Allan Carr, allows readers to self-hypnotize as they read. No willpower needed. One of the authors of this book quit cold turkey after reading the book, and has never had any desire for another cigarette.

The book is available on Amazon for approximately $25.

References

(1) Parsons A. et al., "Influence of smoking cessation after diagnosis of early stage lung cancer on prognosis: systematic review of observational studies with meta-analysis." BMJ 2010 Jan 21;340:b5569. doi: 10.1136/bmj.b5569.

Refined Sugar: Cancer's Source Of Energy

We grow up being admonished not to eat too much sugar because sugar causes tooth decay. As we grow older, we become aware of our weight and at least try to avoid sugar in order to shed pounds. Some people must regulate their sugar intake because they have diabetes, or chose to do so because diabetes runs in their family and they hope to avoid it.   Never do we hear that we should avoid sugar because it enhances the growth of cancer.

This last sentence may cause some surprise, yet sugar fuels the growth of cancer cells more than any other substance. It is, in the opinion of many alternative health practitioners, the best reason to limit the amount of dietary sugar. If you are going to use sugar, use it in reasonable amounts and do not make it a main part of your diet.

Sugar suppresses the immune system so that one is more apt to develop cancer, and directly feeds existing cancer cells. Obesity, linked to the consumption of nutritionless junk food high in starch and sugar, increases the risk for many cancers.

You don't have to go entirely without sugar, just change your source and limit the amount that you use. If you have a craving for sweets, eat some fruit instead of cakes, cookies or candies. While fruits contain a fair amount of fructose, they also contain fiber to slow its uptake (they have a lower glycemic index than refined sugar), as well as antioxidants and phytonutrients.

Some forms of sugar are especially problematic. High fructose corn syrup, ubiquitous in the American diet, is metabolized differently from ordinary sugar, and stimulates the aberrant metabolic pathway used by cancer cells.[1]

Talk to your doctor or nutritionist and ask them to recommend a healthy diet. Learn how to read the labels on packaged foods so that you know if they contain refined sugar or high-fructose corn syrup.

Sugar may be sweet in taste, but what it causes in the way of cancer and other health problems is extremely bitter.

References

(1) Haibo Liuaff, et al., "Fructose Induces Transketolase Flux to Promote Pancreatic Cancer Growth." Cancer Res August 1, 2010 70; 6368

Lack Of Dietary Fiber, Vitamins, & Antioxidants

While recent dietary studies have pointed away from fat intake and moved towards physical inactivity as a potential cause of cancer, certain dietary characteristics are known to increase your cancer risk.

Fortunately, there are good foods in addition to bad foods. Studies have shown that individuals with higher vegetable and fruit intakes have a lowered risk of breast cancer and colon cancer, among others.

Specifically, the antioxidant content of these dietary components seems to be the source of resistannce to cancer formation. In addition, the use of other supplements, such as Vitamin C, Vitamin E, resveratrol, and retinoids have been found to be protective against cancer development.

Vitamin C is thought to prevent the generation of carcinogens, such as nitrosamines, which are linked to cancer. Resveratrol and vitamin E, acting as antioxidants, can scavenge free radicals, which induce DNA damage that predisposes to cancer. Finally, retinoids such as vitamin A prevent the development of head and neck cancers, and may be helpful as an adjunctive treatment. Did you take your vitamins today?

Suppliers

Cheap, mass-marketed multivitamins often lack many essential aantioxidants and trace minerals, and have only a handful of ingredients. A truly complete multivitamin contains all essential vitamins and minerals, enzymes, phytonutrients, and essential fatty acids. One example of a good multivitamin is Mountain Home Daily Advantage.

30 days supply : $49.99

http://www.drdavidwilliams.com

Diets High In Protein

T. Colin Campbell, author of the book "The China Study", claims that a high protein diet promotes tumors. The milk protein casien was fed to animals given the tumor promoter aflatoxin. "Like flipping a light switch on and off, we could control cancer promotion merely by changing levels of protein..The effects of protein feeding on tumor development were nothing less than spectacular. ... [In one experiment] all animals that were administered [the carcinogen] aflatoxin and fed the regular 20% levels of casein [a cow's milk protein] either were dead or near death from liver tumors at 100 weeks. All animals administered the same level of aflatoxin but fed the low 5% protein diet were alive, active and thrifty, with sleek hair coats at 100 weeks. This was a virtual 100 to 0 score, something almost never seen in research."[1]

The amino acid methionine, found in much greater amounts in meat than plant sources, has been linked to increased tumor growth, and methionine-restricted diets, such as veganism, tend to inhibit tumor growth. Methionine is an essential amino acid, and cannot be eliminated altogether, but an excess should probably be avoided.[2]

References

(1) Campbell, T. Colin, and Campbell, Thomas M., "The China Study:The Most Comprehensive Study of Nutrition Ever Conducted and the Startling Implications for Diet, Weight Loss and Long-term Health."BenBella Books, 2006

(2) Cellarier E, et al., "Methionine dependency and cancer treatment." Cancer Treat Rev, 2003 Dec;29(6):489-99

Red, Processed & Overheated Meat

Multiple studies find an association between the consumption of red and processed meat products and cancer, especially colon cancer. However, these are associative studies only, as large and lengthy as some of them are (one of them followed 38,000 middle-aged men for an average of 22 years and 84,000 women for 28 years[1]). These are not randomized studies in which subjects are assigned into different diet groups.

Many of these studies make no distinction between fresh, unprocessed red meat and meat products preserved with nitrates or other toxic substances.

Humans have been consuming meat since the stone age, but the cancer epidemic is a distinctly modern phenomenon. There is a difference in the composition of fatty acids between wild game and free-range livestock, the traditional source of meat in the human diet, and modern, grain-fed factory farmed cattle. Processed or charred meat compared to fresh raw meat is not the same thing at all. The culprit behind the increased disease risk may not be the red meat in its natural state, but rather the way humans process it for storage and consumption.

Prostate cancer is the second most common fatal cancer in men in the United States. Just as cigarette smoking is statistically linked to lung cancer, prostate cancer is linked to a diet rich in red meat, meat fat, and dairy products. Prostate cancer is less common in Asia, where the diet emphasizes vegetables, rice, soy, and tea, rather than the meat and dairy products found in the Western diet. In addition, American meat and dairy cows are treated with steroid drugs which are banned in Europe. In the weeks before slaughter, cows are implanted with a synthetic mixture of estrogen, testosterone, and other hormones to stimulate growth and weight gain.

When added to a petri dish containing cancer cells, these growth-promoting drugs directly accelerate the growth of the cells. Also, in the animal which received the implant, the hormones raise the level of an insulin-like growth factor (IGF-1), which also promotes cancer cell growth.

In rats, the addition of beef fat to the diet increases the activity of genes promoting cancer, and decreases the activity of genes which suppress it. 27 genes were upregulated and 28 genes downregulated by a diet high in beef fat. The genes affected include those which suppress inflammation, allow cells to escape normal controls on growth, promote tissue invasion by cancerous cells, and affect androgen metabolism.[2]

Avoid fried meat of any kind, not just red meat, but also chicken and fish. Cooking meat at high temperatures produces carcinogenic compounds called heterocyclic amines (HCAs). HCAs are created when sugars and amino acids are cooked at higher temperatures for long time periods. Other carcinogens, such as polycyclic aromatic hydrocarbons (PAHs) are created by grilling or smoking meat. Fat from the meat drips onto an open flame, and as it burns the rising smoke leaves deposits of PAHs on the meat. Both HCAs and PAHs are health hazards.

Consumption of red meat, particularly processed or overheated red meat, contributes to cancers of the gastrointestinal tract, including the esophagus,[5] colon[5], as well as the bladder[4,7], liver[5], lung[5], and prostate.[3]
Consumption of processed meat containing nitrates has been linked to cancer of the pancreas, with the risk of the disease increasing by 19% for every 50 grams consumed daily.[8] This is a small amount, equivalent to 2 strips of bacon.

Men who consumed more than 1.5 servings of pan-fried red meat each week increased their risk of advanced prostate cancer by 30%, which increased to 40% in those eating more than 2.5 servings per week. The risk was associated with hamburgers, but not steak, perhaps because hamburgers heat all the way through very quickly and thus accumulate more heat-induced carcinogens.[3]

One study examined the link between meat consumption and bladder cancer. Subjects with the highest red-meat consumption had a 150% increased risk of developing bladder cancer compared to those who ate little red meat. Even fried chicken and fried fish raised the cancer risk. The level of doneness of the meat also had a marked effect, as those whose diets included well-done meats were almost twice as likely to develop bladder cancer as those who preferred rare meats.[4]

In addition to increasing cancer risk, a study from the Harvard School of Public Health found that consumption of processed red meat, but not unprocessed red meat, was associated with a 42% higher risk of heart disease and a 19% higher risk of type 2 diabetes. On average, each 50 gram (1.8 oz) daily serving of processed meat (1-2 slices of deli meats or 1 hot dog) was associated with a 42% increased risk of heart disease and a 19% increased risk of diabetes. In contrast, eating unprocessed red meat was not associated with these diseases.[6]

In summary, do not overheat animal protein, avoid meats preserved with nitrates, and consume red-meat products such as beef in moderation. If you must grill, marinading meat in a combination of oil and vinegar or citrus juice before grilling greatly reduces the production of toxic substances. Baking or cooking meat is a safer preparation method. Cultivate a taste for steak tartar (raw beef) and sashimi (raw fish).

References

(1) An Pan, et al., "Red Meat Consumption and Mortality Results From 2 Prospective Cohort Studies." Archives of Internal Medicine, April 9 2012;172(7):555-563.

(2) Reyes N, et al., "Microarray analysis of diet-induced alterations in gene expression in the ACI rat prostate." Eur J Cancer Prev, 2002 Aug;11 Suppl 2:S37-42

(3) Joshi AD, Corral R, Catsburg C, Lewinger JP, Koo J, John EM, Ingles S, Stern MC. "Red meat and poultry, cooking practices, genetic susceptibility and risk of prostate cancer: results from the California Collaborative Prostate Cancer Study." Carcinogenesis, Jul 20, 2012

(4) Jie Lin, et al., "Meat, especially if it's well done, may increase risk of bladder cancer. Intake of red meat and heterocyclic amines, metabolic pathway genes and bladder cancer risk." Int J Cancer 2012 Jan 19. doi: 10.1002/ijc.27437.

(5) Cross AJ, Leitzmann MF, Gail MH, Hollenbeck AR, Schatzkin A, et al., "A prospective study of red and processed meat intake in relation to cancer risk.," 2007. PLoS Med 4(12): 325.doi:10.1371 /journal.pmed.0040325

(6) Renata Micha, Sarah K. Wallace, Dariush Mozaffarian, "Red and Processed Meat Consumption and Risk of Incident Coronary Heart Disease, Stroke, and Diabetes Mellitus: A Systematic Review and Meta-Analysis." Circulation, 2010

(7) Leah M. Ferrucci, Rashmi Sinha, Mary H. Ward, Barry I. Graubard, Albert R. Hollenbeck, Briseis A. Kilfoy, Arthur Schatzkin, Dominique S. Michaud, and Amanda J. Cross. "Meat and components of meat and the risk of bladder cancer in the NIH-AARP Diet and Health Study." Cancer, 2010

Dairy Products

Professor Jane Plant is a wife, mother, and widely respected scientist, who was made a CBE for her work in geochemistry. When she developed breast cancer in 1987 at the age of 42, her happy and productive existence seemed destined to fall apart.

After suffering through 5 recurrences of cancer, she and her husband studied the worldwide incidence of breast cancer and found conclusive evidence that the reason for the low rate of breast and prostate cancer in China (and the Orient generally) is that the Chinese don't use dairy products.

She stopped using dairy products and was cancer free after 6 weeks.

Through her advice, she also helped cure 63 other women with breast cancer.

http://www.alkalizeforhealth.net/Lnotmilk6.htm

Further confirmation of Dr. Plant's theory comes from the Harvard Medical School. Ganmaa Davaasambuu is a physician (Mongolia), a Ph.D. in environmental health (Japan), an academic fellow at the Radcliffe Institute for Advanced Study, and a working scientist at the Harvard School of Public Health. According to her research, cows from industrial dairy farms produce milk with more than 30 times the amount of estrone sulfate present in dairy cows used by traditional societies. Estrone sulfate is a potent promoter of reproductive tract cancer.

"Among the routes of human exposure to estrogens, we are mostly concerned about cow's milk, which contains considerable amounts of female sex hormones," Ganmaa states. Dairy consumption supplies 60-80% of estrogens in the diet.

The problem originates with the practices of modern dairy farms, where cows are milked for approximately 300 days a year. During most of that time, the cows are pregnant. The later in pregnancy a cow is, the higher the level of hormones secreted in her milk. Milk from a cow in the late stage of pregnancy contains up to 33 times as much estrone sulfate as milk from a non-pregnant cow. In a comparison of modern milk in Japan versus raw milk from Mongolia, the Japanese milk was also found to contain 10 times more progesterone.

In traditional herding societies such as Mongolia, cows are milked for human consumption only five months a year, said Ganmaa, and only in the early stages of pregnancy. As a result, milk hormone levels are much lower.

Skim milk has lower hormone levels, as hormones are secreted in the milk fat.[1]

Ganmaa's other studies bear out the hypothesis that dairy consumption increases the risk of some cancers.

One of her studies of 42 countries compared diet and cancer rates. It found that milk and cheese consumption are strongly correlated to the incidence of testicular cancer in men ages 20 to 39. Rates were highest in countries such as Switzerland and Denmark, where cheese is a national food, and lowest in Algeria and other countries where dairy is less widely consumed.[2]

Another study by Ganmaa found that milk consumption caused breast, ovarian and uterine cancer.[3]

We recommend that cancer patients, especially those with cancers of the reproductive system (breast, ovarian and prostate) abstain from dairy products. Beverages made from nuts, rice and coconut are excellent substitutes.

Soymilk is not a good substitute, as unfermented soy contains phytoestrogens with unproven effects on hormone-sensitive cancers, thyroid-disrupting substances, and anti-nutrients such as phytic acid, which block intestinal absorption of minerals.

Do not use "non-dairy creamers" as these substances usually contain partially hydrogenated oils.

References

(1) Corydon Ireland, "Hormones in milk can be dangerous." Harvard News Office, Harvard University Gazette, Dec 7, 2006; Jonathan Shaw "Modern Milk", Harvard Magazine, May-June 2007

(2) Ganmaa D, Li XM, Qin LQ, Wang PY, Takeda M, Sato A.,"The Incidence and Mortality of Testis and Prostate Cancers in Relation to World Dietary Practices - Dairies are Causatively Related to these Malignancies." Int J Cancer 2002;98:262-7

(3) Ganmaa D., Sato A., "The Possible Role of Female Sex Hormones in Milk from Pregnant Cows in the Development of Breast, Ovarian and Corpus Uteri Cancers." Medical Hypotheses 2005; 65 (6): 1028-37.

Alcohol

Also worthy of mention among the dietary carcinogens is alcohol. Alcohol has been associated with cancers of the gastrointestinal tract and the upper respiratory tract. Some studies also link alcohol consumption with breast cancer, though this finding has been disputed.

Although limited intake of some alcoholic beverages, such as red wine, is known to actually help prevent some forms of cancer and protect against development of heart disease, chronic and excessive alcohol use are detrimental. Furthermore, the anti-cancer benefits of red wine cannot be translated into other alcoholic beverages such as hard liquor.

For example, chronic alcohol use is known to be associated with numerous major forms of cancer such as cancer of the mouth and esophagus. Alcohol and tobacco act synergistically to exponentially increase the risk of cancer development. The American Cancer Society recommends that adults reduce their drinking to no more than 2 alcoholic beverages daily for men and 1 beverage for women.

84

Replace hard liquor with red wine, which contains the anti-aging and anti-cancer substance resveratrol.

Wine has benefits against cancer, dementia, and other age-related diseases. Moderate consumption of red wine (ie, with meals), has been linked in multiple studies to lower death rates from all causes.

Some studies have linked alcohol consumption by women to higher rates of breast cancer. However, according to a new analysis based on the Framingham study, alcohol consumption is associated with lower rates of the disease.[1]

References

(1) Zhang Y, "Alcohol Consumption and Risk of Breast Cancer: The Framingham Study Revisited." Am. J. Epidemiol. (1999) 149 (2): 93-101.

GMO Foods

"Round-up Ready" corn, which is genetically engineered to withstand high doses of the Monsanto herbicide Round-up, causes cancer in rats.

In September 2012 , French scientists at the University of Caen published a study claiming that rats fed a diet containing a glyphosate-resistant Monsanto GMO corn seed called NK603, or given water mixed with glyphosate herbicide at levels permitted in the United States died earlier than rats fed a diet free of GMO corn and glyphosate. The GMO-fed rats developed more and earlier tumors than the control group.[1]

Not surprisingly, the European Food Safety Authority (EFSA, the European counterpart of the American FDA) immediately dismissed the study, claiming that too few animals (only 10 rats of each sex per group, for a total of 40 test subjects) were used for conclusions to be drawn from the data.[2]

Another complaint was that the French researchers used a strain of rats prone to develop tumors. However, the Sprague-Dawley rats used in the study are the standard test subjects for industry studies.

Multiple other scientists have had their careers derailed for raising inconvenient toxicity concerns about GM crops. These researchers include Ignacio Chapela (University of California, Berkeley), Shiv Chopra and Margaret Hayden (Health Canada), Irina Ermakova (Russian Academy of Sciences), Andres Carrasco (University of Buenos Aires Medical School, Argentina), Arpad Pusztai and Susan Bardosc (Rowett Research Institute, Scotland), and Don Huber (Purdue University).

Another group of researchers performed a meta-analysis of 24 animal feeding studies using GM corn, potato, soybean, rice, or triticale, and found no ill effects on animal health. However, these researchers noted a number of problems in the studies they examined. 13 did not indicate their source of funding and 11 were funded by various national institutes. 6 did not use an appropriate number of test animals. 17 did not use isogenic (certifiably non-GMO) lines of crops for their control group diet, so both test and control groups may have been consuming GMO feed. Poor statistical methods were also widely noted.[3]

In addition to scientific studies about the safety of GM crops, there are multiple complaints from farmers who claim that livestock fed GMO corn experienced chronic gastrointestinal distress, sickness and infertility, symptoms which promptly disappeared when the animals were switched back to conventional feed. Slaughtered animals showed intestinal lesions visible to the naked eye.

The most widely consumed GMO products in America are corn and soy, and most of these crops grown in America are GMO. Soy should be avoided for a multitude of other reasons in addition to its GMO status. In light of chronic reported problems with GMO corn, it is probably not safe for consumption either. Unfortunately, it is ubiquitous in the American diet.

When it comes to conventional produce and prepared foods, manufacturers are not required to list the presence of GMO products. However, organic foods are not allowed to contain any genetically modified ingredients. Buy only organic corn, and avoid purchasing conventional products containing either corn or soy.

References

(1) Gilles-Eric Seralini et al., "Long term toxicity of a Roundup herbicide and a Roundup-tolerant genetically modified maize." Food and Chemical Toxicity, Vol 50 issue 11 November 2012, Pages 4221–4231

(2) Review of the Séralini et al. (2012) publication on a 2-year rodent feeding study with glyphosate formulations and GM maize NK603 as published online on 19 September 2012 in Food and Chemical Toxicology, EFSA Journal 2012;10(10):2910

(3) Snell C, Bernheim A, Berge J-B, Muntz M, Pascal G, et al, "An assessment of the health impact of GM plant diets in long-term and multigenerational feeding trials-A literature review." Food Chem Toxicity 2012 50 1134-48

Bisphenol-A (BPA)

Healthy eating may no longer be a matter of just what you eat and drink. It may also depend on the type of container used to store, prepare, and heat those food and beverages.

Scientific research has linked the weak estrogenic compound Bisphenol-A (BPA) to breast cancer.

BPA is the main building block of polycarbonate plastic, a hard plastic widely used to make kitchen utensils, food storage containers, travel mugs, and water bottles. BPA is also a main component of the epoxy linings found in metal food and beverage cans.

Stop eating canned food, and avoid using plastic food containers, especially when heating food. Use Pyrex glassware or regular glass containers instead.

Teflon Cookware

Teflon contains perfluorooctanoic acid, or PFOA. A widely prevelant environmental pollutant, trace amounts of it have shown up in blood samples taken from people across the country. When rats and mice were exposed to PFOA in far greater amounts, they developed brain tumors. Now, an EPA advisory panel reports, "PFOA is a likely carcinogen in humans."

Ceramic non-stick pans are available that do not contain PFOA.

Antibiotics

The overuse of antibiotics to treat viral and minor bacterial infections may be leading to more than just the well-know effect of antibiotic resistance. It may also be causing cancer. This may be due to one or more factors. By eliminating fevers and bursts of hyperactivity by the immune system, opportunities for the body to rid itself of small tumors have also been removed.

Gut bacteria are decimated by antibiotics, and there is a complex feedback mechanism between gut bacteria and the rest of the body, including the immune system.

In addition, some antibiotics, like ciprofloxacin, are directly toxic to body cells as well as bacteria.

A large study compared rates of antibiotic use in 2,266 women with breast and 7,953 women without the disease. Researchers found that women who received more than 25 prescriptions for antibiotics over a 17 year period (more than 500 days of use) had twice as many breast cancers as women who had taken no antibiotics at all. Even 1-25 prescriptions in such a time period were associated with a 50% increased risk.[1]

A Finnish study of 3,112,624 individuals also found antibiotic use directly correlated with an increased risk of multiple types of cancer. In the group of subjects having 2-5 prescriptions for antibiotics, the increased risk of any type of cancer was 27%; in the group receiving more than 6 prescriptions, increased risk was 37%. Separated into cancer types, the average increased risk was 39% for prostate, 14% for breast, 79% for lung, 15% for colon, and 260% for endocrine gland.[2]

Some antibiotics have been associated more than others with an increased risk of cancer. These include Cipro (ciprofloxacin), Flagyl (metronidazole), Garamycin (gentamicin), Grisovin (griseofulvin), and tetracyclines such as Sumycin, Terramycin, Tetracyn, and Panmycin.

However, it should be noted that these were only associative studies. Patients in these studies were not randomly assigned to take antibiotics, or not to take them. It may be that people who did not take antibiotics did not require them because they had uniquely active immune systems capable of handling infections without any help from a prescription. Those who did require multiple prescriptions may have suffered more infections due to innately weak immune systems.

In this case, antibiotic use is a secondary marker for another factor leading to a higher cancer risk, a weak immune system.

While antibiotic use is sometimes unavoidable, it should be used only on the basis of clear evidence of a bacterial infection; and not, for instance, for every minor upper respiratory infection. Use probiotics after completing antibiotic treatment to replenish beneficial bacteria.

References

(1) Velicer CM, Heckbert SR, Lampe JW, Potter JD, Robertson CA, Taplin SH. "Antibiotic Use in Relation to the Risk of Breast Cancer. "Journal of the American Medical Association, Feb. 18, 2004;291(7):827-835

(2) Annamari Kilkkinen, et al., "Antibiotic Use Predicts an Increased Risk of Cancer." Int J Cancer Vol 123 Issue 9, pp 2152-2155, Nov. 1 2008

Hormone-Replacement Therapy & Hormone Imbalance

Hormone replacement therapy has long been known to predispose to specific cancers of hormone-sensitive organs, such as breast & uterine cancers. Hormone replacement therapy with equine (horse) estrogens, derived from the urine of pregnant mares, was initially introduced as a means to counteract the symptoms of low-estrogen following menopause. Synthetic progestins (artificially-synthesized chemicals somewhat similar to natural progesterone) were sometimes used in conjunction. However, evidence soon emerged that showed a greater incidence of breast cancer in women undergoing this form of hormone-replacement therapy.

Bio-identical estrogen and progesterone should not be confused with artificial hormones. Their biochemical effects and risks are quite different.

Natural human estrogen comes in three forms, estrone (E1), estradiol (E2), and estriol (E3). During the reproductive years, estradiol predominates both in terms of serum levels as well as estrogenic activity (80X that of estriol). During pregnancy, estriol predominates. After the ovaries stop producing estradiol during menopause, estrone produced by fat cells and the adrenal glands predominates.

Estrogen supplements usually consist of estradiol, though some include one or both other forms as well. Some researchers have recommended the estriol, rather than estradiol, be used for menopausal estrogen supplementation; however, studies exist claiming it is even more likely than estradiol to cause breast cancer cell proliferation.[1]

Estrogen should *always* be accompanied by natural progesterone. Estrogen and progesterone have complementary effects which balance each other.

Significant research has now been directed towards understanding the hormonal mechanisms linked to breast cancer. Recent studies show that it is the impact of *unopposed* estrogen that seems to mediate this increased cancer risk in hormone-sensitive organs such as the breast or uterus. In contrast, this risk seems to be absent when estrogen and progesterone are given together.[2-10]

This effect is also seen in cases of naturally-occuring hormone imbalance. In one long-term prospective study, researchers followed 1083 women who had been treated for infertility from 1945-1965. The women were catagorized as having infertility due to endogenous progesterone deficiency, or other causes. By 1978, those with low levels of progesterone were found to be 4.5 times as prone to develop pre-menopausal breast cancer, and 10 times more prone to develop all forms of cancer.[11]

According to a 1996 study, serum progesterone levels at the time of breast cancer surgery influence survival rates. Breast cancer patients with progesterone levels of 4 ng/mL or greater at the time of breast cancer surgery had significantly better 18-year survival rates than those with lower serum levels of progesterone at date of surgery. Of those with higher progesterone levels at the time of surgery, approximately 65% were alive 18 years later, compared to only 35% of the women with low levels.[12]

Your doctor will no doubt warn of the danger of hormone supplementation in the case of hormone-sensitive cancers. However, supplementation with natural progesterone may actually improve prognosis. The progesterone creams sold over the counter in America vary widely in content, and may not increase serum levels enough to impact cancer; prescription products such as Prometrium are more appropriate.

Plant estrogens, such as genistein from soy, attach to cellular estrogen receptors and prevent the binding of stronger natural estrogen, effectively acting as estrogen blockers. In high amounts, they may act like estrogen supplements. The effect of phytoestrogens on cancer is a controversial topic, but it is better to be safe than sorry. Avoid soy.

References

(1) Boothby LA, Doering LA. "Bioidentical hormone therapy. a panacea that lacks supportive evidence." Curr Opin Obstet Gynecol 2008;20:400-7.

(2) Ravn SH, Rosenberg J, Bostofte E, "Postmenopausal hormone replacement therapy—clinical implications." Eur J Obstet Gynecol Reprod Biol. 1994 Feb;53(2):81-93.

(3) Samsioe G, "The endometrium: effects of estrogen and estrogen-progestogen replacement therapy." Int J Fertil Menopausal Stud. 1994;39 Suppl 2:84-92.

(4) Beresford SA, Weiss NS, Voigt LF, McKnight B, "Risk of endometrial cancer in relation to use of oestrogen combined with cyclic progestagen therapy in postmenopausal women." Lancet. 1997 Feb 15;349(9050):458-61.

(5) Southcott BM, "Carcinoma of the endometrium." Drugs. 2001;61(10):1395-405.

(6) Mahavni V, Sood AK, "Hormone replacement therapy and cancer risk." Curr Opin Oncol. 2001 Sep;13(5):384-9.

(7) De Vivo I, Huggins GS, Hankinson SE, et al., "A functional polymorphism in the promoter of the progesterone receptor gene associated with endometrial cancer risk." Proc Natl Acad Sci USA. 2002 Sep 17;99(19):12263-8.

(8) La Vecchia C, Brinton LA, McTiernan A, "Cancer risk in menopausal women." Best Pract Res Clin Obstet Gynaecol. 2002 Jun;16(3):293-307.

(9) Medina RA, Meneses AM, Vera JC, et al., "Differential regulation of glucose transporter expression by estrogen and progesterone in Ishikawa endometrial cancer cells." J Endocrinol. 2004 Sep;182(3):467-78.

(10) Creasman WT, "Hormone replacement therapy after cancers." Curr Opin Oncol. 2005 Sep;17(5):493-9.

(11) Cowan LD, Gordis L, Tonascia JA, Jones GS, "Breast cancer incidence in women with a history of progesterone deficiency." Am J Epidemiol. 1981 Aug;114(2):209-17.

(12) Mohr PE, Wang DY, Gregory WM, Richards MA, Fentiman IS, "Serum progesterone and prognosis in operable breast cancer." Br J Cancer. 1996 Jun;73(12):1552-5.

Sleeping Pills

A study which followed 10,529 subjects over a time period of approximately 2.5 years found a dramatically increased cancer rate among those who used sleeping pills of any kind, even if only rarely.

Use of sleeping pills correlated with a 5-fold increase in cancer risk for those who used more than 131 pills per year. Even those who took less than 18 pills per year showed a 3-fold increase. The exact chemical in the pill did not matter, whether the pills contained benzodiazepines, barbiturates or sedative antihistamines.[1]

No biological mechanism for this effect was suggested by the researchers. However, it is known that artificial sleep aids disrupt normal sleep patterns, prevent REM sleep, and likely also suppress natural melatonin secretion. Disruption of sleep patterns decreases the function of the immune system, and melatonin is a potent cancer preventative.

Those who have trouble sleeping should use melatonin, which is a completely natural substance that not only improves sleep, but also prevents and treats cancer.

References

(1) Daniel F Kripke, et al., "Hypnotics' association with mortality or cancer: a matched cohort study." BMJ Open 27 February 2012

Physical Inactivity & Obesity

Although physical inactivity is on everyone's list of "adverse health habits" due to increased risks of cardiovascular and metabolic diseases, it may not quite have made it to your list of cancer-causing factors.

Over the last several decades, speculation has abounded with regards to the impact of a high-fat diet on the risk of cancer. Even though initial studies suggested a link between high-fat diets and cancer, more specific studies found that the cancer-causing risk was mostly associated with what is known as *negative energy expenditure*, that is, obesity. Overweight individuals are at higher risk of developing cancer than those of normal weight, due to higher levels of insulin and insulin-like growth factor (IGF).

Obesity is not only associated with a higher risk of developing cancer; some research suggest it is also associated with a lower survival rate from it.[1,2] Cancer patients who are severely obese should try to lose weight.

The importance of physical activity in maintaining a healthy body cannot be questioned. Obese individuals are also at risk of developing type II diabetes, coronary artery disease, and strokes.

Isn't it time you began addressing this issue by implementing exercise in your lifestyle?

References

(1) Frank A Sinicrope, et al., "Obesity and Breast Cancer Prognosis: Weight of the Evidence." JCO January 1, 2011 vol. 29 no. 1 4-7

(2) Frank Sinicrope, et al., "Obesity Is an Independent Prognostic Variable in Colon Cancer Survivors." Clin Cancer Res 2010 March 15; 16(6) 1884-1893

Exercise & Cancer

When you have cancer, your body needs all the zest and vitality it can get. Moderate exercise is best, as we know it stimulates the immune system. By keeping yourself as fit and healthy as you can, your body will be able to respond to the challenge effectively.

A 2011 study of 243 patients with advanced recurrent gliomas at the Preston Robert Tisch Brain Tumor Center at Duke University showed that exercise increased survival significantly. Patients who engaged in regular exercise, the equivalent of a brisk 30-minute walk five days per week, lived an average of 21.84 months compared to 13.03 months for the most sedentary patients.[1]

Regular physical activity was associated with a 6% reduction in mortality of breast cancer patients. This study followed 2987 nurses diagnosed with stage I, II, or III breast cancer between 1984 and 1998, who were tracked until their deaths or until June 2002, whichever came first. The effect of exercise was more pronounced in hormone-sensitive tumors, perhaps because exercise lowers estrogen levels.[2]

A study of 573 colon cancer patients found the lowest 5-year mortality among those who exercised the most. Patients who engaged in less than 3 hours of activity per week had a mortality of 14.1%. Those in the next category, who engaged in 3-17.9 hours of activity per week, had a mortality of 14.3% (not statistically different). However, those who engaged in 18+ hours of activity per week had a mortality of only 6.2%.[3]

Women diagnosed with breast cancer can prevent relapse and extend their lives by exercising. In fact, just 3 to 5 hours per week is all it takes. And if you are undergoing chemotherapy, the fatigue can be reduced if you are physically active. Being fit can keep the bones strong, pump up your immune system and improve your overall quality of life.

The problem is that you have to be motivated to do something that is basically work, or, at the least, effort in a situation which may be fraught with panic and worries.

Staying motivated is a struggle — our drive is constantly assaulted by negative thoughts and anxiety about the future. Everyone faces doubt and depression. What separates the highly persistent from the exercise dropouts is the ability to keep moving forward. Use your imagination to think about nice things. They don't have to be real, don't forget we create our own reality.

There is no simple solution for a lack of motivation. Even after beating the problem, it can reappear at the first sign of failure. The key is understanding your thoughts and how they drive your emotions. By learning how to focus on positive results, and deal with negative thoughts before they sap your resolve, you can maintain the momentum of your exercise program.

References

(1) Emily Ruden, et al., "Exercise Behavior, Functional Capacity, and Survival in Adults With Malignant Recurrent Glioma." J Clin Oncol. 2011 July 20; 29(21): 2918–2923

(2) Holmes M et al, "Physical activity and survival after breast cancer diagnosis" JAMA 2005;293(20):2479-2486

(3) Meyerhardt JA, Giovannucci EL, Holmes MD, et al. "Physical activity and survival after colorectal cancer diagnosis." Journal of Clinical Oncology 2006 Aug 1;24(22):3527-34. Epub 2006 Jul 5.

Stress

The average person deals with a multitude of stressors on a daily basis, from those that are work-related to those associated with family or relationship events. Sleep deprivation in a significant proportion of the population also adds to this problem. Although stress has not been clearly and uniformly linked to an increased risk of cancer, many studies have shown at least an indirect association.

Individuals exposed to high levels of stress are more likely to seek stress-relieving habits that are often deleterious to their health.

Common examples include smoking, alcohol use, and harmful dietary practices, all of which are strongly associated with an increased risk of cancer. As a result, stress may be one of the most significant risk factors for cancer in human beings. Individuals struggling with cancer can seek the help of health professionals as well as stress-relieving activities, from meditation to yoga.

One of the mechanisms by which stress can lead to cancer is its deleterious effects on sleep. Disruption of the circadian rhythm influences the activity of the immune system, and suppresses the secretion of melatonin.

Make sure to get adequate sleep, in complete darkness. Occlude any light sources during sleep, and avoid the use of night-lights.

Indoor & Outdoor Tanning

On April 13, 2011 the International Agency for Research on Cancer of the World Health Organization classified all wavelengths and categories of Ultraviolet Radiation as a Group 1 carcinogen. This is the most severe designation possible for potential carcinogens, meaning, "There is enough evidence to conclude that it can cause cancer in humans".

While minimal exposure to UVB (5-15 minutes daily) has been recommended by some health authorities as a method of producing vitamin D naturally in the body, excessive sunbathing is definitely harmful.

Sunlight consists of a broad spectrum of radiation types. In addition to visible light, sunlight is also composed of ultraviolet (UV) radiation, which comes in two wavelengths: UV-A and UV-B.

UV-B causes the skin to produce vitamin D, which is a cancer preventative, but this is accomplished with minimal sun exposure only to the point of slight skin reddening, not prolonged sunbathing.

As well as causing cancer, exposure to ultraviolet light, UVA or UVB, from sunlight accounts for 90% of the symptoms of premature skin aging. Many skin changes that were formerly believed to be due to aging, such as easy bruising, are actually the result of prolonged exposure to UV radiation. UV radiation also causes eye disorders such as cataract formation, and suppresses the immune system.

UVB causes superficial damage and burning, while UVA affects mainly the deeper layer of the skin, the dermis, and causes changes that lead to skin cancer. UVC is mostly filtered by Earth's atmosphere, but can be generated artificially, such as in some water sterilization systems.

Although you might be told that UV-B rays are linked to skin cancer, recent studies point to UV-A as also being a potential inducer of skin tumors, as well as the main factor in skin aging. This means that tanning booths are potentially deadly, and sunscreens may not effectively protect you against the skin damage that predisposes to skin cancer. Most sunscreens filter out only UV-B, and work poorly against UV-A.

Skin cancer is, by far, the most common cancer type. Every year nearly 70,000 cases of melanoma are diagnosed in the United States and this number continues to rise at a rate of 5-7% every year in fair-skinned populations.

Although early-stage (Stage Ia) melanomas have a 95% 5-year survival rates, advanced-stage tumors are associated with a dismal 19% survival, making melanoma the deadliest of all skin cancers. UV radiation leads to a signature mutation in cells. Surprisingly, this mutation is absent in 92% of all melanomas. While basal and squamous cell skin carcinomas are linked to chronic longterm UV exposure, melanomas are epidemiologically associated with a single blistering sunburn, often during childhood.

Preventive habits include the avoidance of prolonged sun exposure or tanning booth use as well as the use of sunblock creams with SPF greater than 15. Avoid sunburns.

High-Risk Sexual & Drug Use Behaviors

It is unsurprising that high-risk behaviors are associated with higher risk of death, but you may not be aware that many of the common high-risk behaviors & habits are also associated with increased incidence of cancer.

For example, elevated rates of sexual promiscuity and unprotected sex are classically associated with many sexually transmitted diseases, such as the Hepatitis B and C Virus, the Human Immunodefficiency Virus HIV, and the Human Papillomavirus

(HPV). All of these viruses are associated with increased incidence of cancer formation.

The hepatitis virus is associated with often-lethal hepatocellular carcinoma while HIV is associated with Kaposi's Sarcoma and other cancers. Finally, HPV has been demonstrated to be a major factor in the development of cervical and oropharyngeal cancers.

Asbestos

Asbestos was once widely used as a fire-proof insulator. During WWII, it was considered so vital to the American war effort that it was regarded as a strategically significant war material by the US government. Blue asbestos was even used to line gas masks used in WWII. Unprotected exposure to asbestos was common in the shipbuilding, manufacturing and construction workplace. Since the early 1940s, millions of American workers were exposed to asbestos.

Workers breathed in microscopic fibers of asbestos, which settled in their lungs setting up a permanent inflammatory response leading to incurable tumors called mesotheliomas. They also brought the material home on their clothes, exposing their spouses and children to the toxic dust as well. Whole families were wiped out by mesotheliomas. The disease can manifest decades after exposure to asbestos.

Asbestos is now universally recognized as a deadly health hazard. Even one inhalation of a minute amount of asbestos dust can be fatal, as the body can never remove the toxic fibers.

This toxic substance is completely banned in dozens of countries, and used only in tightly controlled circumstances in America.

However, due to previous widespread use, and the long latency period for mesothelioma to develop, it is still a concern.

Some law firms specialize in lawsuits for workers suffering from mesothelioma, and it may be possible to litigate for financial compensation.

Particulate Air Pollution

If you live beside a busy freeway, or downtown in a large city, air pollution will negatively impact your health. Vehicle exhaust is made up of microscopic particles with a large surface area containing polycyclic aromatic hydrocarbons, transition metals and other petrochemical substances implicated in cancer formation.

Many studies show a link between traffic pollution and lung cancer.

In addition, a Canadian study showed that postmenopausal women living in areas with high levels of traffic-generated air pollution have an increased risk of breast cancer.[1] A Danish study found a 25% increases in Hodkin's lymphoma in children exposed to high levels of traffic fumes in utero.[2] The same researchers also found a link with brain and cervical cancer in adults.[3]

If you live in an area with high levels of smog, move to another location if at all possible. If this is not an option, install a good air cleaner.

References

(1) Dan L. Crouse, et al., "Postmenopausal Breast Cancer Is Associated with Exposure to Traffic-Related Air Pollution in Montreal, Canada: A Case–Control Study." Environ Health Perspect. 2010 November; 118(11): 1578–1583

(2) Ole Raaschou-Nielsen, et al, "Air Pollution from Traffic at the Residence of Children with Cancer." American Journal of Epidemiology Vol 153, No. 5)

(3) Ole Raaschou-Nielsen, et al., "Air pollution from traffic and cancer incidence: a Danish cohort study." Environmental Health 2011, 10:67

Mercury Fillings

Many researchers believe that the highly toxic materials used in dentistry are an important reason for the cancer epidemic of modern times. They also state that some of the leading holistic doctors in Germany refuse to treat patients who have amalgams in their teeth, as they know that no treatment can ever be fully effective unless the toxic fillings are removed.

Use composite fillings instead.

Root Canals

In the 1950's, German physician Dr. Josef Issels heard a lecture by immunotherapist Dr. Max Gerson, and subsequently successfully used alternative treatments in helping many cancer patients. Dr. Issels himself spent some time at the CHIPSA hospital, a legacy medical center founded by Gerson.

While Issels was there, Gerson pointed out the severe damage caused by root canal fillings. He said that he refused to treat any cancer patient who did not allow all "devitalized" (dead) teeth to be removed, as he found that he could not obtain good results without this procedure. This echoes similar findings by dentist Weston Price in the 1920s.

Though root canal therapy has improved tremendously since it was invented in the pre-antibiotic era, a dead tooth has a labyrinth of microtubules where harmful microbes can flourish safe from the body's immune system, since the tubules are too small to admit white blood cells. The bacteria secrete toxins and continually seed themselves throughout the body. This chronic, low-level infection causes a constant inflammatory response that has been linked to atherosclerosis and heart disease as well as cancer.

The same can be said for gum disease (gingivitis/periodontitis). A 2007 study by the Harvard School of Public Health in Boston found a 64% increase in pancreatic cancer for men with severe periodontal disease.[1]

Other researchers found associations between periodontal disease and oral, gastric and pancreatic cancers, which persisted even after statistical control for smoking habits.[2]

Dental implants or dentures are a better solution to irreparable teeth than root canals. Have regular dental cleanings to eliminate gum disease.

References

(1) Michaud DS, "A prospective study of periodontal disease and pancreatic cancer in US male health professionals." J Natl Cancer Institute 2007 Jan 17;99(2):171-5

(2) Mara S. Meyer, "A Review of the Relationship between Tooth Loss, Periodontal Disease, and Cancer, A Review of the Relationship between Tooth Loss, Periodontal Disease, and Cancer." Cancer Causes and Control, Volume 19 Number 9 2008), 895-907, DOI: 10.1007/s10552-008-9163-4

Radiation

Few cancer patients have ever suffered from acute radiation poisoning due to a single high-dose exposure. However, DNA damage caused by radiation is cumulative, and multiple low doses add up.

Radiation exists across a spectrum from very high-energy (high-frequency) radiation to very low-energy (low-frequency) radiation. This is sometimes referred to as the *electromagnetic spectrum*. From highest to lowest energy, the main forms of radiation are:

- Gamma rays
- X-rays
- Ultraviolet rays (UV)
- Visible light
- Infrared rays
- Microwaves
- Radiofrequency waves (radio)
- Extremely low-frequency radiation (ELF)

An important distinction that affects the health risks from radiation is whether the energy is ionizing or non-ionizing.

Ionizing radiation is high-frequency radiation that has enough energy to remove an electron from (ionize) an atom or molecule. Ionizing radiation has enough energy to damage the DNA in cells, which in turn may lead to cancer. Gamma rays, x-rays, some high-energy UV rays, and some sub-atomic particles such as alpha particles and protons are forms of ionizing radiation. Ionizing radiation is definitely linked to cancer.

However, non-ionizing radiation, such as from cell phones, has recently been implicated in cancer development as well. The WHO has implicated heavy cell phone use in the development of brain tumors.

Try to avoid all radiation as much as possible. Rural environments may be less contaminated by electrosmog than urban locations. Avoid the use of cellphones, wireless phones and WIFI.

Ionizing Radiation

Many authorities say there is no "safe" level of radiation, and that radiation exposure, even at low levels, leads to cancer in a predictable, straight-line correlational pattern when cancer rates vs. radiation levels are plotted on a graph.

Other scientists claim there is evidence that radiation actually has a "hormetic" effect; that is, low doses have a protective effect. At doses of 3-5 times (and sometimes even up to 100 times) the level of normal background radiation, cancer rates are actually reduced, leading to a U-shaped graph with an upswing to 100% mortality as one moves past the "protective" zone and into higher, damaging exposures. This phenomenon seems to be due to the fact that low levels of radiation stimulate the body's repair mechanisms.[1,2,3,4] This explains why health tours of radium mines and spas featuring radioactive water were a common custom 100 years ago.

While this is an interesting subject for academic debate, modern Americans are exposed to so much radiation from a myriad of sources that they are far past the bottom of any dip in the exposure/cancer incidence graph, and climbing well up the increasing side of the line.

Avoid ionizing radiation.

References

(1) Cohen BL, "Cancer risk from low-level radiation." AJR 2002 Nov;179(5):1137-43

(2) Cohen BL. "A test of the linear-no threshold theory of radiation carcinogenesis". Environ. Res. 1990 53 (2): 193.

(3) Ruth Sponsler, John R Cameron, "Nuclear shipyard worker study (1980–1988): a large cohort exposed to low-dose-rate gamma radiation." Int J Low Radiation 2005 vol 1 no. 4

(4) Cutler JM, "Health Effects of Low Level Radiation: When Will We Acknowledge the Reality?" Dose Response 2007; 5(4): 292–298.

Sources Of Radiation

Medical Radiation

This category includes medical and dental X-rays, CT scans and mammograms.

The level of radiation emitted by a modern X-ray machine is small, but not insignificant; also, radiation-induced DNA damage is cumulative with every exposure.

Much higher levels of radiation are involved in CAT scans, which use multiple X-ray exposures to create a 3-D picture of the inside of the body. CAT scans can deliver up to 500 times more radiation than a conventional X-ray. As a point of comparison, one chest CT is around 10 millisieverts of radiation and a traditional chest X-ray only 0.02 millisieverts.

The US Nuclear Regulatory Commission recommends that people receive no more than 100 millirems or mr (1 milliSievert or mSv) per year of radiation in addition to normal background radiation. Even at the maximum end of what nuclear experts consider low-dose lifetime exposure, 100 millisieverts, approximately 1 person in 100 will develop cancer, according to biostatisticians at the National Cancer Institute, in Bethesda, Md.

A recent study states that the increased use of CT scans, which use doses of radiation hundreds of times higher than those of ordinary X-rays, are exposing patients to levels of radiation similar to those of Hiroshima survivors. The study concluded, "On the basis of such risk estimates and data on CT use from 1991 through 1996, it has been estimated that about 0.4% of all cancers in the United States may be attributable to the radiation from CT studies. By adjusting this estimate for current CT use, this estimate might now be in the range of 1.5 to 2.0%."[1]

Americans are now exposed to approximately seven times more radiation than they were in 1980. "The increase in medical [radiation] exposure was not a big surprise to anybody," said Kenneth Kase, executive vice president of the National Council on Radiation Protection. "Radiation exposure from these scans is not inconsequential and can lead to later cancers," stated Dr. Len Lichtenfeld, deputy chief medical officer for the national office of the American Cancer Society. "This doesn't mean people shouldn't get CT scans, but it does mean we need to be very careful in how we use these technologies in the future."

The report also found that while CT scans made up only 17% of total radiological procedures CT scans account for 49% of all medical radiation exposure, and 24% of all radiation sources.[2]

Other practitioners feel the risks are much higher than 2%.

Dr. John Gofman, Ph.D, is a Professor of Molecular and Cell Biology at the University of California, Berkeley. In 1999, he published a lengthy meta-analysis of American mortality rates due to cancer and ischemic heart disease (atherosclerosis), and concluded that since 1940, medical X-rays have been a major factor in the majority of these deaths. This is a radical concept for many doctors to accept, as X-rays are routinely and repetitively used, often for minor diagnostic benefit without considering their longterm damage. According to Dr. Gofman, the harm caused by diagnostic radiation is not trivial, and the danger of X-ray exposure is not treated with the concern it deserves.

Atherosclerotic plaques, the hallmark of ischemic heart disease, have more in common with cancer than many people realize. These plaques, overgrowths of tissue which cause narrowing of the arteries, are monoclonal; that is, they are derived from a single cell. They can be viewed as miniature, benign tumors in the walls of arteries.

Using the term "fractional causation," Dr. Gofman stated that both cancer and heart disease were multi-factorial diseases, requiring a certain "threshold" of cumulative exposure before the human body would be so overwhelmed that it could no longer compensate for damage. Subtract the "fraction" of the damage caused by medical radiation, and the sum of other factors (such as cigarette smoking and poor diet) would not reach a cumulative level sufficient to cause disease. According to Dr. Gofman, the majority of cancer and IHD patients would not have developed their disease if they had not been subjected to medical radiation.[3]

Avoid unecessary or "routine" X-rays, and especially try to avoid CT scans. An MRI, or magnetic resonance imager, uses no radiation and is a preferred method of diagnosis.

Ironically, radiation used to cure cancer may be responsible for the later development of more aggressive recurrent tumors.

Researchers at the Department of Radiation Oncology at the UCLA Jonsson Comprehensive Cancer Center found that radiation treatment transforms breast cancer cells into treatment-resistant cancer stem cells, even though it debulks tumors by 50%. These surviving cells were up to 30 times more likely to form tumors as nonirradiated breast cancer cells.[4,5]

Radiation-resistant stem cells also play a role in recurrent prostate cancer.[6]

The phenomenon has been observed in breast, prostate, and head and neck cancer, and glioblastomas. Amazingly, lead researcher Dr. Frank Pajonk, an Associate Professor of Experimental Radiation Oncology, stated that the study still did not discredit the usefulness of radiation therapy. "Patients come to me scared by the idea that radiation generates these cells, but it truly is the safest and most effective therapy there is."[5]

Dental X-rays

Meningiomas are the most common form of primary brain tumor in the United States. People who develop meningiomas are more than twice as likely to report having had at least one bitewing, full-mouth or panorex dental X-ray. Exposure to these X-rays before the age of 10 was associated with a 490% risk increase.[7]

Mammograms

The low-dose radiation from annual mammography screening significantly increases breast cancer risk in women with a genetic or familial predisposition to breast cancer. Among all women in the high-risk group, the average risk of breast cancer increased was 1.5 times higher than that of high-risk women with no history of low-dose radiation exposure. Among high-risk women with 5 or more exposures, or exposure before age twenty, risk was 2.5 times greater.

"For women at high risk for breast cancer, screening is very important, but a careful approach should be taken when considering mammography for screening young women, particularly under age 30," Marijke C. Jansen-van der Weide, Ph.D., an epidemiologist in the Department of Epidemiology and Radiology at the University Medical Center Groningen in the Netherlands, said in a statement to the media. "Further, repeated exposure to low-dose radiation should be avoided."[8]

Women who want to be screened for breast cancer should use breast thermography, which measures tissue temperatures and does not involve X-rays, instead of mammograms.

Radon

Radon is a radioactive gas produced by the breakdown of uranium naturally present in soil. Radon is present in nearly all air. Everyone breathes radon in every day, usually at very low levels. However, people who inhale high levels of radon are at an increased risk for developing lung cancer.

Radon is the second leading cause of lung cancer in America (after smoking) and causes 15,000 to 22,000 lung cancer deaths annually. Studies from both uranium miners and the general populaton exposed to high radon levels in their homes show increased rates of lung cancer.

Invisible and odorless, radon can be detected only with a radon meter. Health authorities promote radon testing and encourage homeowners to take corrective measures in homes where high levels are found.

Radon can enter homes through cracks in floors, walls, or foundations, and collect indoors. It can also be released from building materials, or from water obtained from wells that contain radon. Radon can accumulate at high levels in homes that are well insulated, tightly sealed, and/or built on uranium-rich soil. Because of their closeness to the ground, basement and first floors typically have the highest radon levels.

In order to control ground moisture, current building codes mandate the installation of plastic sheeting over the ground before the basement slab is poured to control ground moisture. This sheeting also serves as an excellent barrier for radon gas and should be extended under the house footings and also under any load-bearing pads. Placing a vapor barrier before a house is built is much cheaper than retrofitting with fans and exhaust systems.

The U.S. Environmental Protection Agency has recommended that indoor radon concentrations not be allowed to exceed 4 pCi/L, a concentration that might be expected to double the risk of lung cancer if inhaled throughout an average lifespan.

If the radon concentration in your home is too high, call a contractor who specializes in correcting this problem.

Radon test meters can be purchased for as little as $20.00.

References

(1) Exposure David J. Brenner, Eric J. Hall, "Computed Tomography — An Increasing Source of Radiation." N Engl J Med Nov 29 2007; 357:2277-2284

(2) Audrey Grayson, "Americans' Radiation Exposure Rises 6-Fold in 29 Years."ABC News Medical Unit, March 3, 2009

(3) John W. Gofman, M.D., Ph. D., "Radiation from Medical Procedures in the Pathogenesis of Cancer and Ischemic Heart Disease: Dose-Response Studies with Physicians per 100,000 Population." First Edition: 1999, C.N.R. Book Division, Committee for Nuclear Responsibility, Inc., Post Office Box 421993,San Francisco, California, 94142 U.S.A.)

(4) Carrie Printz, "Radiation treatment generates therapy-resistant cancer stem cells from less aggressive breast cancer cells." Cancer, Volume 118, Issue 13, page 3225, 1 July 2012

(5) Lagadec C, Vlashi E, Della Donna L, Dekmezian C, Pajonk F. "Radiation-induced reprogramming of breast cancer cells." Stem Cells. 2012;30:833-844

(6) Cho YM, et al., "Long-term recovery of irradiated prostate cancer increases cancer stem cells." Prostate. 2012 Apr 18. Epub 2012 Apr 18.

(7) Elizabeth B. Claus MD, PhD, Lisa Calvocoressi PhD, Melissa L. Bondy PhD, Joellen M. Schildkraut PhD, Joseph L. Wiemels PhD, Margaret Wrensch PhD, "Dental x-rays and risk of meningioma." Cancer, Early Online Edition, 10 APR 2012,DOI: 10.1002/cncr.26625

(8) Marijke C. Jansen-van der Weide, Ph.D, "Mammography May Increase Breast Cancer Risk in Some High-Risk Women." Radiological Society of North America, Press Release, December 1, 2009)

Nuclear Weapons Testing

The world's nuclear powers have conducted more than 2000 tests of nuclear weapons since 1945, leading to a worldwide increase in low-level radiation. Areas where tests were performed, such as Nevada, New Mexico, and the Pacific atolls, have had greater exposure than others. However, due to natural spread by wind and water currents, there is no place on the planet where isotopes from nuclear testing cannot be found.

Many Gulf War veterans have been exposed to weapons coated in depleted uranium, as have residents of the Middle East where these weapons have been used. Uranium miners also have a higher risk of cancer.

Nuclear Power Plants

Fukushima and Three Mile Island are the best-known nuclear power plant disasters, but minor leaks at other plants occur on a chronic basis. "Cancer clusters," statistically unusual patterns of cancer incidence, are found in nearby areas.

Non-Ionizing Radiation

These wavelengths were formerly thought of as being entirely benign, but are now coming under increasing scrutiny. Electromagnetic radiation, even in the so-called "non-ionizing" range, is linked to cancer.

EMR In Your neighborhood

Cell phones are ubiquitous. Evidence implicating cell phones with causing brain tumors has caused the WHO to classify cell phone radiation as "possibly carcinogenic."

It has also been suggested that "smart meters" and other WIFI installations may cause cancer, though this has not been proven.

Microwave towers

Mobile phone transmissions kill trees. What are they doing to humans?

Dutch researchers found high levels of cell phone radiation linked to the growth retardation, deformity and death of trees in urban centers. This supposedly harmless "non-ionizing" radiation damages trees at a cellular level to the point where they actually "bleed".

The results come from 3 sources in the Netherlands: Technical University of Delft, the municipality of Alphen aan de Rijn, and Wageningen University.
A few years ago in some parts of Dutch cities, Dutch civil servants discovered very visible distortions on trees. No obvious cause was found. 70% of the trees in Dutch cities showed the same symptoms, up from 10% only 5 years ago.

There were no viruses or bacteria that could account for the symptoms; however, damage levels correlated directly with the exposure of the trees to cell phone radiation.[1]

Further research showed that the symptoms were occurring at lower levels throughout the whole western world in areas of high cell phone radiation.

There are nearly 800 million cellphone users in India, making the nation the second largest cellphone-using population in the world (after China). In 2010, A 13-member fact-finding committee was established by the union ministry of environment and forests to examine the impact of cellphone towers on humans as well as wildlife such as birds, insects, and animals. Asad Rahmani, director of Bombay Natural History Society, was made chairman of the group.

The committee's results were startling. Out of 919 studies evaluated, a staggering 593 found a negative impact of cellphone towers on plants, birds, bees, wildlife and humans. The experts even cited an international study that blamed cellphone towers for the decline of animal populations. They concluded that there was an urgent need to focus more scientific research on cellphone radiation before it was too late.[2]

Get rid of your mobile phone and move if you are living close to a Microwave tower. If you cannot do without a cellphone, pick a brand with lower levels of radiation (ratings vary widely between brands) and use it as infrequently as possible. Hollow air tubes such as Smart Safe are an accessory which can amplify sound while the cell phone is kept away from the body, thus minimizing radiation exposure.

http://www.amazon.com/Smart-Safe-Hollow-Hands-free-Headset

Dirty Electricity

In theory, electrical power is provided at a safe frequency of 60 Hertz (Hz). In reality, it is becoming increasingly contaminated with surges of radio frequency radiation and other electromagnetic phenomena collectively referred to as "Dirty Electricity". This can contribute significantly to exposure to man-made EMF energy, as it can radiate several feet into a room, even when no nearby appliances are turned on.

Transformers and power supplies convert AC current to the low voltages used in energy-efficient electronics, and in the process these devices chop up the conventional AC 60Hz sine wave to create what are known as electrical "transients". This has become increasingly problematic due to the proliferation of "energy-saving" devices such as dimmer switches, fluorescent tubes, CFL and low-voltage halogen lighting (LED is OK), computers and other electronic entertainment devices. These tend to induce high levels of transients (high frequency spikes) and harmonics (multiples of the fundamental 60Hz frequency) back into a building's electrical system.

These undesirable frequencies propagate through the electrical system, affecting the entire building and even other buildings on the same grid through shared transformers.

Another source of electrical contamination is ground current, which can also feed unpredictable frequencies into a building's AC supply.

Many homes are affected by "plumbing current." This occurs when some of the electricity that should normally return through the service line is instead diverted into the grounding system, where it returns to the transformer through alternate routes such as water pipes and the public water main.

Radio waves from nearby broadcast stations can also be picked up and re-radiated by electrical wiring.

This is not a benign electrical phenomenon, as it has been linked to increased incidence of cancer.[3]

Professional consulting firms will evaluate the level of electrical contamination in a home; or individuals can purchase a device such as the Graham-Stetzer Microsurge Meter and measure it themselves. Products such as Greenwave or Graham-Stetzer filters can then be installed to remove these harmful frequencies.

http://www.greenwavefilters.com

Is Your Mattress A Cancer-Causing Antenna?

The rate of breast cancer in Western countries is 10% higher in the left breast than in the right. Melanoma also tends to occur more often on the left side of the body.

Researchers have suggested a surprising explanation for this -- and for the dramatic increase in rates of breast cancer and melanoma over the past three decades.

In Japan, there is no correlation between the rates of melanoma and breast cancer, and there is no left-side prevalence for either disease. The rate of breast cancer in Japan is also significantly lower than in the West.

This may be due to differences in sleeping habits in Japan and Western countries. Previous research has shown that people prefer to sleep on their right sides, possibly as a way of reducing weight stress on the heart. This is most likely the same in both the East and the West, but the futons used for sleeping in Japan are basically large pillows placed directly on the bedroom floor, in contrast to the elevated box springs and mattress of beds used in the West.

116

According to *Scientific American*:
"... [A] 2007 study in Sweden conducted between 1989 and 1993 ... revealed a strong link between the incidence of melanoma and the number of FM and TV transmission towers covering the area where the individuals lived ...
Consider, however, that even a TV set cannot respond to broadcast transmissions unless the weak electromagnetic waves are captured and amplified by an appropriately designed antenna. Antennas are simply metal objects of appropriate length sized to match the wavelength of a specific frequency of electromagnetic radiation."

In the U.S., bed frames and box springs are made of metal, and the length of a bed is exactly half the wavelength of FM and TV transmissions, which have been on the air continuously since the 1940s. The maximum strength of the field develops 75 centimeters above the mattress, so when sleeping on the right side, the sleeper's left side will be exposed to the highest field strength.

Scientific American explains this quite well:

"Just as saxophones are made in different sizes to resonate with and amplify particular wavelengths of sound, electromagnetic waves are selectively amplified by metal objects that are the same, half or one quarter of the wavelength of an electromagnetic wave of a specific frequency.
Electromagnetic waves resonate on a half-wavelength antenna to create a standing wave with a peak at the middle of the antenna and a node at each end, just as when a string stretched between two points is plucked at the center." [4]

Could this explain why Japan has much lower rates of cancer compared to the US and Europe, and why the Japanese do not have higher rates of left- than right-sided breast cancer?

Futons and foam beds are a good alternative to steel-frame boxsprings and mattresses.

References

(1) Niall Firth, "Is Wi-Fi killing trees? Dutch study shows leaves dying after exposure." Mail Online, UPDATED:10:25 GMT, 25 November 2010. Read more: http://www.dailymail.co.uk/sciencetech/article-1332310/Is-Wi-Fi-killing-trees-Dutch-study-shows-leaves-dying-exposure-Wi-Fi-radiation.html#ixzz23qoyBM00

(2) Dr. Asad Rahmani, et al., "Report on possible impact of communication towers on wildlife including birds and bees" PDF file online: http://www.ee.iitb.ac.in/~mwave/Report%20on%20Possible%20Impacts%20of%20Communication%20Towers.pdf

(3) Samuel Milham, MD, MPH L. Lloyd Morgan, BS, "A New Electromagnetic Exposure Metric: High Frequency Voltage Transients Associated With Increased Cancer Incidence in Teachers in a California School." Am. J. Ind. Med. 2008

(4) R. Douglas Fields, "Left-sided Cancer: Blame your Bed and TV?" Scientific American, July 2, 2010)

Vitamin D & Cancer

History Of Vitamin D

Since its identification in the 1920's, vitamin D has become a staple supplement of the American diet. Currently, numerous fortified food items and over-the-counter dietary products boast their high levels of vitamin D, and together they have significantly reduced vitamin D deficiency-associated diseases in the United States. Rickets, an obvious and once common sign of severe vitamin D deficiency, is rarely seen any more.

Have you ever wondered why many older generations subjected themselves to ingesting a spoonful of cod liver oil daily? In the late

19th century, cod liver oil was noted to prevent the development of rickets in infants and children.

Rickets is a bone disorder characterized by the abnormal calcification of bone matter, which results in decreased bone rigidity and bony deformation such as bowed legs. Children with rickets suffer from abnormal bone development that can lead to lifelong musculoskeletal impairment.

However, it wasn't until the early portion of the 20th century that scientists were able to extract and purify the active agent responsible for rickets cure and prevention. In the 1920s, it was identified, characterized, and subsequently given the name of vitamin D.

Although not a true vitamin, vitamin D is an essential molecule necessary for normal calcium regulation in the human body. Its role in cellular physiology can be traced 750 million years back to planktonic primordial life forms.

Although human beings are able to synthesize all necessary amounts of vitamin D, thus precluding this compound from its vitamin status, its synthesis is heavily dependent on diet and sun exposure.

Vitamin D3, also known as cholecalciferol, is synthesized in the skin from cholesterol in a reaction process that requires ultraviolet radiation. As a result, individuals of darker skin color and those who lack sufficient sun exposure are at increased risk for vitamin D deficiency.

Vitamin D3 is then converted by the liver to produce 25-hydroxyvitamin D, (calcitriol), then changed further by the kidneys to make 1,25-dihydroxyvitamin D, the active form of the vitamin.

Small amounts of vitamin D can be widely obtained from a healthy diet including fatty fish such as sardines and other fortified products such as milk.

Vitamin D Plays Multiple Roles In The Human Body.

Over the last half-century, we have learned much about vitamin D's essential role in human health, but it appears that this molecule has much more in store for us. The discovery of vitamin D has heralded numerous applications that have resulted in disease cures and many beneficial effects on a variety of disorders ranging in nature from cardiovascular to endocrine.

Vitamin D is a key regulator of calcium levels in the human body. It acts as a signaling molecule that instructs the intestinal tract and the kidneys to increase their uptake of calcium. It also increases the uptake of calcium by bone tissue, thereby preventing weakening of bones through demineralization. Low levels of vitamin D cause rickets, osteomalacia, and osteoporosis.

However, vitamin D has numerous other effects as well, which may be as important as maintaining bone structure. Low levels of vitamin D are associated with numerous diseases of the entire body, including auto-immune diseases such as multiple sclerosis, neurological diseases such as Parkinson's and Alzheimer's disease, susceptability to contagious diseases such as influenza, and last but certainly not least, cancer.

Some health authorities are now claiming that the higher rates of cancer, heart disease, autism and autoimmune diseases seen in the Northern hemisphere, as opposed to the tropics, are the results of vitamin D deficiency due to lower levels of sunlight.

Though we have long understood many of the functions of Vitamin D in regards to calcium regulation, it now appears that it can have an even greater impact directly at the cellular level. Vitamin D is capable of binding to a group of cell receptors known as the nuclear receptor superfamily.

These receptors, once bound to vitamin D, can travel directly to the cell's nucleus and direct the transcription of specific cellular genes.

Surprisingly, these receptors are found in a wide variety of tissues unrelated to calcium metabolism.

Because of this, scientists became interested in the potential role of vitamin D in other human diseases, including human cancer. Any compound with the ability to impact the cellular transcription of genes associated with cell division can be implicated in carcinogenesis or cancer prevention.

With its ability to influence numerous cellular functions at the genetic level, vitamin D is less of a vitamin and more of an essential cellular signaling molecule. As such, vitamin D has the potential to affect the activity of dozens, if not hundreds, of genes, many of which are associated with cellular growth, division, and differentiation.

Cellular differentiation refers to the tendency of cells to adopt a specific functional or structural role. For example, intestinal lining cells differentiate into cells capable of absorbing nutrients and electrolytes.

The ability to remain differentiated appears to decrease the ability of a cell to transform into a cancerous entity, because differentiated cells tend to not divide. Factors that push a cell towards differentiation can help prevent or reverse the mechanisms of cancer formation.

Vitamin D has shown to have the ability to induce differentiation of leukemia and other cancer cells. Furthermore, cancers of the colon and prostate display a lack of vitamin D receptors, which blocks the stimulus for differentiation. This apparent vitamin D resistance can render cell lines more prone to cancer transformation. Alternatively, this may also mean that vitamin D supplementation early on can act as a preventive strategy against cancer.

Vitamin D also slows the reproduction of cancer cells, and boosts the function of the immune system.

In a study on the synergistic effects of Vitamin D and curcumin, Vitamin D was found to activate Type II macrophages. Curcumin, found in turmeric, selectively activates Type I macrophages. The researchers were using the two substances to stimulate the immune system to remove amyloid plaques characteristic of Alzheimer's disease; however, the immune system also plays a large role in curing cancer.[1]

As we continue to learn more about this molecule, its applications to human disease are sure to continue to increase.

Vitamin D, An Underrated Cancer Fighter

In-vitro (cell studies) show a direct ability of Vitamin D to inhibit cancer. Epidemiology also shows that populations with low levels of vitamin D have higher cancer rates than populations with high vitamin D levels.

The last three decades have seen the completion of numerous promising studies on the impact of vitamin D on cancer survival and prevention. In 1981, two studies first showed an in-vitro ability of vitamin D to inhibit cancer cell growth and progression in melanoma & leukemia cell lines. Subsequently, additional studies found a protective benefit of vitamin D in patients with colorectal cancer and Hodgkin's lymphoma.

On the other hand, some studies have shown worsened survival associated with increased vitamin D intake in patients with pancreatic & prostate cancers.

Finally, some studies have shown both positive and negative effects of vitamin D in the treatment of breast and skin cancers. So, is vitamin D protective or harmful?

Although a significant amount of evidence appears to be mounting in regards to the therapeutic and preventative use of vitamin D for cancer, many studies have been insufficiently consistent.

One important inconsistency relates to the fact that vitamin D form (D2, D3 or fish liver source), dosages and delivery forms are varied in many such studies. Many of the studies were retrospective and involved estimation of the vitamin D intake based on dietary questionnaires. Without controlling the key variable of vitamin D dosage, it will remain difficult to make an accurate assessment of its impact on human cancer.

In addition, in other investigations, fish sources were utilized, raising the possibility of associated intake of carcinogens known as organochlorines present in certain fish populations.

In the future, trials should attempt to eliminate such confounding factors to test this target molecule. It will also become necessary to move away from the *in vitro* studies and epidemiological analyses and to focus more on randomized clinical trials.

Cancer Prevention

Vitamin D reduces deaths from many chronic diseases, not just cancer. In 2011, vitamin D expert Dr. William Grant concluded that doubling vitamin D blood levels in 6 world regions would increase life expectancy by an average of 2 years. "The predicted reduction in all-cause mortality rates ranges from 7.6% for African females to 17.3% for European females," claimed Grant, who heads the Sunlight, Nutrition and Health Research Center in San Francisco.[2]

In September 2007, the journal Archives of Internal Medicine published an analysis of 18 randomized controlled prospective trials involving 57,311 participants over the age of 50. The study concluded that test subjects taking a daily dose of at least 500 international units (IU) of vitamin D had a 7% reduced risk of death (all causes) compared with those given a placebo. Note that this is a very low dose of vitamin D, which would not affect blood levels significantly.[3]

Another study found no decreased risk for colorectal cancer in women given a 400iu/day vitamin D supplement. Again, this study used a very low dose.[4]

Another prospective study found a 60-77% lower cancer rate in postmenopausal women taking a daily dose of 1,100 IU of vitamin D combined with calcium, compared to women who were given a placebo or calcium by itself. The double-blind clinical study, which lasted four years, involved 1179 healthy women over 55 from rural Nebraska.[5]

In 2007, researchers at the University of California, San Diego suggested that taking 2,000 IU of vitamin D daily combined with 10 to 15 minutes of sun exposure and a healthy diet could reduce the incidence of colorectal cancer by two-thirds.[6]

The same authors discovered that breast cancer rates were decreased by 50% in women with high blood levels of vitamin D.[7]

Researchers concluded, "It is projected that raising the minimum year-around serum 25(OH)D level to 40 to 60 ng/mL (100-150 nmol/L) would prevent approximately 58,000 new cases of breast cancer and 49,000 new cases of colorectal cancer each year, and three fourths of deaths from these diseases in the United States and Canada, based on observational studies combined with a randomized trial. Such intakes also are expected to reduce case-fatality rates of patients who have breast, colorectal, or prostate cancer by half."[8]

Cancer Survival

Cancer patients diagnosed in the summer and fall, when serum vitamin D levels are naturally higher, have better survival rates than those diagnosed in winter and spring, when vitamin D levels tend to be lower. Researchers followed patients with breast, colon, lung and prostate cancer. Strongest effects were seen in female breast cancer patients (14% seasonal difference in survival) and male and female lung cancer patients (5% difference).[9,10]

It has also been suggested that the lower cancer survival rate for African-Americans is due to their lower levels of vitamin D (40% lower than those of Caucasians), since melanin in the skin blocks sunlight and prevents endogenous generation of the vitamin.[11]

Brain Tumors

Alfacalcidol, an active metabolite of vitamin D, has a dramatic curative effect on deadly glioblastoma multiforme, the most common primary brain tumor and the type that killed politician Ted Kennedy. Most patients die within 1-2 years of diagnosis despite any known conventional treatment (median survival time is 21 months). In a Phase II trial of 11 patients with brain tumors, researchers found that high dose vitamin alfacalcidol (0.04 microgram/kg) combined with conventional therapy caused tumor regression in 3 patients (27% of cases) for 4, 5 and 7 years respectively. Researchers proposed that alfacalcidol binds to nuclear receptors which regulated mitotic activity, or cell division.[12]

Alfacalcidol, compared to vitamin D, has a greater impact on calcium metabolism,[13] but lesser effects on parathyroid hormone levels.[14] It causes greater stimulation of the immune system, especially on regulatory T-cells.[15] It has a longer half-life in blood and does not require activation by the kidneys, a process which is limited by a negative feedback mechanism. Alfacalcidol is activated by the enzyme 25-hydroxylase in the liver and in osteoblasts (bone-forming cells). One study suggests it may be a superior form for human supplementation.[16] According to the manufacturer's monograph, it is currently used as an additive in poultry feed.

Breast Cancer

Breast cancer patients with vitamin D blood levels >29ng/ml (72nmol/L) at diagnosis had a 42% lower 15-year death rate, and a 50% decrease in metastasis, compared to patients with levels <20ng/ml (50nmol/L).[17]

According to a 2011 study of breast cancer patients by researchers at the University of Rochester, low serum levels of vitamin D at diagnosis correlate with more aggressive types of tumors (basal-cell-like), and poorer scores on known major biological markers associated with tumor prognosis (such as "triple-negative" status, a lack of receptors for estrogen, progesterone, or HER2 human epidermal growth factor receptor 2). The lead researcher concluded, "Based on these results, doctors should strongly consider monitoring vitamin D levels among breast cancer patients and correcting them as needed."[18]

Serum levels of vitamin D are inversely correlated with risk of recurrence in women already treated for breast cancer. Researchers in Toronto, Canada, studied 512 women diagnosed with early-stage breast cancer during the time period of 1989-1996, and followed them for an average of roughly 12 years.

37.5% of the subjects had vitamin D levels of <50 nmol/L (deficient), 38.5% had levels of 50-72 nmol/L (insufficient), and only 24% had levels >72 nmol/L (sufficient). The women with deficient levels had approximately twice the risk of cancer recurrence and death at the time of the 12-year followup, compared to women with sufficient levels.[19]

Colon Cancer

One large prospective study included 48,115 American women (part of the landmark Nurses' Health Study) who were free of cancer and intestinal polyps at the time they completed a food frequency questionnaire in 1980, and who subsequently underwent endoscopy by 2002. From the questionnaire, researchers estimated their intake of calcium, vitamin D and vitamin A (retinol).

Increased calcium intake was associated with 12% reduced risk of distal colorectal adenoma, and a 27% decrease in large adenomas. Increased vitamin D intake was associated with 21% reduced risk of distal colorectal adenoma, and a 33% decrease in distal colon adenoma.

The combination of high vitamin D and low retinal intake further decreased the risk of developing cancer, compared to the other extreme, low vitamin D and high retinol intake. Retinol intake correlated with a 42% increased risk of colorectal adenoma for women with a vitamin A intake of >6,202 IU/day compared to ≤1,989 IU/day.

Researchers stated, "In particular, higher retinol intake may antagonize the actions of vitamin D because of competition for retinoid X receptors, which are required for vitamin D receptor function." In other words, vitamin A acts as a vitamin D blocker by attaching to its binding sites. They concluded, "Higher total calcium and vitamin D intakes were associated with reduced risk, and the actions of vitamin D may be attenuated by high retinol intake."[20]

Data derived from the EPIC study (a large prospective study with more than 520,000 international participants) found that subjects with high serum vitamin D levels were approximately 40% less likely to develop colon cancer than those with low levels (<25.0 nmol/l compared to ≥100.0 nmol/l). Higher calcium intake was also associated with lower levels of colorectal cancer.

In subjects with low levels of vitamin D (<50 nmol/L), higher levels of vitamin A (retinol) correlated with a reduced risk of cancer; however, in subjects with high levels of vitamin D (>75 nmol/L), higher levels of vitamin A increased the cancer risk.[41]

This may be due to the fact that vitamin A binds to vitamin D receptors and weakly activates them, so in cases where vitamin D is lacking, vitamin A provides at least a minimal vitamin D effect. However, in cases where adequate amounts of vitamin D are present, vitamin A blocks the stronger action of vitamin D with its weaker stimulus.

Lung Cancer

In early Stage Non-Small-Cell Lung Cancer, higher vitamin D serum levels correlated with increased survival; however, survival in late-stage cases was unrelated to vitamin D levels, only to different mutations (forms) of the cellular vitamin D receptor. Different forms of receptors cause different activation of genes involved in cell division, cell adhesion, and function. In other words, in advanced lung cancer cases, what cells do in response to stimulation by vitamin D is more important than the amount of vitamin D present in the bloodstream.[21-24]

Cancer patients with overexpression of a gene called CYP24A1, which encodes the main enzyme metabolizing vitamin D, have lower survival rates. Researchers found CYP24A1 elevated 8- to 50-fold in lung adenocarcinoma tissue. This means these patients have lower levels of circulating vitamin D due to faster breakdown of the substance. This overexpression has also been found in cervical, colon, esophageal, ovarian, and squamous cell skin cancer. In patients with lung adenocarcinoma, 5-year survival was 42% for patients with the highest levels of gene expression, compared to 81% for those with the lowest expression.[25]

Melanoma

In a study of 872 melanoma patients, higher serum vitamin D levels at the time of melanoma diagnosis were associated with both thinner tumors, and better survival independent of tumor thickness. Over a median followup period of 4.7 years, a difference of 20 nmol/L increase in vitamin D serum level was associated with a 21% lower rate of recurrence. Researchers concluded, "Patients with melanoma, and those at high risk of melanoma, should seek to ensure vitamin D sufficiency. Additional studies are needed to establish optimal serum levels for patients with melanoma."[26]

Cod liver oil is not a beneficial source of vitamin D in the case of melanoma. A Norwegian study found that the risk of melanoma in women was increased by consumption of both polyunsaturated fat and cod liver oil.[27]

Pancreatic Cancer

Individual variations in cellular vitamin D responsiveness affects cancer outcomes. A genetic variation (rs2853564) of the cellular vitamin D receptor which increases the response to vitamin D is associated with increased survival of pancreatic cancer patients.[28]

One study found that higher vitamin D serum levels (>65.5 nmol/L compared to <32.0 nmol/L) were associated with a 3-fold increased risk for pancreatic cancer[29]; however, another study found no evidence of higher risk at higher levels, and concluded that higher levels acted as a preventative.[30]

The difference may be due to the fact that the first study was done in Finland, and the second was done in America. Scandinavians have a cultural habit of consuming cod liver oil as a vitamin D supplement. Cod liver oil contains vitamin A, which blocks the anti-cancer effects of vitamin D even in moderate doses. Subjects with high vitamin D levels may also have had high vitamin A levels; however, the study did not address this factor.

Prostate Cancer

Like breast cancer, prostate cancer survival is correlated with increased exposure to sunlight (and presumably, with vitamin D levels).[31]

Higher levels of vitamin D correlated with lower occurrence of metastasis.[32]

A study of 44 patients with low-risk prostate cancer who were given 4000iu/day of vitamin D produced moderately successful results, measured in PSA levels and cellular grading at repeat biopsy. 24/44 (55%) showed decreased disease progression; 5/44 (11%) were unchanged; and 15/44 (34%) showed increased disease markers.[33] Other studies on prostate cancer are more cautionary.

A Norwegian study checked the vitamin D serum levels of 622 prostate cancer patients and found that both low (</=19 nmol/l) and high (>/=80 nmol/l) levels were associated with a higher cancer risk. On a graph of prostate cancer risk vs. vitamin D level, this would appear as a U-shaped pattern, with the lowest risk of cancer in the mid-range of vitamin D levels.

The proposed biological mechanism for this is that very low levels produce low tissue concentration and weakened control of mitosis in cancer cells, wheras extremely high levels lead to vitamin D resistance through increased inactivation by the cellular enzyme 24-hydroxylase. Researchers concluded, "It is recommended that vitamin D deficiency be supplemented, but too high vitamin D serum levels might also enhance cancer development."[34]

Also, this is another Scandinavian study, so high levels of vitamin A may have been a confounding factor.

Another study of 749 American subjects who were diagnosed with prostate cancer 1-8 years after blood drawing found higher serum levels of vitamin D directly correlated with an increased rate of aggressive prostate cancer (stage III-IV), with no protective effect at all. Researchers concluded, "The findings of this large prospective study do not support the hypothesis that vitamin D is associated with a decreased risk of prostate cancer; indeed, higher circulating 25(OH)D concentrations may be associated with increased risk of aggressive disease."[35]

Ongoing Studies

A new five-year study was begun in 2009 to determine whether vitamin D and fish oil can lower the risk of cancer, heart disease or stroke. The $20-million study, sponsored by the U.S. National Cancer Institute along with the National Heart, Lung and Blood Institute and other federal agencies, will follow 20,000 healthy test subjects who will be randomly assigned to take vitamin D, fish oil, both nutrients or placebo pills for 5 years.

Participation in the study is limited to women 65 or older and men 60 or older with no history of heart attacks, stroke or a major cancer. One-quarter of the participants will be African-American. Blacks do not produce much vitamin D from sunlight, and researchers want to know if that is why they have elevated rates of cancer, heart disease, and stroke.

Further evidence will need to be acquired before conclusions can be reached about the exact effects of vitamin D on specific cancers. At this point, however, it seems clear that the benefits of vitamin D are numerous and far outweigh any possible risks.

An Epidemic Of Vitamin D Deficiency

Most people are severely Vitamin D deficient,according to a 2009 study published in the *Archives of Internal Medicine*. Between 1988 and 1994, 18,883 people were examined as part of the federal government's National Health and Nutrition Examination Survey. Only 45% of them had vitamin D blood levels of 30 nanograms per milliliter or greater, the level considered sufficient for health. A decade later, only 23% of 13,369 people surveyed achieved this level.[36]

How To Achieve Optimum Vitamin D Levels

How can you maximize your dietary intake of vitamin D? There are numerous natural sources of vitamin D as well as fortified and/or supplemental forms commercially available.

Natural sources include fatty fish such as tuna, salmon, and sardines. Other products, such as eggs, liver and beef are also rich in vitamin D. Milk is artificially fortified with Vitamin D, though sometimes it is the less effective form, D2.

For vegetarians, additional options are available, which include cereal (vitamin D fortified) and mushrooms. Individuals who adopt strictly vegetarian diets may require additional supplementation of vitamin D with over the counter products.

Most ordinary multivitamin supplements contain only the vitamin D necessary to prevent rickets (the RDI is 400 IU), and also an insufficient dose and a number of other necessary vitamins and minerals.

As a result, the Institute of Medicine currently recommends that individuals consume at least 600 international units of vitamin D per day regardless of their degree of sun exposure. The Canadian Cancer Society advises Canadians to consume 1,000 IU of vitamin D daily during the fall and winter months, in consultation with a health-care provider.

However, these organizations are extremely conservative, and other health authorities recomment much higher doses, at least 4,000 – 5,000 IU daily, for optimum health. The vitamin D council, a non-profit group dedicated to educating the public about the importance of vitamin D, maintains a website with detailed information and advice.

http://www.vitamindcouncil.org/

If you do not receive proper sun exposure and/or supplements with adequate amounts of vitamin D3, odds are you are vitamin D deficient. The only way to know for sure is to have your blood vitamin D levels tested. You can buy an accurate Vitamin D test on the web for $75 from ZRT Laboratories. This is also available from the Vitamin D council. Buy it online and take the results to your health care provider.

If you do not order the test online and plan to use a test from your health care provider, be sure to ask for one which measures 25-hydroxyvitamin D, or 25(OH)D. Do not ask simply for a "vitamin D test" as doctors sometimes order a 1,25-dihydroxyvitamin D test, an incorrect test which cannot determine vitamin D deficiency. Make sure your health care provider is using the correct test.

The safest way to achieve a healthy vitamin D blood level is to test your vitamin D levels, then increase your vitamin D intake, and test again until you reach your desired levels.

ZRT test results are given in nanograms per milliliter (ng/mL) and reflect total serum 25(OH)D.

Total serum 25(OH)D is the total amount of vitamin D in your blood, both vitamin D3 and vitamin D2:

Total 25(OH)D = 25(OH)D3 + 25(OH)D2

Since vitamin D2 is not naturally present in the human body, if you do not use anything that contains vitamin D2 your results will only show vitamin D3. This is fine, since vitamin D3 is the preferred form.

Along with vitamin D, it is important to take other elements that help it work in the body, such as magnesium, vitamin K, zinc, boron and vitamin A. Magnesium is a cofactor. Vitamin K allows calcium from the bloodstream into cells. Zinc helps vitamin D bond to the cellular receptor. Boron boosts the effect of vitamin D.

Cod liver oil, the traditional natural source of vitamin D, also contains high levels of vitamin A, which can negate the anti-cancer effect. This occurs at levels of >3000 IU/day of vitamin A intake, which is the amount contained in only 1 teaspoon of cod liver oil.

Current standards severely underestimate the extent of vitamin D deficiency in the population. This is the result of using an outdated 25(OH)D blood level threshold of 30 ng/mL (70 nmol/L) for determining deficiency. Beneficial effects are not seen at levels below 40 ng/mL (120 nmol/L), which indicates a need to revise the official standards of what constitutes a vitamin D deficiency.

Serum levels of at least 50 ng/mL (125 nmol/L) or higher are needed for therapeutic benefit. Using this standard, the percentage of the Western urban population determined to be deficient would likely reach 90% or more, especially in winter due to lack of sun exposure.

For cancer patients, recommended blood levels are 70-100 ng/ml.

For average size females, it will usually take a supplement of at least 4000 IU to reach therapeutic blood levels. For average size males, a dose of 5000 IU is recommended. For children the dose is 35 IU/lbs of body weight. Variations in body size, sun exposure and metabolism can affect individual needs. Some people may require an intake as high as 8000 IU per day to achieve correct blood levels.

Regular blood testing of vitamin D levels is important because a chronic overdose of vitamin D can have deleterious health effects. Vitamin D toxicity can lead to calcinosis, which is the deposition of calcium salts in soft tissues such as the heart, blood vessels, kidneys and lungs; and hypercalcemia, high blood levels of calcium. Symptoms of excessive vitamin D intake include heart arrhythmias, mental status deterioration and confusion, muscle pain, eye irritation, gastric symptoms such as loss of appetite and vomiting, weight loss, as well as fever and chills.

However, studies have shown this is only a risk at extremely high levels of vitamin D consumption, 20,000 IU or more daily for several months. Toxicity is highly unlikely to occur at supplementation levels of 4,000-5,000 IU per day. Although vitamin D toxicity is rare, you may be at greater risk if you have health problems, such as liver or kidney conditions, or if you take thiazide-type diuretics. As always, make sure your doctor is aware of any vitamins or supplements you take.

Forms Of Vitamin D

Be sure to supplement with the bioidentical Vitamin D3 (cholecalciferol), not the synthetic vitamin D2 (ergocalciferol). Like the synthetic form of vitamin E, it has markedly less biological activity than its natural counterpart, interferes with the activity of the natural form of the vitamin, and can actually increase mortality.

Drisdol is the brand name of the synthetic form of vitamin D2, and this is the form of vitamin D typically prescribed by doctors. Because it is cheap, it is also sometimes used to fortify foods.

A recent study by the Cochrane Database analysed mortality rates for people who supplemented their diets with D2 compared with others who used D3. The results of 50 random controlled clinical trials, with 94,000 test subjects, showed a 6% risk reduction in those who used D3, but a 2% increased health risk in those taking D2.[37]

Chemotherapy & Vitamin D

Chemotherapy lowers vitamin D levels, and patients undergoing this form of treatment should re-test their vitamin D levels, as a higher level of supplementation may be required.[38,39,40]

Caution

Use vitamin D supplements with caution if you have sarcoidosis.

There is some question about the effect of very high levels of vitamin D and pancreatic and prostate cancer. Until this issue is completely clarified, it may be wise to maintain moderate serum levels of vitamin D.

Vitamin A at levels >3000 iu per day blocks the anti-cancer effects of vitamin D. Avoid cod liver oil, as it contains high levels of vitamin A.

Instructions

Have blood levels taken. Usual dose to maintain proper blood levels is 35 iu per pound of body weight.

Suppliers

Widely available online and in stores.

References

(1) Mizwicki MT et al., "Genomic and Nongenomic Signaling Induced by 1α,25(OH)2-Vitamin D3 Promotes the Recovery of Amyloid-β Phagocytosis by Alzheimer's Disease Macrophages." J Alzheimers Dis, 2012 Jan 1;29(1):51-62

(2) Grant W.B., "An estimate of the global reduction in mortality rates through doubling vitamin D levels." European Journal of Clinical Nutrition (2011) 65, 1016–1026

(3) Autier P, Gandini S, "Vitamin D supplementation and total mortality: a meta-analysis of randomized controlled trials." Archives of Internal Medicine 2007 Sep 10;167(16):1730-7

(4) Wactawski-Wende J, et al. "Calcium plus vitamin D supplementation and the risk of colorectal cancer." N Engl J Med 2006;354:684-96.

(5) Joan M Lappe, Dianne Travers-Gustafson, K Michael Davies, Robert R Recker and Robert P Heaney,"Vitamin D and calcium supplementation reduces cancer risk: results of a randomized trial." American Journal of Clinical Nutrition, Vol. 85, No. 6, 1586-1591, June 2007

(6) Gorham ED, Garland CF, Garland FC, Grant WB, Mohr SB, Lipkin M, Newmark HL, Giovannucci E, Wei M, Holick MF, "Optimal vitamin D status for colorectal cancer prevention: a quantitative meta analysis." Am J Prev Med, 2007 Mar;32(3):210-6.

(7) Garland CF, Gorham ED, Mohr SB, Grant WB, Giovannucci EL, Lipkin M, Newmark H, Holick MF, Garland FC, "Vitamin D and prevention of breast cancer: pooled analysis." J Steroid Biochem Mol Biol., 2007 Mar;103(3-5):708-11

(8) Garland CF, Gorham ED, Mohr SB, Garland FC. "Vitamin D for cancer prevention: global perspective." Ann Epidemiol 2009 Jul;19(7):468-83.

(9) Lim HS, et al., "Cancer survival is dependent on season of diagnosis and sunlight exposure." Int J Cancer 2006 Oct 1;119(7):1530-6

(10) Robsahm TE, et al., "Vitamin D3 from sunlight may improve the prognosis of breast-, colon- and prostate cancer (Norway). Cancer Causes Control 2004 Mar;15(2):149-58.

(11) William B. Grant and Alan N. Peiris, "Lower Vitamin-D Production from Solar Ultraviolet-B Irradiance May Explain Some Differences in Cancer Survival Rates." Dermato-Endocrinology 2012 Vol 4, issue 2, pp 85-94

(12) P Trouillas, et al., "Redifferentiation therapy in brain tumors: long-lasting complete regression of glioblastomas and an anaplastic astrocytoma under long term 1-alpha-hydroxycholecalciferol." J Neurooncol 2001 Jan;51(1):57-66.

(13) "Biological effects of various regimes of 25-hydroxyvitamin D3 (calcidiol) administration on bone mineral metabolism in postmenopausal women." Clin Cases Miner Bone Metab. 2009 May–Aug; 6(2): 169–173;

(14) Moe S, et al., "Oral calcitriol versus oral alfacalcidol for the treatment of secondary hyperparathyroidism in patients receiving hemodialysis: a randomized, crossover trial." Can J ,Clin Pharmacol Vol 15 (1) Winter 2008:e36 -e43; January 9, 2008;

(15) Zold E, et al.,"Alfacalcidol treatment restores derailed immune-regulation in patients with undifferentiated connective tissue disease." Autoimmunity Reviews, August 2010;

(16) Ruti R, et al., "Superiority of alfacalcidol compared to vitamin D plus calcium in lumbar bone mineral density in postmenopausal osteoporosis." Rheumatol Int. 2006 Mar;26(5):445-53. Epub 2005 Nov 10

(17) Goodwin P, Ennis M, Pritchard K, Koo J, Hood N, Lunenfeld S, et al. "Vitamin D deficiency is common at breast cancer diagnosis and is associated with a significantly higher risk of distant recurrence and death in a prospective cohort study of T1-3, N0-1, M0 BC." J Clin Oncol. 2008;26(Suppl): Abstract 511

(18) Peppone LJ, Rickles AS, Janelsins MC, Insalaco MR, Skinner KA, "The Association Between Breast Cancer Prognostic Indicators and Serum 25-OH Vitamin D Levels." Ann Surg Oncol, 2012 Aug;19(8):2590-9. Epub 2012 Mar 24.

(19) Goodwin PJ et al. "Prognostic effects of 25-hydroxyvitamin D levels in early breast cancer." J Clin Oncol. 2009; 27(23):3757

(20) Oh K, Willett WC, Wu K, Fuchs CS, Giovannucci EL. "Calcium and vitamin D intakes in relation to risk of distal colorectal adenoma in women." Am. J. Epidemiol. (2007) 165 (10): 1178-1186.

(21) Zhou W, Suk R, Liu G, et al., "Vitamin D is associated with improved survival in early stage non-small cell lung cancer patients." Cancer Epidemiol Biomarkers Prev 14:2303-2309, 2005.

(22) Zhou W, Heist RS, Liu G, et al., "Circulating 25-hydroxyvitamin D levels predict survival in early stage non-small cell lung cancer patients." J Clin Oncol 25:479-485, 2007.

(23) Zhou W, et al., "Circulating 25-Hydroxyvitamin D, VDR Polymorphisms, and Survival in Advanced Non–Small-Cell Lung Cancer," J Clin Oncol. 2008 December 1; 26(34): 5596–5602.

(24) Nakagawa K, Kawaura A, Kato S, et al., "1a-25-dihydroxyvitamin D is a preventive factor in the metastasis of lung cancer." Carcinogenesis 26:429-440, 2005.

(25) Chen G et al., "CYP24A1 is an independent prognostic marker of survival in patients with lung adenocarcinoma." Clin Cancer Res 2011 Feb 15;17(4):817-26. Epub 2010 Dec 17.

(26) Newton-Bishop JA, "Serum 25-hydroxyvitamin D3 levels are associated with breslow thickness at presentation and survival from melanoma." J Clin Oncol 2009 Nov 10;27(32):5439-44. Epub 2009 Sep 21.

(27) Veierød MB, et al "Diet and risk of cutaneous malignant melanoma: a prospective study of 50,757 Norwegian men and women." Int J Cancer 1997 May 16;71(4):600-4.

(28) Jeremy Moore, "Genetic marker in vitamin D receptor gene associated with increased pancreatic cancer survival." NCI Press Release, date: 19-Jun-2012

(29) Stolzenberg-Solomon RZ, A prospective nested case-control study of vitamin D status and pancreatic cancer risk in male smokers. Cancer Res 2006 Oct 15;66(20):10213-9.

(30) Wolpin BM, et al., "Plasma 25-hydroxyvitamin D and risk of pancreatic cancer." Cancer Epidemiol Biomarkers Prev 2012 Jan;21(1):82-91. Epub 2011 Nov 15.

(31) Lagunova Z, Porojnicu AC, Dahlback A, Berg JP, Beer TM, Moan J. "Prostate cancer survival is dependent on season of diagnosis." Prostate. 2007;67:1362–1370.

(32) William B. Grant,"Vitamin D May Reduce Prostate Cancer Metastasis by Several Mechanisms Including Blocking Stat3," Am J Pathol. 2008 November; 173(5): 1589–1590.

(33) David T Marshall, et al., "Vitamin D3 Supplementation at 4000 International Units Per Day for One Year Results in a Decrease of Positive Cores at Repeat Biopsy in Subjects with Low-Risk Prostate Cancer under Active Surveillance." The Journal of Clinical Endocrinology & Metabolism July 1, 2012 vol. 97 no. 7 2315-2324

(34) Tuohimaa P, "Both high and low levels of blood vitamin D are associated with a higher prostate cancer risk: a longitudinal, nested case-control study in the Nordic countries." Int J Cancer 2004 Jan 1;108(1):104-8.

(35) Ahn J, et al., "Serum vitamin D concentration and prostate cancer risk: a nested case-control study." J Natl Cancer Inst 2008 Jun 4;100(11):796-804. Epub 2008 May 27.

(36) Ginde, M. C. Liu and C. A. Camargo Jr., "Demographic Differences and Trends of Vitamin D Insufficiency in the US Population, 1988-2004." Archives of Internal Medicine, Vol. 169, No. 6, 2009, pp. 626-632

(37) Bjelakovic G, "Vitamin D supplementation for prevention of mortality in adults." Cochrane Database Syst Review 2011 Jul 6;(7):CD007470.

(38) Fakih MG, et al., "Chemotherapy is linked to severe vitamin D deficiency in patients with colorectal cancer." Int J Colorectal Dis 2009 Feb;24(2):219-24. Epub 2008 Oct 2

(39) Fakih MG, et al., "A prospective clinical trial of cholecalciferol 2000 IU/day in colorectal cancer patients: evidence of a chemotherapy-response interaction." AntiCancer Res 2012 Apr;32(4):1333-8.

(40) Jacot W. "Increased prevalence of vitamin D insufficiency in patients with breast cancer after neoadjuvant chemotherapy." Breast Cancer Res Treat 2012 Jul;134(2):709-17. Epub 2012 May 6.

(41) Jenab M et al. "Association between pre-diagnostic circulating vitamin D concentration and risk of colorectal cancer in European populations: a nested case-control study." BMJ 2010;340:b5500

9. Clean Up Your Internal Environment

Coffee Enemas

Coffee enemas used to be considered part of mainstream medicine, and were even mentioned in the Merck Manual until the 1970s, when the topic was dropped mainly out of space considerations. Currently, they are used mainly by alternative medical practitioners.

Undergoing an enema involves using a bag of water and a tube to fill the colon with enough water to stimulate contraction of the walls of the colon - the idea is to force the colon into expelling waste materials out through the anal sphincter.

It is the liver and small intestine which neutralize the most common tissue toxins: ammonia, polyamines, toxic nitrogen compounds, and free radicals. These detoxification systems are stimulated enhanced by coffee enemas. Physiological Chemistry and Physics has stated that "caffeine enemas cause dilation of bile ducts, which facilitates excretion of toxic cancer breakdown products by the liver and dialysis of toxic products across the colonic wall."

One-time enemas seem to be quite useful in cleaning the inside environment.

Be careful to not become dependent on enemas, because they can stretch the wall of the colon too much.

People with chronic constipation and problems with hemorrhoids or anal fissures can usually benefit from clearing out their colon and rectal pouch with an enema. Be sure to use organic coffee.

If you are unsure of your own proficiency, some alternative health clinics perform colon cleansing and coffee enemas.

At the same time start eating more fruits and vegetables which will improve constipation. Avoid white rice and white flour.

Make Your Internal Environment Slightly Alkaline

To oxygenate properly, the body needs a slightly alkaline environment, and therefore you must change the body's pH slightly.

Many people believe that an alkaline pH can not only protect the body against cancer, but can even help to cure it once it has developed.

In-vitro studies have shown that cancer cells and tumors thrive and grow in a more acidic environment. When the level of acid is lowered, tumors grow much more slowly.

It stands to reason that cancer cells in the body would also be detrimentally affected by an overall alkaline environment. It would also make sense that if the body's pH is acidic, the growth of cancer cells and tumors would be encouraged.

By eating mainly foods that make the body's pH more alkaline, there would be less of a chance for cancer cells to develop and grow. So, by adjusting the diet, it is actually possible to create a less hospitable environment for cancer cells, thus improving the chances of experiencing good health.

An alkaline diet usually involves eating very little meat, no dairy products, no white flour or white sugar, because these foods have a very acidic reaction on the body's pH level.

Instead, the diet usually focuses heavily on fresh fruits and vegetables, and nuts such as almonds.

Consumption of small amounts of baking soda can also help neutralize excess acidity. Place a pinch (1/8 tsp) of baking soda (sodium bicarbonate) in your mouth, and use your tongue to swish it around your gums and teeth before swallowing it. Do this 3 times daily, and also drink a glass of water containing a teaspoon of baking soda before going to bed each night.

You can also buy 1 liter of alkalinized water for $2 in most vitamin stores or you can buy a Santevia water filter that will turn the filtered water slightly Alkaline. (www.santevia.com)

Anti-Cancer Newsletter 2007

Supposedly, the Johns Hopkins Hospital sent out a newsletter in 2007 containing brief pointers on the main tenets of alternative cancer treatment. It was widely circulated on the internet. Subsequently, Johns Hopkins said the newsletter did not originate from their institution. Its exact origin and author are unkown. However, it still contains very good advice:

1. Every person has cancer cells in the body. These cancer cells do not show up in the standard tests until they have multiplied to a few billion. When doctors tell cancer patients that there are no more cancer cells in their bodies after treatment, it just means the tests are unable to detect the cancer cells because they have not reached the detectable size.

2. Cancer cells occur between 6 to more than 10 times in a person's lifetime.

3. When the person's immune system is strong the cancer cells will be destroyed and prevented from multiplying and forming tumors.

4. When a person has cancer it indicates the person has multiple nutritional deficiencies. These could be due to genetic, environmental, food and lifestyle factors.

5. To overcome the multiple nutritional deficiencies, changing diet and including supplements will strengthen the immune system.

6. Chemotherapy involves poisoning the rapidly-growing cancer cells and also destroys rapidly-growing healthy cells in the bone marrow, gastro-intestinal tract etc, and can cause organ damage, like liver, kidneys, heart, lungs etc.

7. Radiation while destroying cancer cells also burns, scars and damages healthy cells, tissues and organs.

8. Initial treatment with chemotherapy and radiation will often

reduce tumor size. However prolonged use of chemotherapy and radiation do not result in more tumor destruction.

9. When the body has too much toxic burden from chemotherapy and radiation the immune system is either compromised or destroyed, hence the person can succumb to various kinds of infections and complications.

10. Chemotherapy and radiation can cause cancer cells to mutate and become resistant and difficult to destroy. Surgery can also cause cancer cells to spread to other sites.

11. An effective way to battle cancer is to starve the cancer cells by not feeding it with the foods it needs to multiply.

CANCER CELLS FEED ON:

a. Sugar is a cancer-feeder.
By cutting off sugar it cuts off one important food supply to the cancer cells. Sugar substitutes like NutraSweet, Equal, Spoonful, etc are made with Aspartame and they are harmful. A better natural substitute would be Manuka honey or molasses but only in very small amounts. Table salt has a chemical added to make it white in color. Better alternative is Bragg's amino or sea salt.

b. Milk causes the body to produce mucus, especially in the gastro-intestinal tract. Cancer feeds on mucus. By cutting off milk and substituting with unsweetened soya milk cancer cells are being starved.

c. Cancer cells thrive in an acid environment.
A meat-based diet is acidic and it is best to eat fish, and a little chicken rather than beef or pork. Meat also contains livestock antibiotics, growth hormones and parasites, which are all harmful, especially to people with cancer.

d. A diet made of 80% fresh vegetables and juice, whole grains, seeds, nuts and a little fruit help put the body into an alkaline environment.

About 20% can be from cooked food including beans. Fresh vegetable juices provide live enzymes that are easily absorbed and reach down to cellular levels within 15 minutes to nourish and enhance growth of healthy cells. To obtain live enzymes for building healthy cells try and drink fresh vegetable juice (most vegetables including bean sprouts) and eat some raw vegetables 2 or 3 times a day. Enzymes are destroyed at temperatures of 104 degrees F (40 degrees C).

e. Avoid coffee, tea, and chocolate, which have high caffeine. Green tea is a better alternative and has cancer-fighting properties. Water- it is best to drink purified water, or filtered, to avoid known toxins and heavy metals in tap water. Distilled water is acidic, avoid it.

f. Meat protein is difficult to digest and requires a lot of digestive enzymes. Undigested meat remaining in the intestines becomes putrefied and leads to more toxic build-up.

g. Cancer cell walls have a tough protein covering. By refraining from or eating less meat it frees more enzymes to attack the protein walls of cancer cells and allows the body's killer cells to destroy the cancer cells.

h. Some supplements build up the immune system (IP6, Floressence, Essiac, anti-oxidants, vitamins, minerals, EFAs etc.) to enable the body's own killer cells to destroy cancer cells. Other supplements like vitamin E are known to cause apoptosis, or programmed cell death, the body's normal method of disposing of damaged, unwanted, or unneeded cells.

i. Cancer is a disease of the mind, body, and spirit. A proactive and positive spirit will help the cancer warrior be a survivor. Anger, unforgiveness and bitterness put the body into a stressful and acidic environment. Learn to have a loving and forgiving spirit. Learn to relax and enjoy life.

j. Cancer cells cannot thrive in an oxygenated environment. Exercising daily, and deep breathing help to get more oxygen down to the cellular level. Oxygen therapy is another means employed to destroy cancer cells.

k. Avoid toxins from plastic:

1. No Plastic Bottles

2. No water bottles in freezer.

3. No plastic wrap in microwave.

Overcome Cachexia

People normally don't die directly of cancer; instead, they waste away and starve to death, a process called cachexia.

Cancer cells require up to 15 times as much energy as regular cells to survive, and get this energy by robbing normal cells of their nutrition.

Formal definition of cachexia is the loss of body mass that cannot be reversed nutritionally. In fact, simply overfeeding cancer patients actually shortens their lives further.

In 1981, one randomized study funded by the NCI attempted to overcome cancer cachexia by increasing patients' intake of calories and other nutrients, through either tube feeding or oral supplementation. The increased consumption did not lead to replenished body mass. The patients retained water and grew a small amount of fat, but had no increase in lean body mass. Worse, all the cancer patients subjected to extra feeding, and colon cancer patients in particular, died much sooner than those not supplemented.

Survival time for the fed patients with advanced colon cancer was approximately 80 days, compared to 360 days for patients who were simply left alone, a huge difference.[1]

Obviously, there is more to the development of cachexia than simple inadequate intake of nutrition. There is an underlying metabolic error causing the starvation.

Ironically, there is evidence that fasting (consumption of water only) for 2 days before and 1 day after chemotherapy can increase the effectiveness of the chemo and minimize damage to normal tissue. In mouse experiments, "the combination of fasting cycles plus chemotherapy was either more or much more effective than chemo alone," according to researcher Valter Longo, professor of gerontology and biological sciences at the University of Southern California.[2]

How Does Starvation Occur?

Starvation occurs when the body cannot make enough ATP, which is used by the body to produce energy. After only 24 hours of not eating properly, the body is nearly depleted of its ATP reserves. The body must make more ATP in order for the body to function at all. The body goes into an energy conservation mode, called starvation, at this time. Liver and pancreatic enzyme production is significantly lowered to insufficient amounts during this conservation mode. The body then takes the energy it requires for ATP manufacture from itself, and begins to digest its organs and muscles.

References

(1) Nixon D.W. "Total parenteral nutrition as an adjunct to chemotherapy of metastatic colorectal cancer." Cancer Treat Rep 1981;65 Suppl 5:121-8

(2) Changhan Lee, Lizzia Raffaghello, Sebastian Brandhorst, Fernando M. Safdie, Giovanna Bianchi, Alejandro Martin-Montalvo, Vito Pistoia, Min Wei, Saewon Hwang, Annalisa Merlino, Laura Emionite, Rafael de Cabo, and Valter D. Longo. "Fasting Cycles Retard Growth of Tumors and Sensitize a

Range of Cancer Cell Types to Chemotherapy." Science Translational Medicine, Feb 8, 2012

Hydrazine Sulfate

Hydrazine sulfate traces its origin back to the mid-1970s, when it was promoted as a cancer treatment by US physician Joseph Gold. By the middle 1980s, scientific research teams in both the Soviet Union and Harbor-UCLA Medical Center independently corroborated each other's clinical results on HS, both concluding that this drug represented a promising new therapeutic agent.

Later on, it was popularized as a cancer treatment in Penthouse Magazine. The treatment was used by Kathy Keeton, the wife of Bob Guccione to treat her breast cancer until her demise in 1997. Kathy and other proponents of hydrazine sulfate claimed that the US government hid the beneficial results of the treatment.

Hydrazine sulfate (HS), an inexpensive, mass-produced chemical compound used for many industrial applications, was first proposed as an anticachexia agent based on its inhibition of the gluconeogenic enzyme, phosphoenolpyruvate carboxykinase (PEP CK). Gluconeogenesis is the metabolic process that creates glucose from other metabolic substances. Glucose is the main fuel for the body's cells.

Tumor energy (ATP) gain and host energy loss (resulting from cancer-induced excessive gluconeogenesis) are functionally connected. By indirect and non-toxic means, HS inhibits tumor growth by preventing cancer cells from creating food for themselves. HS stops tumors from consuming the rest of the body to support their own excessive growth.

There may be an additional mechanism for the anti-cancer action of hydrazine sulfate. It blocks tumor necrosis factor-alpha (TNF-alpha), a substance frequently elevated in cancer patients. TNF-alpha is manufactured by white blood cells to fight infections and tissue damage. It causes anorexia, tiredness and breakdown of muscle tissue. As muscle tissue is destroyed, it produces sugar which feeds the cancer. By blocking TNF-alpha, hydrazine sulfate stops these effects.

Early *in-vivo* (animal) studies demonstrated that HS inhibited weight loss (cachexia) and tumor growth in a variety of transplanted mouse and rat models, could add to the antitumor effects of chemotherapy drugs, and was free of significant side effects or direct cytotoxicity. These results strongly suggest that HS is a new means of non-toxic cancer chemotherapy.

Like Laetrile, hydrazine sulfate is a controversial drug. The National Cancer Institute evaluated it in the 1980s and stated that there is little evidence for its effectiveness, and that Russian studies proved it to be worthless. However, criticism of the NCI studies includes familiar allegations of deliberate sabotage of experiments by giving patients drugs known to interact with hydrazine sulfate, and misrepresentation of results.

As for the Russian research, the summary states, "Clinical observations enabled us to state a definite therapeutic effect of hydrazine sulfate in patients with lymphogranulomatosis [Hodgkin's and non-Hodgkin's lymphomas] and malignant tumors of various localizations, when other measures of specific therapy failed."[1]

Details of the controversy are available in an article by Dr. Jeseph Gold, M.D.

May 28, 2009

THE TRUTH ABOUT HYDRAZINE SULFATE - DR. GOLD SPEAKS - 2 **MedTruth Blog** A commentary on truth in medicine

Studies

Multiple clinical trials of hydrazine sulfate have been done and published in peer-reviewed medical journals with worldwide circulation. Results have been generally positive, with patients either gaining or maintaining body weight.[2]

Hydrazine sulfate was shown to improve nutritional status and to increase survival in patients with non-small-cell lung cancer.[3] Hydrazine sulfate normalized carbohydrate metabolism in cancer patients.[4]

However, a few studies showed a decrease in survival and quality of life in patients with non-small-cell lung cancer and advanced colorectal cancer.[5,6]

Clinical trials in Russia show HS to be extremely effective in more than 50% of patients with AIDS and cancer.

Caution

In high doses, HS is carcinogenic as well as toxic to mammalian cells. However, at therapeutic doses, side effects are mainly gastrointestinal, such as nausea/vomiting, or neurological, such as dizziness and tingling of the extremities.

HS may lead to a decrease in blood sugar levels.

One case of fatal liver and kidney failure has been reported. However, this case is anecdotal and no evidence existed that this patient ever actually consumed hydrazine sulfate.

Do not mix with tranquilizers – this can have fatal results. HS interacts with alcohol, barbiturates, and tranquilizers. Patients receiving hydrazine sulfate must avoid these substances while undergoing treatment.

Instructions

One 60 mg capsule every day for the first 3 days, with or before breakfast.

No other medications for a half hour afterwards.

One 60 mg capsule twice a day for the next 3 days, before breakfast and before dinner.

One 60 mg capsule three times a day thereafter, approximately every 8 hours beginning with breakfast.

Stop after 45 days for 1 to 2 weeks to prevent side effects.

Supplier

1-Bottle (60mg) 100 Caps $43.95

http://www.positive-works.com/hydrazine

References

(1) Seits, J.F., Gershanovich, M.L., Filov, V.A., et al. "Experimental and clinical data on the antitumor action of hydrazine sulfate." Vopr. Onkol. 21:45-52, 1975

(2) Chlebowski RT, Bulcavage L, Grosvenor M, et al. "Hydrazine sulfate in cancer patients with weight loss. A placebo-controlled clinical experience." Cancer 59 (3): 406-10, 1987

(3) Chlebowski RT, et al., "Hydrazine sulfate influence on nutritional status and survival in non-small-cell lung cancer."J Clin Oncol, 1990 Jan;8(1):9-15

(4) Chlebowski, "Influence of hydrazine sulfate on abnormal carbohydrate metabolism in cancer patients with weight loss." Cancer Res, 1984 Feb;44(2):857-61

(5) Loprinzi CL, Goldberg RM, Su JQ, et al.: "Placebo-controlled trial of hydrazine sulfate in patients with newly diagnosed non-small-cell lung cancer." J Clin Oncol 12 (6): 1126-9, 1994

(6) Loprinzi CL et al., "Randomized placebo-controlled evaluation of hydrazine sulfate in patients with advanced colorectal cancer." J Clin Oncol,1994 Jun;12(6):1121-5.

Megestrol Acetate

Megestrol acetate (MA) is a progestational drug (an artificial analog to the hormone progesterone, called a progestin) currently known as an extremely effective appetite stimulant in patients suffering from cancer-induced anorexia/cachexia syndrome.

According to researchers, it causes an increase in appetite and food intake, and can lead to substantial nonfluid weight gain in some patients with cachexia. The only side effects are mild edema.[1]

Oral megestrol acetate improved appetite and quality of life in patients with advanced cancers and cachexia.[2]

Another study showed no improvement in cachexia in patients with advanced gastrointestinal cancer treated with megestrol alone, but improvement did occur in patients treated with a combination of megestrol and ibuprofen.[3]

Dose

In a study comparing the effectiveness of different doses of megestrol acetate, patients were given either 160 mg, 320 mg or 480 mg/day. Patients given the higher doses showed slightly more improvement than those given low doses, but the difference was not judged to be statistically significant. Researchers felt that dosages of more than 480 mg/day would offer no advantage. A stepped program of medication dosage was recommended, with dosages starting at lower levels and being increased if no response was seen. Most patients responded to the treatment within 15 days.[4]

Other studies have used up to 800 mg per day megestrol acetate per day.

References

(1) Loprinzi C., et al., "Controlled trial of megestrol acetate for the treatment of cancer anorexia and cachexia." J Natl Cancer Inst, 1990 Jul 4;82(13):1127-32.

(2) Tomiska M, "Palliative treatment of cancer anorexia with oral suspension of megestrol acetate." Neoplasma, 2003;50(3):227-33.

(3) McMillan DC, "A prospective randomized study of megestrol acetate and ibuprofen in gastrointestinal cancer patients with weight loss." Br J Cancer 1999 Feb;79(3-4):495-500.

(4) Gebbia V et al., "Prospective randomised trial of two dose levels of megestrol acetate in the management of anorexia-cachexia syndrome in patients with metastatic cancer." Br J Cancer,1996 Jun;73(12):1576-80.

10. Most Effective Treatments

After taking care of the external causes of cancer, cleansing the intestines, and alkalinizing, it is time to attack the cancer itself. Cancer patients increase their chances of survival by using as many credible approaches as possible. Cancer is a formidable enemy, but it is not unbeatable. No cure comes with a 100% guarantee, but these treatments will help create odds in favor of survival.

The most widely applicable treatments are listed first, followed by categories of miscellaneous cures.

The Budwig diet seems to be effective for all cancers, and is a very inexpensive home therapy.

Melatonin, green foods and resveratrol are completely safe, cause no side effects and have proven health benefits for everyone.

Low-dose naltrexone has a proven record of success, is very safe, and has no serious side effects.

Paw-paw is one of the few therapies specifically effective on drug-resistant tumors.

A Note on Suppliers

The alternative therapies listed also include suppliers of the products mentioned. These are included as examples only; we have not tested and do not endorse any particular brands.

Some large online supplement retailers (such as Vitamins.com, Vitacost.com and Iherb.com) tend to have consistently lower prices than other websites. Often, there are hundreds of suppliers online for any given product.

Ebay is sometimes a good source for bulk powders. For large quantities, buyers may want to deal directly with manufacturers through global trading sites such as Alibaba.com.

Items may also be available in local stores, though almost certainly for a higher price.

The Johanna Budwig Flaxseed Diet

Oxygen Therapy

Cancer cells generally use anaerobic glycolysis rather than respiration (oxidative phosphorylation) to produce energy. Otto Warburg was awarded the Nobel Prize in 1931 for this discovery. When the body is not able to fully oxygenate, the cells must either die of asphyxiation and toxic build-up, or regress to a more primitive state of existence where they can live and grow without requiring much oxygen.

Under conditions of low oxygen, mitochondria, intracellular organelles which produce energy aerobically, shut down. However, mitochondria also control apoptosis, or normal cell death. When the mitochondria cease to function properly, their control of apoptosis is also lost, and cells then begin to multiply uncontrollably. Viewed in this fashion, cancer is not a disease in and of itself, but rather an unfortunate side effect of a cellular survival mechanism.

This process is not irreversible. It is possible to restart aerobic metabolism in cancer cells, at which point the mitochondria resumes control of the cell's life cycle, and the cell undergoes apoptosis.

Cancer cells do not thrive in well-oxygenated environments. Daily exercise and deep breathing help to deliver oxygen to body's cells.

Some treatments, such as the Budwig Diet, do this indirectly by changing the cell membrane to improve transport of oxygen and nutrients. Others, such as DCA, directly effect the mitochondria.

History

This diet was designed in 1951 by Dr. Johanna Budwig, a German Ph.D (biochemistry) who performed major studies in the field of cancer and its relationship to dietary fats. Dr. Budwig felt that the diet was not only an excellent preventative of cancer, but was also an actual cure for cancer.

Dr. Budwig reported that her studies revealed that while some fats such as hydrogenated oils are disastrous to human health, other fats such as essential fatty acids are successful preventatives of cancer and other degenerative diseases. Today, terms such as "hydrogenated oils" and "trans fatty acids" are popular topics even in supermarket tabloids, but Dr. Budwig first raised the alarm about "bad fats" 50 years ago. The fat we eat becomes part of cell membranes and affects cell functions.

Dr. Budwig claimed that her scientific studies showed that the blood of people afflicted with cancer was significantly lower in substances known as phosphatides and lipoproteins, compared to the blood of healthy people.

According to Dr. Budwig, in her paper written in 1952 which bears the title *On Fat Biology V. Paper Chromatography of Blood Lipoids, the Tumour Problem and Fat Research,* she stated, "It is basically proven that highly unsaturated fatty acids are the heretofore undiscovered decisive factor in respiratory enzyme function."

It was Dr. Budwig's contention that if the phosphatides and lipoprotein levels in the blood of people with cancer were raised, their cancer would disappear.

She was the first researcher to understand the importance of what we today call essential fatty acids. In a speech given on November 2, 1959 in Zurich, Switzerland, Dr. Budwig is quoted as saying, "Without these fatty acids, the respiratory enzymes cannot function and the person suffocates, even when he is given oxygen-rich air. A deficiency in these highly unsaturated fatty-acids impairs many vital functions. First of all, it decreases the person's supply of available oxygen. We cannot survive without air and food; nor can we survive without these fatty acids. That has been proven long ago."

In layman's terms, Dr. Budwig's diet allows cancerous cells to start breathing again, thus interrupting the functional disorder that lies at the heart of cancer, anaerobic metabolism.

It is a simple cure. It allows the body to heal itself, rather than depending upon the more invasive and unnatural treatments of chemotherapy, radiation and drugs as well as the most invasive of all, surgery.

Dr. Budwig was declared by Germany's Federal Institute for Fats Research as "the world's leading authority on fats and oils", a high honor indeed, since this designation came from leading professionals who also had made similar studies or had seen the results of Dr. Budwig's treatments for themselves.

In her efforts to reach out to other professionals as well as to the general public, Dr. Budwig wrote a large number of books in which she shared her findings, including *Cancer: the Problem and the Solution, The Fat Syndrome, The Death of the Tumor,* and *Flax Oil*

As A True Aid Against Arthritis, Heart Infarction, Cancer And Other Diseases.

Since only a few of Dr. Budwig's books have been translated into English, she has not always experienced the fame in English speaking countries that she has in her own country, although that is beginning to change.

Although she was seven times nominated for a Nobel Prize for her work, Dr. Budwig also came under major attack by some of the more traditional medical professionals. Dr. Budwig was prosecuted several times for malpractice in Germany, even though all her patients had cancers untreatable by conventional means. In every case, she was exonerated by the court because patient case histories supported the benefits of her treatment methods.

According to Dr. Budwig, a number of medical professionals came to Germany to study her methods and were quite impressed, until they found that she was unwilling to enter into an agreement with them, even though it would have made them all quite wealthy. At this point, they lost interest in promoting her work.

Dr. Budwig also met opposition from food manufacturers due to her opinion that toxic fats caused sickness. This was a direct attack on many standard food production methods, which involved the use of refined, oxidized and hydrogenated fats. If her ideas were to be followed on a large basis, it would mean a serious financial cost to the processed food industry.

Dr. Budwig based her treatments on a special diet, the therapeutic basis of which consisted of flaxseed oil and cottage cheese. The diet also stressed the consumption of organic fruits, vegetables, and fiber. It banned animal fats, butter, sugar, processed oils such as salad oils, and especially margarine. After 3 months on this diet, some cancer patients had smaller tumors, some had no tumors left, and all felt subjectively better.

While flaxseed oil and cottage cheese may seem like a strange combination, not carrying the prestigious, mysterious sounding names of many "cures", Dr. Budwig claimed to have documented over one thousand cases in which cancer literally disappeared.

One can only wonder if the millions of people who have died of cancer in the almost sixty years that have followed the writing and publishing of her books have done so needlessly. Perhaps their lives could have been saved by the use of the Budwig Diet, simply by consuming a common food product.

Flaxseed is the number one richest vegetable source of what we call omega three fatty acids, linoleic acid and alpha-linolenic acid. Alpha-linolenic acid (ALA) is converted by the body into eicosapentaenoic acid (EPA) and docosahexaenoic acid (DHA), the omega-3 fatty acids found in fish oil. Individuals have varying abilities to make this conversion, and in some cases fish oil has been added to the program along with the flax oil.

Generally, women convert ALA to essential fatty acids EPA and DHA at a higher rate due to the presence of estrogen. Research has shown that young women convert 21% of ALA to EPA (compared to 8% conversion in males) and 9% to DHA (0-4% conversion in males).[1]

A major component of flax is lignan, which contains antioxidants as well as phytoestrogens that act as mild estrogens and displace stronger human estrogen from its cellular receptor site.

Enterodiol and enterolactone, produced by fermentive biotransformation of flax in the colon, are weak estrogens which block stronger human estrogen from its binding sites on cells. This is of vital importance in the case of hormone-sensitive cancers, such as breast, ovarian or prostate cancer.

Flax meal also contains nitrilosides, compounds related to amygdalin/Laetrile/vitamin B17 which have also been used as cancer treatments by themselves.

Dr. Budwig combined this with the type of sulphurated protein found in cottage cheese. It seems that this particular protein emulsifies the flaxseed oils to make them water soluble without putting a strain on the body, particularly the liver, by making it break down the unsaturated fats through its own efforts. Dr. Budwig made it clear that both of these food substances needed to be taken together, not just one or the other, in order for this diet to be effective. Making substitutions, such as using yogurt instead of cottage cheese, diminishes the effectiveness of the diet because it is missing the exact sulphurated protein found in cottage cheese.

She also stressed the need for the person taking the treatment to expose themselves to sunlight, to have a positive mental attitude, a positive spiritual attitude (spiritual meaning whatever it means to the person themselves), and the right emotional attitude concerning their cancer and the treatment which she recommended.

In her writings, Dr. Budwig also recommended the use of what she calls Electron Differentation Oil to massage the body, and also as an enema. It was Dr. Budwig's belief and claim that the use of flaxseed oil and cottage cheese on the inside of the body, combined with the Electron Differentation Oil on the outside, led to the elimination of all toxic substances in the body.

Cancer patients worldwide who have followed Dr. Budwig's diet claim that they have found themselves to be entirely cured of cancer. Many of these claims are further supported by medical professionals who had earlier been treating these patients.

Studies

In 2005, a study was performed on breast cancer patients who consumed a muffin containing 25 gram flaxseed daily over the course of 32 days. After observing decreased tumor markers and increased apoptosis (programmed cell death) in the patients treated with flaxseed, researchers concluded, "Dietary flaxseed has the potential to reduce tumor growth in patients with breast cancer."[2]

A 2008 study showed a decrease in tumor cell proliferation in men with prostate cancer who consumed a flaxseed supplement for at least 21 days prior to prostatectomy. The study concluded, "Findings suggest that flaxseed is safe and associated with biological alterations that may be protective for prostate cancer."[3]

Instructions

To start the diet, you will need to have 3 appliances:

A coffee grinder for the flaxseeds. Do not buy pre-ground flaxseeds, as the oils oxidize and become rancid very quickly.
A hand-held immersion blender (a stick-shaped mixer). Hand mixing will not blend the mixture sufficiently.

A Juice Machine. A masticating type juicer gives higher-quality juice than a centrifugal type.

Ingredients : Cottage Cheese or Quark, and Organic Flax Seeds and Flax Oil
Each tablespoon of Flaxseed Oil is mixed with 2 or more tablespoons of low-fat organic Cottage Cheese or quark. Be sure to buy the low-fat product so that the flax oil does not have to compete with dairy fat for absorption.

To make the Budwig Muesli, blend 3 Tablespoons of flaxseed oil with 6 Tbsp of Quark or Cottage Cheese with a hand-held immersion blender for up to a minute. If the mixture is too thick and/or the oil does not disappear, you may need an additional 2-3 Tablespoons of milk, preferably goat milk.

Do not add water or juices when blending this mixture. It should resemble rich whipped cream with no separated oil.

When possible, always use organic food products.

Now once the oil and cottage cheese are well mixed, grind 2 Tbsp flaxseeds and add them to the mixture.

Ground flaxseeds should be used within 20 minutes after being ground or they will become rancid. *Do not pre-grind flaxseeds or buy ground flaxseed.*

Next, mix in by hand or with the blender 1 teaspoon of honey, preferably raw and unpasteurized.

At this point, other ingredients may be added such as chopped fruit, applesauce, chopped nuts, vanilla, etc. Do not add peanuts as they may contain high levels of aflatoxin that strain the liver. Not more than 1 cup of fruit or other foods should be added.

(Optional) Add ground up *Apricot kernels* (no more than 6 kernels/day). Or you may decide to eat these apricot kernels by themselves.

Some people develop nausea from the ground flaxseeds, this may be counteracted by consuming a small bowl of papaya immediately afterwards. The papaya can be added to the muesli too, as the enzymes in the papaya aid digestion.

The Basic Rule with the Budwig diet is, *"if God made it then it's fine and try to eat it in the same form that God made it"*. The following foods are acceptable to the Budwig Diet:

- Stevia, raw non-pasteurized honey, figs, dates, fruit and berry juices serve as sweeteners - no other sweeteners are permitted
- Herbs in natural form
- Raw unroasted nuts are allowed with the exception of peanuts
- Seeds especially sunflower seeds
- Shredded, unsweetened coconut
- Raw unprocessed cocoa
- Small amounts of cold pressed sunflower oil, which according to Dr. Budwig was better than olive oil
- Organic beef or chicken (NO pork)
- Black tea is accepted, coffee is not recommended
- Flour of any type except corn, as long as it is 100% whole grain. Corn has problems with mold/fungus and is frequently GMO.

- 2-3 slices of health food store pickles, as long as they are free of preservatives.

Freezing these ingredients is OK, but freezing quark or cottage cheese will cause it to separate and affects it ability to emulsify oil.

VERY IMPORTANT: Always store flaxseed oil in the refrigerator. It will stay fresh for 12 months in the freezer. Buy as directly as possible from a reputable manufacturer (like Barlean's), and refrigerate as soon as possible. Otherwise, ask a local health food store to keep a supply in the refrigerator for you.

Drink only purified water, distilled water or reverse osmosis is best

Avoid the following products entirely:

- hydrogenated oils, trans-fats or animal fats
- pork, processed meat, shellfish
- products made with white flour. Spelt pasta and bread are better choices than wheat as many cancer patients are intolerant of wheat. Whole oat, rye, or multigrain bread is allowed. Corn is very much discouraged (because of mold and genetic modification issues).
- dairy products (other than the cottage cheese and some cheese)
- white sugar, molasses, maple syrup, or artificial sweeteners,
- processed foods and preservatives
- soybean products, except fermented (ie, natto)
- pesticides and chemicals, even those in cleaning products and cosmetics. Vinegar and baking soda are non-toxic substitutions.
- microwaved food
- Teflon or aluminium cookware or aluminium foil. The Budwig Center recommends enamel cookware. Use stainless steel, cast iron, ceramic, glass or corningware.

Do not combine the Budwig diet program in conjunction with other therapies because they may interfere with it. Chemotherapy, Oxygen therapies, vitamin C infusions, Laetrile (Vitamin B17 injections), and most supplements should not be used at the same time. Check with the Budwig Center if you are not sure.

Warning: if you cannot follow the above diet exactly, contact
http://www.budwigcenter.com/anti-cancer-diet.php

You can buy a personally tailored distance program directly from the Budwig Centre for as little as EU 1000.

For more than 120 testimonials that the Budwig diet works check out this website:
http://cancerfighter.wordpress.com

Controversy Regarding ALA

There is some controversy regarding the effect of certain fats on prostate cancer.

According to one meta-analysis of several dietary studies from different countries, there is evidence that high levels of ALA (alpha-linolenic acid), the plant fat found in flax seed, can increase the risk of prostate cancer by 70%. However, the risk was not present in all countries studied, and a few studies actually found a protective effect on prostate cancer from ALA. The effect was unrelated to the source of the ALA, whether it had been derived from meat or plants. The researchers who performed the analysis concluded that the relationship of prostate cancer to dietary ALA warrants further studies. Fish oils did not have a negative effect on prostate cancer incidence in any studies surveyed, and may have a positive effect.[4]

This is a paradoxical finding, since other studies previously mentioned found a positive effect on pre-existing prostate cancer from eating ground whole flaxseed. Of course, flaxseed contains many more ingredients other than just oil.

In addition, test subjects were probably not getting their ALA from flax or cold-pressed flax oil. They were more likely obtaining it either from red meat or the rancid, deodorized and over-processed vegetable oils (such as soy oil) found in a myriad of commercial food products.

Udo Erasmus, an expert on health and fats, published a long article about the controversy, stating that multiple issues were involved, such as oxidation of fats and dietary balance of omega-3 versus omega-6 fats.

http://www.udoerasmus.com/articles/

There is no evidence that cold-processed flax oil has negative health effects, and the Budwig diet has been proven successful against prostate cancer.

References

(1) Burdge GC, et al., "Conversion of alpha-linolenic acid to eicosapentaenoic, docosapentaenoic and docosahexaenoic acids in young women." Br J Nutr, 2002 Oct;88(4):411-20.

(2) Lilian U Thompson, Jian Min Chen, Tong Li, Kathrin Strasser-Weippl, Paul E Goss "Dietary flaxseed alters tumor biological markers in postmenopausal breast cancer." Clin Cancer Res. 2005 May 15;11(10):3828-35.)

(3) Wendy Demark-Wahnefried et al., "Flaxseed supplementation (not dietary fat restriction) reduces prostate cancer proliferation rates in men presurgery." Cancer Epidemiol Biomarkers Prev. 2008 Dec;17(12):3577-87.)

(4) Brouwer I., et al., "Dietary α-Linolenic Acid Is Associated with Reduced Risk of Fatal Coronary Heart Disease, but Increased Prostate Cancer Risk: A Meta-Analysis." J. Nutr. April 1, 2004 vol. 134 no. 4 919-922)

Green Foods

Chlorella

Chlorella was first identified in 1890 by a Dutch microbiologist, Martinus W. Beijerinck. It has probably been studied more than any other algae known throughout human history. It has been researched by Stanford Research Foundation, the Rockefeller Foundation, NASA, the Carnegie Institute, and the Japan Chlorella Research Center.

Chlorella is the top selling health food supplement in Japan, and is consumed by over 30% of the Japanese population. Approximately 10 million people worldwide eat Chlorella regularly.

Chlorella is a genus of single-celled green algae, belonging to the phylum chlorophyta. It is round and lacks flagella. Chlorella contains the green photosynthetic pigments chlorophyll-a and -b in its chloroplast.

Chlorella contains the highest chlorophyll level concentration of any plant, as much as 7% of its total weight, which is 5 to 10 times more chlorophyll than spirulina, and 10 times more than alfalfa. Chlorella does not contain the biliprotein phycocyanin, which is found in blue-green algae such as spirulina. Each green product has its own unique benefits.

It also contains protein (roughly 60%) and all essential amino acids, carbohydrates (15%), all the B vitamins except for B-12 (trace amounts only), beta-carotene, vitamins C and E, essential fatty acids, enzymes and rare trace minerals. Chlorella is both nutritious and immunosupportive.

Chlorella also contains a unique nucleotide-peptide complex of substances called Chlorella Growth Factor. This substance includes amino acids, nucleic acids, peptides, polysaccharides, and beta glucans.

Cancer cells develop in all of our bodies, even in those of us who have never been diagnosed with cancer. When these cancer cells develop, our immune systems naturally and efficiently destroy them before cancer symptoms appear.

However, when our immune systems are not functioning properly, cancer cells can proliferate. It is therefore absolutely necessary to keep our immune systems in perfect condition. Chlorella does just that. It helps protect the body in its fight against both infections and cancer.[1]

The Japanese have studied Chlorella intensively, and have used it in treating patients after Nagasaki and Hiroshima. The Japanese consider Chlorella a food product and consume it on a regular basis. It may be one reason why the Japanese have one of the lowest rates of cancer in the world.

Dr. Ralph W. Moss stated in *Cancer Therapy*, "Japanese scientists studied Chlorella pyrenoidosa as a biological response modifier... Since chlorella does not directly kill cancer cells, the scientists concluded that its effects were caused by boosting the immune response."[1]

In the Japanese study, scientists placed lab mice on a chlorella regimen for ten days, then injected the mice with either breast, ascites, or leukemic cancer cells. According to Dr. Moss, more than 70% of the mice fortified with chlorella did not develop cancer, while all of the untreated mice died of cancer within 20 days.[2]

A series of studies during the 1980s showed that tumor growth in mice could be reduced or stopped by injecting them with a water solution of chlorella, [3,4] or by feeding them chlorella.[5]

Human studies also exist. One experiment with Chlorella was done at the Medical College of Virginia in 1990. A research team led by Dr. Randall Merchant gave Chlorella to patients with various types of deadly brain tumors, including malignant glioblastomas. These patients all had advanced cancer and were considered to be terminal cases, incurable by conventional medicine. After two years of follow-up, 7 of 20 patients (35%) were still alive and their tumors had not recurred.[6]

This is highly unusual for these types of tumors, which normally have a survival rate of less than 10% after two years.

After Dr. Merchant's research grant expired in 1990, official tracking of the patients ceased. However, Dr. Merchant encountered one patient in 1994, still alive and continuing her consumption of chlorella. She was still living as of 1996.

Chlorella can be used in conjunction with surgery, chemo and radiation. It has been used in the treatment of radiation poisoning. It helps prevent damage to the immune system caused by chemotherapy.

Caution

Chlorella can cause gastric upset and photosensitivity.

Instructions

3 grams per day is the usual maintenance dose, for therapeutic effects take at least 5-7 grams per day. One teaspoon equals approximately 2 grams.

Suppliers

It is probably best to buy thin-cell-walled chlorella, as it is the most absorbable form. There are two new strains of thin-cell-wall chlorella, one derived from *Chlorella Vulgaris* and another variety called *Chlorella Sorokiniana.*

Older strains with thicker cell walls must be processed to have their cell walls broken in order to become digestible. One example is Sun Chlorella, a well-known, reputable brand from Japan.

Avoid purchasing ordinary thick-cell-walled *Chlorella Vulgaris,* which is closely related to common pond algae. This older strain has less Chlorella Growth Factor and fewer nutrients than the cultivated thick-cell wall variety, *Chlorella Pyrenoidosa*

Here are 3 reliable chlorella suppliers:

Thin-cell-wall chlorella
www.Znaturalfoods.com

Broken-cell-wall chlorella

www.Sunchlorellausa.com

www.Mercola.com

References

(1) Fumiko Kunishi, et al. "Enhanced resistance against Escherichia coli infection by subcutaneous administration of the hot-water extract of Chlorella vulgaris in cyclophosphamide-treated mice." Cancer Immunol Immunother 1990;32(1):1-7

(2) Miyazawa, Y., et al. "Immunomodulation by a unicellular green algae (Chlorella pyrenoidosa) in tumor-bearing mice." Journal of Ethnopharmacology. 24(2-3):135-146, 1988.

(3) Kuniaki Tanaka et al., "Augmentation of antitumor resistance by a strain of unicellular green algae, Chlorella Vulgaris," Cancer Immunology, Immunotherapy Volume 17, Number 2 (1984), 90-94, DOI: 10.1007/BF00200042

(4) Fumiko Konishi et al., "Antitumor effect induced by a hot water extract of Chlorella vulgaris (CE): Resistance to meth-A tumor growth mediated by CE-induced polymorphonuclear leukocytes." Cancer Immunology, Immunotherapy Volume 19, Number 2 (1985), 73-78, DOI: 10.1007/BF00199712

(5) Tanaka K et al., "Oral administration of Chlorella vulgaris augments concomitant antitumor Immunity," Immunopharmacol Immunotoxicol. 1990;12(2):277-91.

(6) Merchant R.E., Rice C.D., Young H.F., "Dietary Chlorella pyrenoidosa for Patients with Malignant Glioma: Effects on Immunocompetence, Quality of Life, and Survival." Phytotherapy Research, volume 4, issue 6, pages 220–231, December 1990)

Spirulina

Spirulina is a blue-green algae found naturally in alkaline, warm-water lakes. Like chlorella, it is cultivated for commercial use in specially designed algae farms.

It is rich in beta-carotene and other carotenoids. Spirulina is a rich source of the blue pigment phycocyanin, a biliprotein which has been shown to inhibit cancer-colony formation

Spirulina has a 62% amino acid content, it is the world's richest plant source of vitamin B-12, and contains a whole spectrum of natural mixed carotene and xanthophyll phytopigments. Spirulina has a soft cell wall made of complex sugars and protein, and is different from most other algae in that it is easily digested without processing.

Spirulina is especially effective against oral cancers.

In a study conducted in 1995 by biologist Padmanabhan Nair of the USDA-ARS Beltsville Human Nutrition Research Center in Maryland, a 1-gram capsule of spirulina capsule was given daily for a year to 44 tobacco and betel nut chewers with precancerous lesions of the mouth, a common illness in southwestern India. The lesions regressed completely in 20 of 44 (45%) subjects on the supplement and in only 3 of 43 (7%) consuming a placebo.[1]

Spirulina was found to be an effective preventative of liver cancer in rats treated with carcinogenic chemicals. The incidence of liver tumors was dramatically decreased from 80% to 20% in rats treated with a cancer-inducing nitrosamine compound. Survival time of animals which developed tumors was also increased by C-phycocyanin, the main blue-green pigment in spirulina.[2]

A 2009 study found that selenium-enriched spirulina extract caused apoptosis (programmed cell death) of MCF-7 human breast cancer cells implanted in rats.[3]

Spirulina protects the kidneys from being damaged by the chemotherapy drug cisplatin.[4]

It is also a protective agent against radiation, and has been used to treat victims of Chernobyl. As such, it is a useful adjunct to conventional cancer treatment.

Instructions

Dosage is about the same as for chlorella. 3 grams per day is the usual maintenance dose, for therapeutic effects take at least 5-7 grams per day. One teaspoon equals approximately 2 grams.

Suppliers

Spirulina is sold on EBay for as little as $10 per pound. Cheap generic chlorella and spirulina usually comes from Asian sources. It varies in quality and purity.

Probably the best quality spirulina is produced by Cyanotech in Hawaii, because of the intense sunlight, clean seawater and low-temperature processing. However, it is at least twice as expensive as spirulina from other sources.

References

(1) Padmanabhan Nair et al., "Evaluation of Chemoprevention of Oral Cancer by Spirulina Fusiformis." Nutr Cancer 24, 197-202, 1995

(2) Ismail MF, "Chemoprevention of rat liver toxicity and carcinogenesis by Spirulina." Int J Biol Sci 2009; 5(4):377-387

(3) Chen T et al., "Induction of G1 cell cycle arrest and mitochondria-mediated apoptosis in MCF-7 human breast carcinoma cells by selenium-enriched Spirulina extract." Biomed Pharmacother 2009 Oct 27 Epub.

(4) Mohan IK, et al., "Protection against cisplatin-induced nephrotoxicity by Spirulina in rats." Cancer Chemother Pharmacol 2006 Dec;58(6):802-8. Epub 2006 Mar 22.

Barley Grass

Barley grass is another green "superfood", with anti-inflammatory [1] and antioxidant [2] properties, containing a unique compound (called P4-D I by scientists who discovered it) which stimulates repair of damaged cellular DNA.[3]

Barley grass is a concentrated source of many vitamins and minerals, especially beta-carotene, and vitamin C, the B vitamins, folate, chlorophyll, and eighteen amino acids, including all nine essential amino acids. It also contains superoxide dismutase (SOD) an anti-inflammatory enzyme.

Studies

The anti-tumor activity of barley grass has been studied extensively by Dr. Allen L. Goldstein, Ph.D., head of the biochemistry department at George Washington University's School of Medicine and Health Sciences in Washington, D.C. According to Dr. Goldstein, multiple anti-oxidants including alpha-tocopherol succinate, a potent biochemical relative of alpha-tocopherol (vitamin E) may be responsible for its effects against cancer cells.

Barley grass has been shown in-vitro to inhibit several types of cancer, including leukemia, brain tumors, and prostate cancer. In a

2010 experiment, Dr. Goldstein exposed leukemic cancer cells to dehydrated barley grass extract, and almost all were killed. In subsequent trials, the extract eliminated 30-50 % of brain cancer cells, and 90-100% of three cell lines of prostate cancer.

Dr. Allan L. Goldstein, Ph.D, George Washington Univ. Medical Center stated, "Barley grass leaf extract dramatically inhibits the growth of human prostatic cancer cells grown in tissue culture...It may provide a new nutritional approach to the treatment of prostate cancer."[4]

Instructions

Concentrated barley grass extract is recommended, at least 5 grams daily.

Suppliers

Puritan's Pride (vitamins.com) supplies 120 Tablets x 2 bottles for $9.99. However, these are whole, dried barley green, inactive cellulose included.

http://www.puritan.com/food-supplements

More concentrated, and more expensive, products are made of pure barley green juice.

One example of such a product is Green Supreme, formulated by Dr. Yoshihide Hagiwara. There are more than 3,000 different types of enzymes in the human body. Green barley contains all 3,000 of them, according to Dr. Hagiwara.

Green Supreme comes in a 200 tablet bottle for $14.99.

Cancer patients need to take 17 V-Caps or 20 tablets per day, according to cancer researcher Bill Henderson.

www.greensupreme.net

Barley juice powder is also sold by Znaturals, a company which also features thin-cell-wall chlorella.
http://www.znaturalfoods.com

References

(1) Kubota K, Matsuoka Y, Seki H, "Isolation of Potent Anti-Inflammatory Protein From Barley Leaves." The Japanese journal of Inflammation, 1983 Vol. 3, No. 4.

(2) Osawa T, et al., "A Flavonoid With Strong Antioxidative Activity Isolated From Young Green Barley Leaves." J. Agric. Food Chem., 1992, 40 (7), pp 1135–1138

(3) Food Phytochemicals for Cancer Prevention IL 1994 Edited by Chi-Tang Ho, Toshihiko Osawa, Mou-Tuan Huany, and Robert T. Rosen. Washington, D.C: ACS Symposium Series. American Chemical Association.

(4) Hotta, Y. 1984. "Stimulation of DNA Repair-synthesis by P4-D I, One of the Novel Components of Barley Extracts." Lecture given in Honolulu, Hawaii.

(5) M. Badamchian and Allan L. Goldstein, "Biochemical Characterization of the Novel Molecule(s) in Barley Leaf Extract That Inhibits Growth of Human Prostate Cancer Cells. Preliminary report." Dept. of Biochemistry and Molecular Biology. George Washington Univ. Medical center

Low Dose Naltrexone (LDN)

Dr. Bernard Bihari, who is currently also working with Artemisia compounds, pioneered the use of low-dose naltrexone to treat HIV/AIDS, autoimmune diseases, and cancer.

Since 1984, Naltrexone has been used in high doses (50 mg per day) for opiate addiction. At this dose, it acts as an opiate blocker.

Scientists believe LDN works through three mechanisms.

First, it increases levels of metenkephalin (an endorphin produced in large amounts in the adrenal medulla) and beta-endorphin in the blood stream.

Second, it increases the number and density of opiate receptors on cancer cell membranes, making them more responsive to the growth-inhibiting effects of endorphins, which directly induce apoptosis in the cancer cells. If activation of opiate receptors occurs while a cancer cell is dividing, it dies. In-vitro tests show that relatively low concentrations of metenkephalin added to cultures of human pancreatic cancer cells or human colon cancer kills both cell types.

Before being used to treat cancer, LDN was used to treat HIV/AIDS. A double-blinded placebo-controlled study in 1986 showed that naltrexone provided significant immune system protection from HIV. The use of LDN was based on its ability to induce increases in the endorphin levels in the body. Endorphins are the primary homeostatic regulators of the immune system, representing 90% of its hormonal control. 90% of daily endorphin production by the pituitary and adrenal glands occurs between 2 a.m. and 4 a.m.

Third, LDN-mediated increases in endorphins boost the number and activity of natural killer (NK) cells and lymphocyte-activated CD8 cells, which destroy cancer cells.

Doses ranging from 1.75 to 4.5 milligrams (much less than the 50 mg dose given to opiate addicts) trigger endorphin production during sleep. Except during exercise, endorphins are made by the body only during the sleep cycle, usually between 2-4 a.m. The brain signals the adrenal and pituitary glands to make endorphins. Giving patients a small dose of naltrexone three to five hours before bedtime causes the brain to make the signal much stronger.

LDN doses lower than 1.5 mg have no effect on endorphin production. Doses higher than 4.5 mg produce no greater release of endorphins, but block endorphins for a significantly longer time period, thus reducing the benefit of the higher levels.

The only drug interaction is with narcotics, such as Demerol, morphine, and Percocet, which it briefly blocks.

More information about LDN:

http://www.ldninfo.org/
http://www.ldnscience.org/

Studies

There are multiple animal studies showing that the administration of endorphins, metenkephalins, beta-endorphins or low dose Naltrexone to mice with transplants of human cancer cells produced remission of disease.

Paradoxically, naltrexone has both stimulatory and inhibitory effects on tumor growth, depending on the dosage. In mouse test subjects implanted with neuroblastoma cells, the lower dose of naltrexone provided therapeutic advantages, whereas the higher dose actually worsened the disease.

Compared to a control group receiving no treatment, at low doses (0.1 mg per kg of body weight) naltrexone caused a 33% decrease in tumor incidence, a 98% delay in the time before tumor appearance, and a 36% increase in survival time. However, mice receiving a high dose of naltrexone (10 mg per kg) showed 100% tumor incidence, a 27% reduction in the time before tumor appearance, and a 19% decrease in survival time.[1]

According to Dr. Bihari, who originated the LDN protocol, LDN has caused remission of incurable, metastatic cancers in hundreds of patients, including virtually incurable cancers such as neuroblastoma, multiple myeloma, and pancreatic cancer.

In an interview given in September 23, 2003 with Dr. Kamau B. Kokayi, Dr. Bihari stated he had used LDN to treat 420 patients with various types of cancer. In cases of very advanced cancer, he also added intravenous metenkephalin (an endorphin) three times weekly. In approximately 2/3 of patients, cancers stopped growing. In roughly half of that group, about 1/3 of the total group of patients, the cancer disappeared entirely after several months.

As the interviewer, Dr. Kokayi, said, "That's phenomenal. I don't think there's any chemo or radiating oncologist with numbers like that."

Dr. Bihari's results differ from the two usual cancer treatment outcomes: either eventual death from the cancer, or a total cure. LDN therapy creates a viable third outcome, long-term stabilization of the tumor and/or gradual shrinkage. It reduces cancer to a manageable chronic disease without the side effects of conventional therapy. Best results are seen when the therapy is implemented in the early stages of the disease.[2,3]

LDN has been combined with alpha lipoic acid by one practitioner, Dr. Burton Berkson. He published a report on the treatment of a patient with metastatic pancreatic cancer, using intravenous alpha-lipoic acid (300-600mg) 2 days per week, and low-dose naltrexone (LDN), 4.5 mg orally at bedtime. In addition, the patient was given oral antioxidants, alpha-lipoic acid (600 mg daily), selenium (200 mcg twice daily), and silymarin (300 mg 4 times daily). At the time the report was published, 78 months after the patient had been diagnosed, the patient felt subjectively well, and a CT scan showed shrinkage of the original tumor as well as the liver metastasis. Since pancreatic cancer, especially stage IV, is almost always fatal within a year of diagnosis, this represents a near-miraculous cure.[4,5]

Similar positive results occurred in a patient with B-cell lymphoma.[6]

In patients with high-grade malignant gliomas (brain tumors), use of naltrexone with radiotherapy resulted in a significant 1-year survival advantage, though increased tumor-shrinking effects were not obvious immediately post-treatment. 5/10 patients given the combination treatment were still alive after 1 year, compared to 1/11 of those given only radiotherapy. The LDN therapy was well-tolerated.[7]

Two recent human studies in Mali found that LDN helped to stabilize immunocyte counts in AIDS patients.[8]
LDN is currently being evaluated by the NCI, and clinical studies are underway for its use in irritable bowel and multiple sclerosis.

Caution

May briefly interfere with opiate pain medication.

Instructions

4.5 mg 3-5 hours before bedtime. Some alternative practitioners recommend 2 doses of 3-4.5 mg, 12 hours apart.

Suppliers

LDN is available by prescription for addiction treatment, and doctors may be willing to prescribe it for off-label use to treat cancer. It may also be obtained from internet pharmacies, usually in 50mg tablets, and diluted with water or other substances down to 4.5mg doses.

References

(1) Zagon IS, McLaughlin PJ. "Naltrexone modulates tumor response in mice with neuroblastoma." Science. 1983;221:671-673.

(2) Bihari B. LDN and cancer. http://www.lowdosenaltrexone.org/ldn_and_cancer.htm. Accessed December 8, 2005.

(3) Bihari B. Keynote address. Presented at: first annual Low Dose Naltrexone Conference at the New York Academy of Sciences; June 11, 2005; New York, NY.

(4) Berkson, BM, Rubin D, Berkson AJ. "The long-term survival of a patient with pancreatic cancer with metastases to the liver after treatment with the intravenous alpha-lipoic acid/low-dose naltrexone protocol." Integr Cancer Ther. 2006;5:83-89.

(5) Burton M. Berkson, MD, MS, PhD; Daniel M. Rubin, ND, FABNO; and Arthur J. Berkson, MD, "Revisiting the ALA/N (a-Lipoic Acid/Low-Dose Naltrexone) Protocol for People With Metastatic and Nonmetastatic Pancreatic Cancer: A Report of 3 New Cases." Integrative Cancer Therapies 2009, 8(4) 416 –422

(6) Berkson, BM, Rubin D, Berkson AJ. "Reversal of signs and symptoms of a B-cell lymphoma in a patient using only low dose naltrexone." Integr Cancer Ther. 2007;6:293-296.

(7) Lissoni P, Meregalli S, Fossati V, et al. "Radioendocrine therapy of brain tumors with the long acting opioid antagonist naltrexone in association with radiotherapy." Tumori. 1993;79:198-201.

(8) Abdel K. Traore, Oumar Thiero, Sounkalo Dao, Fadia F. C. Kounde, Ousmane Faye, Mamadou Cisee, Jaquelyn B. McCandless, Jack M. Zimmerman, Karim Coulibaly, Ayouba Diarra, Mamadou S. Kieta, Souleymane Diallo, Ibrahima G. Traore and Ousmane Koita, "Single cohort study of the effect of low dose naltrexone on the evolution of immunological, virological and clinical state of HIV+ adults in Mali." Journal of AIDS and HIV Research Vol. 3(10), pp. 180-188, October 2011; "Impact of low dose naltrexone (LDN) on antiretroviral therapy (ART) treated HIV+ adults in Mali: A single blind randomized clinical trial." Journal of AIDS and HIV Research Vol. 3(10), pp. 189-198, October 2011;

Melatonin

Melatonin is a primary regulator of the immune system and is a powerful anti-oxidant (free-radical fighter). It has been said to have the potential to increase immune response dramatically, help in the treatment of cancer and AIDS, lower cholesterol and blood pressure, improve mood and reduce symptoms of PMS, induce sleep as effectively as a prescription drug (without side effects), and prevent the free radical damage that underlies aging.

Melatonin inhibits cancer cell growth, and can kill directly many different types of human tumor cells.

Melatonin directly kills tumor cells by causing apoptosis (cancer cell auto-destruction), and stops angiogenesis (the development of new blood vessels to supply the tumor). It blocks the stimulation of hormone-sensitive tumors by estrogen. Melatonin prevents tumor growth through several mechanisms, such as through the inhibition of epidermal growth factor receptors on cancer cells. Melatonin stimulates the immune system and boosts the activity of monocytes, macrophages, T-helper cells, natural killer cells, and eosinophils, which are active in cancer cell destruction. Melatonin is also an anti-oxidant, and blocks the inflammation that fuels tumor growth.

Studies

Melatonin is produced by the human pineal gland during deep sleep, and disruption to sleep patterns causes a lowering of melatonin levels, giving those with disturbed sleep patterns, such as night shift workers, a higher risk of developing cancer.[1,2,3,4]

Light blocks the secretion of melatonin,[5] and researchers speculate that the modern, 24-hour day with its ubiquitous artificial lighting are causing disturbances in biological circadian rhythm and melatonin secretion, leading to higher rates of cancer.

The low-level magnetic fields of household wiring can also suppress melatonin secretion.[6]

Exposure to 50-Hz magnetic fields, such as those generated by power lines, has been linked to an increased incidence of breast cancer,[7] and it is postulated that this may be due to lowered levels of melatonin. Levels of other hormones were unaffected.[8]

In 1985, researchers found that prostate cancer patients have an abnormal melatonin secretion pattern, and that this may be related to the growth of their cancer.[9] In 1992, the same research team found abnormally low levels of melatonin in prostate cancer patients.[10]

People living north of the Arctic circle, which has long, dark nights during winter have a lower incidence of hormone-dependent cancers, such as breast and prostate cancer. Researchers postulated that this is due to increased secretion of melatonin.[11]

Much of the early research on melatonin was performed by Georges Maestroni, director of the Center for Experimental Pathology in Switzerland. In the early 1980s he first discovered that melatonin affected the immune system when he learned that animals that had been deprived of their pineal glands, the source of melatonin, had atrophied thymus glands. Thymus glands are part of the body's immune system, and if the presence of melatonin is required for them to remain functional, then melatonin is fundamental to healthy immunity.

In one of his many articles he wrote that melatonin is not only produced by the pineal gland, but also by many other organs and tissues of the body, particularly those of the lymphoid system such as the bone marrow, thymus and lymphocytes.[12]

Studies on rodents show that removal of the pineal gland increases tumor growth[13], that administration of melatonin inhibits the growth of chemically induced mammary tumors[13,14], and that continual light exposure enhances the growth of chemically induced tumors.[15]

In 2005, researchers at the University of Texas treated both androgen-sensitive and androgen-insensitive prostate cancer cells with pharmaceutical doses of melatonin, and found the treatment substantially reduced the number of cancer cells, and prevented the growth of new tumor cells. It also prompted cellular differentiation; that is, the cells functioned more like normal prostate cells.[16]

Chinese researchers treated a patient with terminal, metastatic prostate cancer and rising PSA levels with 5 mg/day of melatonin (taken at 8 PM), and this therapy stabilized his disease for 6 weeks as indicated by stable PSA levels.[17]

A 1996 study tested the effects of melatonin on 30 patients with glioblastoma, a brain tumor which is nearly always fatal. 14 patients were given radiotherapy plus a daily dose of 20 mg of melatonin, while 16 were given radiotherapy alone. A year later, 6 of the 14 patients given melatonin were still alive, compared with only 1 of the 16 patients given radiotherapy alone. Also, side effects of conventional treatment were lessened by melatonin, thus improving both the length and quality of life in these patients.[18]

A 2003 study by the same researcher tested the effects of melatonin plus chemotherapy versus chemotherapy alone on 100 patients with non-small-cell lung cancer. After 2 years, all 51 patients treated with chemotherapy alone had died; however, even after 5 years, 3 of 49 patients treated with chemotherapy plus 20 mg/day of melatonin were still alive. Chemotherapy was also better tolerated by patients treated with melatonin.[19]

In a review of 8 randomized, controlled clinical trials, researchers found that 20 mg of melatonin combined with chemotherapy, versus chemotherapy alone, increased the rate of partial or complete remissions by almost 50%, increased 1-year survival by 45%, and decreased the usual side effects of chemotherapy such as fatigue, low platelet count, and neuropathy by 65%, 89%, and 83% respectively. These effects occurred in all types of cancer tested. No side effects from melatonin were reported. Researchers concluded, "Melatonin as an adjuvant therapy for cancer led to substantial improvements in tumor remission, 1-year survival, and alleviation of radiochemotherapy-related side effects."[20]

Caution - Who Should Not Take Melatonin

The only people who should avoid melatonin, or who should only take it very carefully under the care of a physician, are patients with leukemia, lymphomas, or other immune system cancers, or who have auto immune diseases such as lupus or rheumatoid arthritis. Such patients need to be careful about taking melatonin because it is a strong immune system stimulant, which is beneficial for most people, but can cause problems in patients whose immune system has gone awry.

There is also some evidence from a rodent trial suggesting that patients with ovarian cancer should **not** take melatonin, as melatonin stimulated endogenous (murine) ovarian cancer in the mouse test subjects. However, studies on human ovarian cancer cells indicates that melatonin does not stimulate tumor growth, and potentiates the effect of chemotherapy, so this animal study is likely not applicable to humans.[21]

The only other people who should be careful about taking melatonin are women who are pregnant, or who want to become pregnant. The reason for this is that melatonin is involved in the control of reproductive function, and studies are underway to use it as a contraceptive. Even though much higher doses of melatonin are being used in these studies than are used for anti-aging purposes, caution should be exercised.

Instructions

Take 20 mg melatonin every night before bedtime.

Do not keep electrical appliances close by the bed during sleep. It may be worthwhile to buy a meter to measure electromagnetic fields in the bedroom, and fix or avoid sources of "dirty electricity" (ie, electricity contaminated by frequency spikes and resonant frequencies), which generates EM fields.

Suppliers

Melatonin is usually sold in 3mg strength to aid sleep. Seven of these can be taken each evening before bedtime, or you can buy the less common 10 or 20 mg strength. Vitamins.com sells 10 mg capsules, and Iherb.com sells 20 mg capsules.

http://www.iherb.com/

References

(1) Jasser, SA, et al. "Light during darkness and cancer: relationships in circadian photoreception and tumor biology." Cancer Causes Control, Vol. 17, No. 4, May 2006, pp. 515-23

(2) Stevens, RG. "Artificial lighting in the industrialized world: circadian disruption and breast cancer." Cancer Causes Control, Vol. 17, No. 4, May 2006, pp. 501-07

(3) Bartsch, C and Bartsch, H. "The anti-tumor activity of pineal melatonin and cancer enhancing life styles in industrialized societies." Cancer Causes Control, Vol. 17, No. 4, May 2006, pp. 559-71

(4) Hansen, J. "Increased breast cancer risk among women who work predominantly at night." Epidemiology, Vol. 12, January 2001, pp. 74-77

(5) Lewy AJ, "Light suppresses melatonin secretion in humans." Science 12 December 1980: Vol. 210 no. 4475 pp. 1267-1269

(6) Davis, S, et al. "Residential magnetic fields, light-at-night, and nocturnal urinary 6-sulfatoxymelatonin concentration in women." American Journal of Epidemiology, Vol. 154, October 1, 2001, pp. 591-600

(7) Kliukiene, J, et al. Residential and occupational exposures to 50-Hz magnetic fields and breast cancer in women: a population-based study. American Journal of Epidemiology, Vol. 159, May 1, 2004, pp. 852-61

(8) Davis, S, et al. "Effects of 60-Hz magnetic field exposure on nocturnal 6-sulfatoxymelatonin, estrogens, luteinizing hormone, and follicle-stimulating hormone in healthy reproductive-age women: results of a crossover trial." Ann Epidemiol, January 31, 2006

(9) Bartsch, C, et al. "Evidence for modulation of melatonin secretion in men with benign and malignant tumors of the prostate: relationship with the pituitary hormones." J Pineal Res, Vol. 2, No. 2, 1985, pp. 121-32

(10) Bartsch, C, et al. "Melatonin and 6-sulfatoxymelatonin circadian rhythms in serum and urine of primary prostate cancer patients: evidence for reduced pineal activity and relevance of urinary determinations." Clin Chim Acta, Vol. 209, August 31, 1992, pp. 153-67

(11) Erren, TC and Piekarski, C. "Does winter darkness in the Arctic protect against cancer? The melatonin hypothesis revisited." Med Hypotheses, Vol. 53, July 1999, pp. 1-5

(12) Georges J Maestroni et al., "Immunomodulation by melatonin: its significance for seasonally occurring diseases." Neuroimmunomodulation,15 (2):93-101 (2008) PMID 18679047

(13) Tamarkin L, Cohen M, Roselle D, Reichert C, Lippman M, Chabner B., "Melatonin inhibition and pinealectomy enhancement of 7,12-

dimethylbenz(a)anthracene-induced mammary tumors in the rat." Cancer Res 1981;41:4432–6.

(14) Blask DE, Pelletier DB, Hill SM, Lemus-Wilson A, Grosso DS, Wilson ST, et al., "Pineal melatonin inhibition of tumor promotion in the N-nitroso-N-methylurea model of mammary carcinogenesis: potential involvement of antiestrogenic mechanisms in vivo." J Cancer Res Clin Oncol 1991;117:526–32.

(15) van den Heiligenberg S, Depres-Brummer P, Barbason H, Claustrat B, Reynes M, Levi F, "The tumor promoting effect of constant light exposure on diethylnitrosamine-induced hepatocarcinogenesis in rats." Life Sci 1999;64:2523–34.

(16) Sainz RM, et al., "Melatonin reduces prostate cancer cell growth leading to neuroendocrine differentiation via a receptor and PKA independent mechanism." Prostate, 2005 Apr 1;63(1):29-43.

(17) Shiu SY, et al, "Melatonin slowed the early biochemical progression of hormone-refractory prostate cancer in a patient whose prostate tumor tissue expressed MT1 receptor subtype." J Pineal Res, 2003 Oct;35(3):177-82.

(18) Lissoni P, et al., "Increased survival time in brain glioblastomas by a radioneuroendocrine strategy with radiotherapy plus melatonin compared to radiotherapy alone." Oncology, 1996 Jan-Feb;53(1):43-6.

(19) P. Lissoni, M. Chilelli, S. Villa, L. Cerizza, G. Tancini, "Five years survival in metastatic non-small cell lung cancer patients treated with chemotherapy alone or chemotherapy and melatonin: a randomized trial." J Pineal Res, Aug 2003 Vol 35, Issue 1, pages 12-15

(20) Wang YM, et al., "The efficacy and safety of melatonin in concurrent chemotherapy or radiotherapy for solid tumors: a meta-analysis of randomized controlled trials." Cancer Chemother Pharmacol 2012 May;69(5):1213-20. Epub 2012 Jan 24.

(21) Futagami, "Effects of melatonin on the proliferation and cis-diamminedichloroplatinum (CDDP) sensitivity of cultured human ovarian cancer cells." Gynecol Oncol. 2001 Sep;82(3):544-9.

Noni

On the Pacific islands of Hawaii and Tahiti, a popular cure-all is the fruit of the Noni plant (*morinda citrifolia*). Noni is known anecdotally as the "Aspirin of the Pacific" due to its multiple uses in traditional Polynesian medicine.

Noni is a small, flowering shrub native to the Pacific islands, Polynesia, Asia, and Australia. It grows to a height of up to 10 feet, with dark green, oval leaves. The flower heads mature into translucent off-white fruits with a pungent, cheese-like odor.

Noni is endowed with a wider array of health-giving phytochemicals than almost any other plant. It has analgesic, immunosupportive, anti-viral and anti-cancer activity.

Studies

Noni has been extensively studied by the U.S. Department of Agriculture.

500 different tropical plant extracts were tested for their ability to inhibit K-ras NRK cells (precursors to certain types of cancer). One particular compound found in Noni, damnacanthal, was found to be most effective in inhibiting Ras function among the 500 extracts tested.[1]

In 1992, a team of researchers led by Annie Hirazumi at the University of Hawaii School of Medicine introduced lung cancer cells called Lewis Lung Carcinoma into a group of mice especially bred to be highly susceptible to this type of cancer. The mouse test subjects were divided into 2 groups. The mice in the first group were left untreated, while the mice in the second group were given five doses of Noni extract.

Within 9 to 12 days the control group of mice which were given no Noni were all dead as a result of tumor growth. However, the mice given Noni were still alive and doing well.

At the end of 24 days, the Noni treated mice were all still alive, a 100% increase in survival time. Actually, 40%, that is 9/22 mice given the Noni, survived for more than 50 days. This is a lifespan more than 4 times greater than the longest living mouse not receiving the Noni.

To be sure that these amazing results were not a fluke, the experiment was repeated with similar results. The research team stated that Noni juice acts as an anti-tumor agent through enhancement of the cancer host's immune system of macrophages and/or lymphocytes.[2]

Noni is a ubiquitous folk remedy in Hawaii, and Annie Hirazumi had first become interested in it after two personal experiences. In one instance, her father gave Noni juice to a sick friend; and later, she administered Noni juice to a dying pet dog. The dog miraculously recovered, and Ms. Hirazumi became determined to learn more about the amazing healing properties of this tropical fruit.

Perhaps the most amazing thing about Noni juice is how fast it works. There are anecdotal cases of terminal cancer patients who claim to have been cured in as little as 10-12 days.

Instructions

30-60 mls noni juice daily is the maintenance dose; double or triple doses may be used for therapeutic effect. Take the noni twice daily on an empty stomach.

Use the higher dose of noni daily for at least 3 months, after that if results are seen go to maintenance dose.

A few rare cases of acute hepatitis (liver toxicity) have been reported in association with the consumption noni juice. However, these cases are anecdotal and retrospective, and in-vitro tests on hepatocytes (liver cells) failed to find any toxicity of noni.

Suppliers

High quality Hawaiian Noni juice and capsules:

http://estatenoni.com

References

(1) Hiramatsu, T.; et al., "Induction of normal phenotypes in ras-transformed cells by damnacanthal from Morinda citrifolia." Cancer Letters 1993; 73, 161-166

(2) Hirazumi, A., "Antitumor Activity of Morinda citrifolia on IP Implanted Lewis Lung Carcinoma in Mice." Proceedings, Annual Meeting of the American Association for Cancer Research 1992; 33, 515.

Pawpaw: One Of The Last Resorts For Multi Drug Resistant Cancer

Pawpaw has been used as a fruit and medicine for centuries. The fruit is not confined to one geographic location or ethnic group. As such, it is very commonly used as a food product in many households. The scientific name for paw-paw is *Asimina triloba*. It is in the same botanical family, Annonaceae, as the graviola or soursop (*Annona muricata*), which has also been investigated for its anti-cancer potential.

The pawpaw tree is a conical deciduous tree with a narrow trunk that manifests no branches. Instead, its dark green oblong leaves grow on stalks that rise from the trunk. In natural conditions, the pawpaw tree will grow to a height of about 12 to 20 feet After flowering, which happens during March to May, the tree bears the paw paw fruit, which is the largest edible fruit found in America. A mature fruit is shaped like a mango and weighs between 4 to 17 ounces.

Origin of Pawpaw

Before being cultivated and adapted to different environments, pawpaw flourished in the temperate woodlands of the Eastern United States. American aboriginals are credited with spreading the fruit throughout the Eastern part of the U.S. and later to Texas and Kansas. The fruit was cultivated from the Great Lakes to the Gulf. Subsequently, the pawpaw fruit is readily available.

Pawpaw as a treatment for Cancer

Paw Paw is one of the few alternative cancer treatments that can pass the blood/brain barrier. The other alternative cancer treatments that can cross this barrier are Cantron and Protocel, which work in much the same manner as paw-paw.

Purdue University researcher Jerry McLaughlin, working with doctoral student Nicholas Oberlies, has found compounds in the bark of the paw-paw tree that show preliminary success in fighting drug-resistant cancers. Research done by Dr. McLaughlin in the 1980s through 90s received funding of $5,000,000 from the National Cancer Institute. Dr. McLaughlin has received numerous honors and awards during his career. He has published more than 330 research papers, and his work is protected by several patents.

Where other cancer treatments have failed, you can count on an inexpensive and natural cure: the pawpaw. To understand how pawpaw works against cancer, you need to understand basic cell biology first.

How It Works

For human body cells to survive, multiply, and live, they need energy. No real surprise here. When we eat food, it is broken down through a process known as digestion to form blood sugar, technically known as glucose. The cells then absorb this glucose to stay alive. However, the cells cannot use glucose in its entirety. It must be broken down into its constituents to produce energy. The process involved is known as metabolism and takes place in specialized microscopic organelles known as mitochondria.

The energy produced is known as ATP, short for adenosine triphosphate.

The usefulness of pawpaw comes in at this stage. Cancer cells use up to 15 times as much ATP as healthy cells. It is possible to cure cancer by utilizing this metabolic difference, by starving the cancer cells of their life-sustaining ATP without killing the normal cells.

Pawpaw extract contains substances known as acetogenins, which greatly reduce the amount of ATP produced by the mitochondria. When ingested, acetogenins are transported in the blood stream to the body's cells.

Cancer cells absorb acetogenins at a higher rate than normal cells. Acetogenins selectively modulate the production of ATP in cancer cells, and are non-toxic to normal cells. Decreasing the production of ATP affects the viability of tumors and the growth of blood vessels that nourish them. The drop in ATP production in cancer cells adversely affects their metabolism to the point where they die off.

Paw Paw Kills Multi-Drug-Resistant Cancer Cells.

Acetogenins also support and enhance the effectiveness of conventional medical approaches.

After the majority of cancer cells have been killed by chemotherapy, a small core of Drug Resistant cancer cells remain, which then spread again. Unlike the original tumor cells, they can no longer be killed by chemotherapy.

Cancer cells which survive chemotherapy often develop resistance to the drug originally used as treatment, along with resistance to other, even unrelated, medications. This phenomenon is referred to as "multi-drug resistance (MDR)." It occurs when a small percentage of cancer cells develop a biochemical mechanism called a "P-glycoprotein mediated pump" which transports cytotoxic drugs out of the cell before they can be effective. It takes a great deal of energy to run this pump, and anything that depletes the energy supply of the cancer cell prevents the operation of this defence mechanism.

Annonaceous acetogenins exhibit their effects through depletion of cellular ATP, the energy source used by cells, and thus offer a special advantage in the treatment of MDR cancers. Deprived of the energy needed to extrude chemotherapy drugs, cancer cells become susceptable to chemotherapy once again. The lack of ATP also kills tumor cells directly by starving them.

Three separate laboratories have shown that acetogenins interfere with the mitochondrial electron transport systems of cells, including tumors, and inhibit ATP production. Annonacin, the main component of graviola, is described as a lipophilic inhibitor of mitochondrial complex I. Mitochondria are intracellular organelles which produce the life energy needed to sustain cells, so disrupting this process would be expected to have disastrous effects on cell function.

Acetogenins also block angiogenesis, the formation of new blood vessels to feed tumor growth

In addition to its anti-cancer activity, paw-paw also benefits viral illnesses such as cold sores, shingles, as well as fungal illnesses such as toe nail fungus, athletes' foot, and eczema. It has been formulated in capsules, lotions and salves. As a pesticidal agent, it has even been used as a treatment for head lice.[1]

Active Compounds In Paw-Paw

Asimicin, bullatacin, trilobacin, bullatalicin have been identified as some of the most important acetogenins in paw-paw. Acetogenins are derivatives of long-chain fatty acids with 0 to 3 tetrahydrofuran rings in their structure. Those with 2 rings have the most powerful anti-tumor action, followed by the 1-ring form.

In his investigation of the different acetogenins, Dr. McLaughlin also examined related plants such as graviola. However, he found that commercial products of graviola contained only 2-4% the concentration of acetogenins as paw-paw extract, and that the content from batch to batch varied widely due to lack of standardization. In addition, the acetogenins contained in graviola are only those with the less potent 1-ring structure.

Dr. McLaughlin produces a standardized extract called Paw-Paw Cell-Reg, a mixture of over 50 acetogenins. The standardization process eliminates the high variation normally found in plant extracts. In the case of paw-paw, this is extremely important because the acetogenin content can vary greatly from tree to tree, and season to season.

For more information about paw-paw, visit the website:

http://www.pawpawresearch.com/

Studies

More than 100 scientific studies have been published regarding the biochemistry of pawpaw-derived substances, including positive effects during in-vitro anti-cancer tests.[2,3,4,5]

In an in-vitro test, 14 different Annonaceous acetogenins, representing three main classes of chemical compounds (bis-adjacent, bis-nonadjacent, and single-THF ring), were tested for their ability to prevent the growth of adriamycin resistant human breast adenocarcinoma cells (MCF-7/Adr). This multidrug-resistant cell line survives treatment with common chemotherapy drugs adriamycin, vincristine, and vinblastine. One of the compounds tested showed as much as 250 times the potency of adriamycin. Researchers concluded, "The acetogenins may, thus, have chemotherapeutic potential, especially with regard to MDR tumors."[6]

Dr. McLaughlin's article entitled, "A novel mechanism for the control of clinical cancer: Inhibition of the production of adenosine triphosphate (ATP) with a standardized extract of paw paw" details the biochemical action of paw-paw extract, and patient histories from an informal and unpublished clinical trial of 94 terminal cancer patients.

Of the total of 94 patients enrolled in the study, 20 patients were treated personally by one of the researchers, Dr. James Forsythe of the Reno Cancer Screening and Treatment Center in Nevada. These 20 patients were given paw-paw extract (12.5 mg four times daily with meals), and 13/20 were still alive 18 months after starting treatment, with reduced tumor sizes and tumor markers, minimal side effects, and increased survival time. 10 case studies are described in detail in the report.[7]

Caution

Do not used pawpaw extract with substances which increase the production of cellular energy, such as alpha lipoic acid, coenzyme Q-10, thyroid stimulators such as iodine, creatine, nutritional algae like chlorella, anti-oxidants, etc. These products counteract the effects of the paw-paw. It is best to discontinue all vitamin and nutritional supplements while taking paw-paw.

AVOID VITAMIN C. Taking vitamin C along with paw-paw will cause treatment failure.

Because it only acts against cancer cells, pawpaw extract is not a preventative, and should only be consumed by cancer patients. Patients with Parkinson's Disease should also avoid paw-paw unless alkaloids have been removed from the extract. Pregnant women should not take paw-paw as it may damage the rapidly growing cells of the fetus.

Instructions

ALWAYS take with a full stomach to avoid serious gastric upset. Use the EXACT SAME TIME INTERVAL (down to the minute, if possible) between doses for maximum effect. Do NOT SKIP doses. This is very important as this substance works by slowly starving cancer cells, and any drug-free time window gives them a chance to re-accumulate ATP.

Most cancer patients are using Paw Paw in conjunction with conventional cancer treatments.

Paw-Paw Cell Reg contains 8.5 mg of standardized paw paw extract per capsule. Take 2 capsules with food three times daily.

Supplier

Paw-Paw Cell Reg, the recommended standardized extract developed by Dr. McLaughlin, is available at:

http://www.theherbsplace.com

http://www.healthy-sunshine.com/

Price: $39.95 for a month's supply. Most cancer patients need 2-3 months of treatment.

References

(1) McCage, CM; Ward, SM; Paling, CA; Fisher, DA; Flynn, PJ; McLaughlin, JL (2002). "Development of a paw paw herbal shampoo for the removal of head lice". Phytomedicine 9 (8): 743–8

(2) He, K., Zhao, G. X., Shi, G., Zeng, L., Chao, J. F., and McLaughlin, J. L. "Additional bioactive annonaceous acetogenins from Asimina triloba (Annonaceae)." Bioorg.Med.Chem. 1997;5(3):501-506.

(3) Alali, F. Q., Liu, X. X., and McLaughlin, J. L. "Annonaceous acetogenins: recent progress." J Nat Prod 1999;62(3):504-540.

(4) Kim EJ, Suh KM, Kim DH, et al. "Asimitrin and 4-hydroxytrilobin, new bioactive annonaceous acetogenins from the seeds of Asimina triloba possessing a bis-tetrahydrofuran ring." J Nat Prod 2005;68(2):194-197.

(5) McLaughlin, Jerry L. "Paw Paw and Cancer: Annonaceous Acetogenins from Discovery to Commercial Products". Journal of Natural Products 2008 71 (7): 1311–21

(6) Nicholas Oberlies, Ching-jer Chang, Jerry McLaughlin "Structure–Activity Relationships of Diverse Annonaceous Acetogenins against Multidrug Resistant Human Mammary Adenocarcinoma (MCF-7/Adr) Cells."J. Med. Chem., 1997, 40 (13), pp 2102–2106

(7) Jerry McLaughlin, Gina Benson, John Forsythe "A novel mechanism for the control of clinical cancer: Inhibition of the production of adenosine triphosphate (ATP) with a standardized extract of paw paw (Asimincz triloba, Annonaceae)." PDF article available online

Resveratrol & Grape Juice

These two inter-related subjects are placed together because resveratrol is one of the main therapeutic chemicals derived from grapes, though grapes contain other useful tumor-fighting compounds in addition to it.

Resveratrol is the first natural medicine to have solid evidence behind it showing that it blocks or stops many stages of cancer. Resveratrol not only prevents cancer, it functions as a treatment.

Here is some anecdotal evidence of the power of grape juice as it appears on the Internet.

She Did Not Give Up - Nor Should You

http://cancerhealingstory.blogspot.com

"When she was baptized Ursula Barbara Michael in 1907 at the Dorseyville Lutheran Evangelical Reformed Church, just over the hill from her farm, no one could have imagined that 92 years later she would be waging a winning battle with ovarian cancer.

She called it "God's Miracle". I overheard her gynecological oncologist tell a group of medical students, "Now I will show you *my miracle."* Please understand, I would never discount the power of God, or the abilities of this prominent doctor. But I want to introduce yet another possible factor…"

Due to acites (accumulation of fluid due to widespread ovarian cancer), this elderly woman's abdomen had expanded to the size of a full-term pregnancy. Her doctor suggested a low-dose chemotherapy regime, for palliative purposes only, of cisplatin at 20% of normal dose, given monthly, not weekly as it is usually administered.

Tests of tumor markers two months later showed the chemotherapy to be ineffective. However, her son refused to give up and found on the Internet information about resveratrol and its effect on cancer. Apparently, resveratrol potentiates the effect of chemotherapy. Long before resveratrol was identified by chemists, the Amish knew about its healing powers against cancer. "The Amish Cancer Cure," an old form of folk medicine, basically involved the consumption of large quantities of red grape juice, a concentrated source of resveratrol.

On her son's advice, this woman consumed a gallon and a half of Welch's Red Grape Juice the day before, the day of, and the day after her third session of chemotherapy.

Approximately one week after this, her abdomen suddenly became flat, and tests showed her tumor markers were down. Her doctor was amazed, and after 3 more sessions of low-dose chemotherapy and grape juice, CAT scans revealed no trace of her tumor.

Concord grape juice, and to a lesser extent red grape juice, is a concentrated source of polyphenols including resveratrol, a compound currently being promoted as an anti-aging supplement, general anti-oxidant and heart disease preventative. It should be noted that the skins and the seeds, rather than the translucent meat of the grape, is the most concentrated source of phytochemicals.

Constituents of grape juice include:

- Amygdalin, also called Laetrile or Vitamin B17 (seeds)
- beta-carotene
- catechin
- caffeic acid and/or ferulic acid
- ellagic acid
- gallic acid
- lutein
- lycopene
- pterostilbene
- pycnogenol, also called oligomeric proanthocyanidins (OPC) or procyanidolic oligomers (PCO), (seeds)
- quercetin
- resveratrol (skin coloring of purple grapes)
- selenium

These chemicals appear to have potent anti-tumor effect, without any of the cytotoxic effects of standard chemotherapy. This may have been the secret ingredient behind this story of a miraculous cure.

The Brandt Cancer Cure

This diet was popularized in the 1920s by Johanna Brandt, a South African immigrant to America. Related to the "Amish Cancer Cure," it involves 12-hour periods of water-only fasting followed by the ingestion of concord grape juice. Sugar is the main food of cancer cells, and the periods of fasting are intended to starve the cancer cells, so that they take up more of the sugary grape juice along its cancer-killing phytochemicals.

Use purified, **non-chlorinated** water only during the fasting periods. Do not use distilled water. It is important to use only **organic** concord grapes, as these fruits are heavily treated with pesticide if grown by conventional agriculture.

Resveratrol Induces Cell Death and Growth Inhibition in Ovarian Cancer Cells.

Ovarian cancer is notoriously resistant to conventional treatment and has an extremely high mortality rate. Resveratrol suppresses the growth of this form of tumor both in-vitro and in-vivo.[1]

Resveratrol appears to cause the death of ovarian cancer cells through autophagocytosis (self-digestion) rather than apoptosis, though some biochemical markers for apoptosis are also found. Treatment of A2780 ovarian cancer cells with resveratrol caused cell death within 24 hours. Cell cultures were observed over 72 hours of continuous treatment, during which time there was no further growth. To determine whether the cytotoxic response to resveratrol was unique to A2780 cells, researchers also tested four additional cell lines of ovarian cancer. Resveratrol induced cell death in each one.[2]

Resveratrol has been shown to best sensitize ovarian cancer cells to chemotherapy drugs when applied 2 hours before chemotherapy. Lesser effects are seen when resveratrol is administered concurrently with the chemo drug.[3]

Other Studies

Resveratrol induces apoptosis in tumor cells,[4] with or without the P53 tumor suppressor gene [5], or hormone receptors.[6,7] It can cause breast cancer cell death through apoptosis or necrosis, depending on the cell line.[7]

The body converts vitamin D3 to a steroid which inhibits the growth of breast cancer cells. Research at the University of Notre Dame found that resveratrol boosts this effect.[8]

Resveratrol enhances the effects of chemotherapy drugs. It increases the susceptability of drug-resistant non-Hodgkin's lymphoma cancer cells to chemotherapies such as cisplatinum, Gemcetabine, Navelbine, Paclitaxel, and TRIAL.[9]

An Austrian study found that resveratrol blocks by a factor of 30-71% the biochemical mechanism used by tumor cells to metastasize to bone. The greatest effects were seen in pancreas, breast, and kidney cancer. Tumors of the prostate and colon were affected to a lesser extent.[10]

The standard Western diet promotes cancer cell growth due to its high containment of a fat called linoleic acid. Linoleic acid is converted by the body to arachidonic acid, which in turn fuels the production of pro-inflammatory hormone-like substances (ie, leukotriene B4 and prostaglandin E2) that can promote tumor growth. The Western diet can induce colon cancer in rodents without the presence of any cofactor.[11]

A Japanese study found that resveratrol inhibited the growth of breast cancer cells, and blocked the tumor-promoting effects of linoleic acid derived from the Western diet.[12]

A 2012 study on the use of anti-oxidants as cancer therapy screened 4000 substances and found 22 active compounds. Resveratrol, genistein, and baicalein all stopped cell division in rapidly dividing cells without causing genetic mutations, a major drawback of conventional cancer therapy. In addition, resveratrol and genistein killed multidrug-resistant cancer cells. Researchers concluded, "We therefore propose that resveratrol, genistein, and baicalein are attractive candidates for improved chemotherapeutic agents."[13]

Resveratrol acts against a wide variety of tumor cells, including breast, leukemia, mouse papilloma,[14] and pancreatic cancer cells.[15]

Despite numerous in-vitro studies, curative doses for animal subjects inoculated with cancer have not been established, and results have been mixed, with some studies showing positive results,[16] while others showed no effect.[17] No human trials have been performed.

Caution

An animal study was performed on the effects of resveratrol on ischemic (hypoxic) heart damage due to 30 minutes of ischemia followed by 2 hours of re-perfusion. A hormetic effect was noted in the use of pure resveratrol by itself, but not of the supplement Longevinex, a formula of resveratrol combined with other antioxidants (quercetin and ferulic acid) and an iron chelator.

In the case of resveratrol alone, a low dose was found to be protective against cell damage, while high doses were found to be more toxic than no treatment at all. Longevinex showed no toxicity even at doses of 100 mg/kg, while the same dose of pure resveratrol was 100% toxic. In the use of resveratrol alone, 2.5 mg/kg improved survival, 25/mg/kg produced roughly the same survival as an untreated control group, while 100 mg/kg worsened cell damage.[18]

In rat studies, 300 mg/kg resveratrol daily (the equivalent of 21 grams daily in a 70 kg human) was found to be completely safe.[19]

A small Phase I human study found that a single dose of up to 5 grams of trans-resveratrol caused no serious negative effects in healthy test subjects.[20]

Instructions

No established dosage guidelines exist, but it has been suggested by some alternative health practitioners that at least 3-5 gm resveratrol per day are needed to achieve blood levels high enough to fight cancer.

Take it before, during and after chemotherapy to potentiate the effect of the chemo drugs.

If adding grape juice to the regime, be sure to use only **organic** grapes, and mix the whole grape, seeds and all, in a blender. Do not buy seedless grapes, as the seeds themselves contain bioactive compounds. Buy **dark purple concord** grapes, not white or red grapes.

Suppliers

Due to its many health benefits, resveratrol is widely consumed and widely available, with literally hundreds of brands for sale. However, brands vary widely in potency, with some containing hardly any of the active ingredient.

The substance occurs as two isomers, cis- and trans-resveratrol. Trans-resveratrol is the active component, and refined products containing only this substance may be cheaper per mg of active ingredient. Unrefined products contain a 50/50 mix. Unlike the unrefined form, which is brown and has a tannin-like taste, trans-resveratrol is a white, mild-tasting powder.

Purified (98-99%) trans-resveratrol powder is widely available on the internet and on Ebay. Bulk powder is the most economical.

The anti-aging supplement Longevinex is a more expensive, but clinically tested product, which combines resveratrol with other synergistic ingredients, antioxidants (quercetin and ferulic acid), an iron chelator (IP6), vitamin D, and nucleotides. $37 for 30 capsules:

http://www.longevinex.com/

References

(1) Mee-Hyun Lee, et al, "Resveratrol Suppresses Growth of Human Ovarian Cancer Cells in Culture and in a Murine Xenograft Model: Eukaryotic Elongation Factor 1A2 as a Potential Target." Cancer Res September 15, 2009 69; 7449

(2) Opipari AW, "Resveratrol-induced Autophagocytosis in Ovarian Cancer Cells.," Cancer Res January 15, 2004 64; 696

(3) Nessa MU, "Combinations of resveratrol, cisplatin and oxaliplatin applied to human ovarian cancer cells." Anticancer Res, 2012 Jan;32(1):53-9.

(4) Cal, C. et al. "Resveratrol and cancer: chemoprevention, apoptosis, and chemoimmunosensitizing activities." Curr. Med. Chem-Anti-Cancer Agents 2003;3:77-93

(5) Narayanan, B.A. et al. "Interactive gene expression pattern in prostate cancer cells exposed to phenolic antioxidants." Life Sci. 2002;70:1821-39

(6) Lu, R. et al. "Resveratrol, a natural product derived from grape, exhibits antiestrogenic activity and inhibits the growth of human breast cancer cells." J. Cell. Physiol. 1999;179:297-304

(7) Pozo-Guisado, E. et al. "The antiproliferative activity of resveratrol results in apoptosis in MCF-7 but not in MDA-MB-231 human breast cancer cells: cell-specific alteration of the cell cycle." Biochem. Pharmacol. 2002;64:1375-86

(8) Wietzke, J.A. et al. "Phytoestrogen regulation of a vitamin D3 receptor promoter and 1.25-dihydroxyvitamin D3 actions in human breast cancer cells." J. Steroid Biochem. Mol. Biol. 2003; 84:149-57

(9) Cal, C. et al. "Resveratrol and cancer: chemoprevention, apoptosis, and chemoimmunosensitizing activities." Curr. Med. Chem-Anti-Cancer Agents 2003;3:77-93

(10) Ulsperger, E. et al. "Resveratrol pretreatment desensitizes AHTO-7 human osteoblasts to growth stimulation in response to carcinoma cell supernatants." Int. J. Oncol. 1999;15:955-59

(11) Lipkin, M. et al. "Dietary factors in human colorectal cancer." Annu. Rev. Nutr. 1999;19:545-86.

(12) Nakagawa, H. et al. "Resveratrol inhibits human breast cancer cell growth and may mitigate the effect of linoleic acid, a potent breast cancer cell stimulator." J. Cancer Res. Clin. Oncol. 2001;127:258-64

(13) Fox JT et al., "High-throughput genotoxicity assay identifies antioxidants as inducers of DNA damage response and cell death." Proc Natl Acad Sci USA, 2012 Mar 19)

(14) Pervaiz, S. "Resveratrol–from the bottle to the bedside?" Leuk. Lymphoma 2001;40:491-8.

(15) Ding, X.Z. et al. "Resveratrol inhibits proliferation and induces apoptosis in human pancreatic cancer cells." Pancreas 2002;25:e71-e76.

(16) Kimura Y, Okuda H (June 2001). "Resveratrol isolated from Polygonum cuspidatum root prevents tumor growth and metastasis to lung and tumor-

induced neovascularization in Lewis lung carcinoma-bearing mice". J. Nutr. 131 (6): 1844–9

(17) Niles RM, Cook CP, Meadows GG, Fu YM, McLaughlin JL, Rankin GO (October 2006). "Resveratrol is rapidly metabolized in athymic (nu/nu) mice and does not inhibit human melanoma xenograft tumor growth." J. Nutr. 136 (10): 2542–6.

(18) Juhasz B et al. "Hormetic response of resveratrol against cardioprotection." Exp Clin Cardiol 2010 Winter;15(4):e134-8.
(18) James A Crowell, et al., "Resveratrol-Associated Renal Toxicity." Toxicol Sci. (2004) 82 (2): 614-619.

(19) Boocock DJ, Faust GE, Patel KR, Schinas AM, Brown VA, Ducharme MP, Booth TD, Crowell JA, Perloff M, Gescher AJ, Steward WP, Brenner DE (June 2007). "Phase I dose escalation

11. Other Cancer Cures

Immune System Boosters

Agaricus subrufescens/Agaricus blazei/ABM Mushroom

Agaricus subrufescens is a medicinal mushroom also known as almond mushroom, mushroom of life, mushroom of the sun, God's mushroom, royal sun agaricus, *jisongrong* or *himematsutake* (Japanese for "princess matsutake"). It has been incorrectly identified as *Agaricus blazei*, *Agaricus blazei* Murrill, *Agaricus brasiliensis* and *Agaricus rufotegulis*.

Like AHCC hybridized mushrooms, it is an immune system stimulator. The active ingredients are alpha and beta glucans. Researched compounds derived from *Agaricus subrufescens* include blazeispirol A, LMPAB, ABM-FD, and ABPC.

This mushroom was first described in 1893 by American botanist Charles Horton Peck. During the late 19th and early 20th century, it was cultivated as a food item in the eastern US. It was rediscovered again in Brazil in the 1970s, where it was misidentified as a related species Agaricus blazei Murrill which is native to Florida, and marketed as a health product under this name. People who ate the mushroom in Brazil were noted for their long life and a relative lack of cancer, high blood pressure, diabetes, hepatitis, Alzheimer's disease and arthritis.

This mushroom has also been found growing in Hawaii, California, Holland, Great Britain, Taiwan, the Philippines and Brazil.

Within the last decade it has been reclassified and renamed. However, despite the various names under which it has been sold and studied, it is the same identical mushroom.

It has been reported that as much as 300,000 kg of dehydrated *Agaricus subrufescens* are produced annually in Japan. These extracts have been used by up to 500,000 people for anticancer activity.

Recently, Watanabe and collegues published a report in the *Biological and Pharmaceutical Bulletin* about the antioxidant activity of a new hybrid of *A. subrufescens* called *Basidiomycetes-X* (BDM-X). A US patent was issued on a hybrid of Agaricus with another medicinal mushroom, resulting in a new hybrid claimed to exhibit 10 to 3000 times the potency of similar but unpatented mushrooms.[1]

Studies

There are hundreds of studies about the medicinal properties of this mushroom. Only a few are presented here.

Agaricus stimulates the production of active immune cells in the bone marrow. Cytokines are activated which stimulate production of interferon and other molecules that enhance the immune system. Tumor necrosis factor (TNF), which can destroy certain tumor cells, is released and white blood cells that attack cancer cells are activated. There is evidence from some studies that the extract can cause apoptosis of tumor cells directly. Agaricus also shows antioxidant activity.

In animal studies, Agaricus cures both implanted tumors as well as tumors induced by carcinogenic toxins.

Treatment of tumors grafted onto mice with Agaricus extract caused infiltration of the tumor and its distant metastasis by Natural Killer (NK) cells in-vivo, and also directly caused apoptosis in tumor cells in-vitro. Normal cells were unaffected.[2]

Reserachers found no direct anti-tumor activity of Agaricus extract in-vitro, but did see a strong anti-tumor action in-vivo, leading them to conclude that the extract's effect was due to activation of the immune system.[3]

Researchers used sarcoma grafts in mice to investigate the antitumor properties of LMPAB, a component of Agaricus. They found tumor growth inhibition of 33.0% after administration of LMPAB at 200 mg/kg/day for 2 weeks. Angiogenesis was also suppressed.[4]

Agaricus extract also causes tumor cell apoptosis directly by caspase 3 activation and reduces telomerase activity, possibly through regulation of Akt signaling.[5,6]

One hundred cervical, ovarian, and endometrial cancer patients being treated with standard chemotherapies were given oral supplements of Agaricus extract, and compared with a placebo group. In the group given the mushroom extract, natural killer cell activity was increased significantly, and chemotherapy-associated side effects such as anorexia, alopecia, emotional stability, and general weakness were all improved. Researchers concluded, "this suggests that ABMK treatment might be beneficial for gynecological cancer patients undergoing chemotherapy."[7]

Ten patients with acute non-lymphocytic leukemia (ANLL) were treated with chemotherapy and Agaricus extract. The extract increased bone marrow hemopoiesis (production of blood cells), enhanced the effect of chemotherapy, and significantly increased the levels of hemoglobin, white blood cells and platelets in peripheral blood. It also increased the concentration of lgM (a component of the immune system), albumin and A/G ratio and decreased the concentration of globulin in plasma. Researchers concluded that Agaricus Blazei promoted immune system functioning and had an inhibitory effect on leukemia cells.[8]

Agaricus vs. Other Fungal Products

Around the time Agaricus was introduced to Japan, Dr. Shoji Shibata, a professor in the Pharmacological Department of Tokyo University, and Dr. Tetuo Ikegawa of the National Cancer Center, jointly researched the medicinal properties of Agaricus. Their findings were presented at the general convention of the Japan Pharmacological Association and the Japan Cancer Association.

In a study performed by the Medical Department of Tokyo University, The National Cancer Center Laboratory and the Tokyo College of Pharmacy, Agaricus Blazei Murill was found to be the greatest anticancer activity of 5 well-known fungal cancer treatments. The rate of complete regression within test animals was as high as 90%, and 99.4% of test subjects experienced some anti-tumor effect. In other words, only 0.6% of test animals experienced no anti-cancer benefits whatsoever.

A line of tumor cells, Sarcoma 180, was injected in guinea pigs. Without treatment, this causes test animals to die of cancer within 4-5 weeks. Agaricus mushroom activated the immune systems of the test animals, and when cancer invaded normal tissue, it was eliminated through macrophage and interferon production. Agaricus also prevented the growth, metastasis and re-occurrence of cancer.

A dose of only 10 mg/kg of Agaricus was used, compared to 30 mg/kg of other fungi. Popular medicinal mushrooms produced the following results:
Agaricus Blazei Murill 90.0% (complete recovery) / 99.4% (partial response), Shiitake 54.5% / 80.7%, Coriolus Versicor 50.0% / 77.5%, Tree Oyster Mushroom 45.5% / 75.3% and Reishi (Ganoderma Lucidum) only 20.0% / 77.8%.

The only other fungus that produced comparable results was Grifola umbellate, not commonly available as a medicinal mushroom supplement in the U.S. or Canada.

Interestingly enough, Agaricus Blazei's complete remission rate compared to Coriolus Versicolor (on which Japan's PSK cancer drug is based) was dramatically better, 90% compared to 50%. Reishi, the most widely marketed mushroom in North America, produced only a 20% complete recovery rate.

Another comparative test was performed with 13 popular fungal therapies, using mouse test subjects implanted with Sarcoma-180 tumor cells. Trametes versicolor topped the list, with a 100% response rate. Agaricus came a close second. Administration of Agaricus polysaccharide at 10 mg/kg produced a complete remission in 87.5% of the test subjects and partial response in 93.6%.

This study was presented by professors Hitoshi Ito, Keishiro Shimura and Sensuke Naruse of the Mie University medical school at the the 39th General Meeting of the Japanese Cancer Academy in 1980.

Since the presentation, clinical reports from various hospitals and researchers claim that ABM mushroom is effective against cancer of the breast, colon, liver, lung, and ovary, as well as Ehrlich's ascites carcinoma.

Caution

Until 2006, no side effects due to ABM had been reported in Japan, where it has been in wide use since the mid 1990s. However, a recent report links ABM to liver failure in 3 cancer patients. 2 of the 3 died of acute hepatitis several days after commencing the supplement, and the third patient recovered after ceasing to consume ABM. As soon as that patient restarted the mushroom extract, liver function began to deteriorate again.[9]

It is unclear whether this problem may potentially occur with all ABM supplements, or if it is linked to the particular brand of supplement these patients were using (marketed as "Himematsutake" in Japan). Also, the patients had been using chemotherapy and other medications which weaken the liver.

A well-known alternative practitioner, Dr. Ray Sahelian, recommends limiting consumption of agaricus to a maximum of 3 times weekly, with a week off each month.

Instructions

It is recommended to buy whole mushrooms rather than powder, as powder may be adulterated, and is more prone to oxidization.

Daily dose for normal health maintenance is about 6 grams (about ¼ of a dry mushroom) or 40 grams (aprox. 2 mushrooms) for serious illness. Tea is also a popular way of consuming the mushroom. Use about 1 mushroom per liter (1 quart) and boil it for an hour. Drink one cup a day.

Vitamin C is said to boost the beneficial properties of the mushroom.

Suppliers

http://www.iherb.com

References

(1) US patient 6120772, Ito, Hitoshi; Sumiya, Toshimitsu, "Oral drugs for treating AIDS patients." issued 19 September 2000

(2) Fujimiya Y, Suzuki Y, Oshiman K, Kobori H, Moriguchi K, Nakashima H, Matumoto Y, Takahara S, Ebina T, Katakura R (May 1998). "Selective tumoricidal effect of soluble proteoglucan extracted from the basidiomycete, Agaricus blazei Murill, mediated via natural killer cell activation and apoptosis." Cancer Immunol Immunother (Springer Verlag) 46 (3): 147–159.

(3) Gonzaga ML, Bezerra DP, Alves AP, et al. (January 2009). "In vivo growth-inhibition of Sarcoma 180 by an alpha-(1-->4)-glucan-beta-(1-->6)-glucan-protein complex polysaccharide obtained from Agaricus blazei Murill." Nat Med (Tokyo) 63 (1): 32–40.

(4) Niu YC, Liu JC, Zhao XM, Wu XX (January 2009). "A low molecular weight polysaccharide isolated from Agaricus blazei suppresses tumor growth and angiogenesis in vivo." Oncol. Rep. 21 (1): 145–52.

(5) Gao L, Sun Y, Chen C, et al. "Primary mechanism of apoptosis induction in a leukemia cell line by fraction FA-2-b-ss prepared from the mushroom Agaricus blazei Murill." Braz J Med Biol Res. Nov 2007; 40(11):1545-1555.

(6) Jin CY, Moon DO, Choi YH, et al."Bcl-2 and caspase-3 are major regulator in Agaricus blazei-induced human leukemic U937 cell apoptosis through dephosphorylation of Akt." Biol Pharm Bull. Aug 2007; 30(8):1432-1437.

(7) Ahn WS, Kim DJ, Chae GT, Lee JM, Bae SM, Sin JI, Kim YW, Namkoong SE, Lee IP (July–August 2004). "Natural killer cell activity and quality of life were improved by consumption of a mushroom extract, Agaricus blazei Murill Kyowa, in gynecological cancer patients undergoing chemotherapy." Int J Gynecol Cancer 14 (4): 589–94.

(8) Tian, X., et al.; (1994). "Clinical Observation on Treatment of Acute Non Lymphocytic Leukemia with Agaricus Blazei Murrill.", Journal of Lanzhou University (Medical Sciences) 1994 20: 169–171.

(9) Mukai H, Watanabe T, Ando M, Katsumata N. Division of Oncology/Hematology, National Cancer Center Hospital East, 6-5-1, Kashiwanoha, Kashiwa-shi, Chiba, Japan. "An Alternative Medicine, Agaricus blazei, May Have Induced Severe Hepatic Dysfunction in Cancer Patients." Japan J Clinical Oncology. 2006 Dec;36(12):808-10.

Antrodia Camphorata

Antrodia camphorata, known in China as Niu-Chang, has been used in traditional Chinese medicine for many years. Aside from its use as a cancer treatment, it is also used to treat itching, allergies, and as a liver protectant. It is relatively unknown outside of Taiwan. It has immunosupportive and antioxidant effects and is directly cytotoxic to tumors.

Claims have been made that the mushroom is becoming increasingly more difficult to obtain due to deforestation, as much of it is wild-harvested. Attempts are being made to increase cultivated supplies.

Antrodia contains more than 78 bioactive compounds consisting of benzenoids, benzoquinones, lignans, terpenoids, succinic and maleic derivatives, and polysaccharides.

Terpenoids, which have also been found in a small number of other mushrooms make up approximately half of the chemicals isolated. Triterpenoids with ketonic functional groups have potent cytotoxic activity against a number of cancer cell lines.

Polysaccharides from Antrodia are a variety of monosaccharides, galactose, glucose, mannose, glucosamine and galactosamine. The mushroom also contains β-D-glucans (β-(1→3)-D-glucopyranans and β-(1→6)-D-glucosyl branches).

Antrodia is usually used alongside conventional chemotherapy.[1]

Studies

Antrodia camphorata caused apoptosis in estrogen non-responsive human breast cancer cells (cell line MDA-MB-231) both in-vitro and inoculated into mice. The mushroom extract decreased the proliferation of tumor cells by arresting progression through the G1 mitotic (reproductive) phase of the cell cycle. Also, development of tumors was delayed and size of tumors was reduced.[2]

Similar anti-tumor results have been obtained from studies using colon, liver, lung and prostate cancer cells.

Cancer was inhibited in a dose-dependent manner, that is, higher doses had more effect than low doses.

Interactions between different components of Antrodia produce a synergistic effect, making the whole mushroom more effective than its isolated compounds against tumor cells.

Anti-inflammatory, anti-viral, antioxidant, hepatoprotective, neuroprotective and antihypertensive activity was also noted.[3]

Antrodia also showed in-vitro activity against ovarian cancer cells.[4]

Instructions

Antrodia Camphorata Polysaccharide Capsules usually contain 500 mg.

Take 2 capsules once daily with warm boiled water on an empty stomach, no alcohol.

Suppliers

Antrodia is said to be the world's most expensive medicinal mushroom.

Sold by Asian suppliers for approximately $700.00 for ½ pound. Vitalsail Antrodia Camphorata is grown using a proprietary, patented technology by Well Shine Biotech that results in a cultivated mushroom that is 99.97% chemically identical to natural specimens growing in the wild (in triterpenoids pattern, polysaccharides, phenyl and biophenyl compounds).

http://www.myasianstore.com/products/

Also sold as "Ruby Mushroom" by Simpson Biotech.

http://simpsonbioteche.so-buy.com

References

(1) Madamanchi Geethangili and Yew-Min Tzeng, "Review of Pharmacological Effects of Antrodia camphorata and Its Bioactive Compounds." Evidence-Based Complementary and Alternative Medicine, Volume 2011 (2011), Article ID 212641.

(2) Hseu YC, Chen SC, Chen HC, Liao JW, Yang HL. "Antrodia camphorata inhibits proliferation of human breast cancer cells in vitro and in vivo." Food Chem. Toxicol, August 2008.

(3) Madamanchi Geethangili and Yew-Min Tzeng, "Review of Pharmacological Effects of Antrodia camphorata and Its Bioactive Compounds." Evidence-Based Complementary and Alternative Medicine, Volume 2011 (2011), Article ID 212641.

(4) Liu F.S. "Antrodia camphorata induces apoptosis and enhances the cytotoxic effect of paclitaxel in human ovarian cancer cells." Int J Gynecol Cancer, 2011 Oct;21(7):1172-9

Beta 1,3D Glucan

Beta-glucans are polysaccharides (sugar compounds) of D-glucose connected by beta-glycosidic bonds. Different beta-glucans are described by a pair of numbers that indicate which carbons in each of the glucose units form the link.

There are many different molecules within this chemical group that vary with respect to viscosity, solubility, molecular mass, and three-dimensional structure. They occur most commonly as cellulose in plants, the bran layer of grains, yeast cell walls, and they are also found in some mushrooms (reishi, shiitake and maitake), fungi and bacteria.

Beta-glucans derived from yeast and mushrooms are known to boost the immune system. The fiber-like, insoluble (1,3/1,6) beta-glucan has more of a biological effect than the soluble (1,3/1,4) beta-glucans.

Beta(1,3)D-glucan supplements are often derived from the cell wall of baker's yeast (Saccharomyces cerevisiae). These are more effective than the beta-glucans derived from mushrooms or cereal grains.

Beta-glucan has been used to control cholesterol levels as well as boost the immune system. It has been studied as an aid to allow the immune system to fight infection as well as cancer.

Beta-glucans are known as "biological response modifiers" due to their activation of the immune system. A receptor on the surface of neutrophils called the Complement Receptor 3 (CR3) binds to the beta-glucans. This causes activation of the neutrophils, which then attack cancer cells or infectious agents. Neutrophils comprise 50-60% of the body's immune system cells, along with Natural Killer (NK) cells, lymphocytes and macrophages.

In Japan, beta-glucan is an officially-recognized immunostimulant for cancer treatment. It is considered a primary treatment for cancer throughout Asia. Beta-glucans can help reverse immunosuppression resulting from radiation and chemotherapy.

One of the first clinical experiments with beta glucan was performed in 1975 by Dr. Peter Mansell of the National Cancer Institute. He injected beta glucan into subcutaneous nodules of malignant melanoma and noted with satisfaction that they were "strikingly reduced in as short a period as five days" and in some instances "resolution was complete"[1]

A 1986 Japanese study showed increased survival times for patients with advanced gastric or colorectal cancer who were given beta-1,3 glucans derived from shiitake mushrooms, along with chemotherapy.[2]

Both animal and human studies show beta-glucan boosts the action of the immune system against infectious agents as well as cancer. Administration of beta-glucan decreases post-operative infections in high-risk colorectal surgery by 39%.[3]

An animal study by the Canadian Department of Defence using mice exposed to Anthrax found that beta-glucans increased survival with or without addition of antibiotics. 80-90% of mice treated with beta-glucan survived after 10 days of exposure to B. anthracis, compared with 30% of the untreated control group. Mice treated with antibiotics alone did not survive.[4]

Due to activation of macrophages, beta-glucan also helps wound healing and increases tensile strength of scars. It is a helpful product to aid in recovery from cancer surgery.

Beta-glucan is widely available on the Web, but quality and strength varies greatly. The milligram dose and the percentage of active linkages are two separate variables.

In 2007, the *Journal of American Nutraceuticals Association* published an evaluation of commercially available Beta 1, 3 Glucans. Due to differences in purity, commercially available brands tested contained 18-88% chemically active linkages, with the majority containing 70% or less. This would produce a wide range of biological activity, with some brands being completely ineffective.

Some of the least effective brands tested came from large, well-known vitamin manufacturers. Beta glucan #300 by Southeastern Pharmaceutical was shown to be the best product evaluated.[5,6]
http://www.ana-jana.org/Journal/

Instructions/Suppliers

Beta glucan #300 by Southeastern Pharmaceutical has been shown to be effective by independent testing, and due to the wide variation between beta-glucan products, we recommend this brand. The dose suggested by the manufacturer is 2 1000mg capsules daily.

http://www.beta-glucan.com/

References

(1) Mansell PW, Ichinose H, Reed RJ, et al., "Macrophage-mediated destruction of human malignant cells in vivo." J Natl Cancer Inst. 1975 Mar; 54(3): 571-80).

(2) Wakui A., "Randomized study of lentinan on patients with advanced gastric and colorectal cancer. Tohoku Lentinan Study Group." Gan To Kagaku Ryoho 1986 Apr;13(4 Pt 1):1050-9.)

(3) Dellinger EP, et al., "Effect of PGG-glucan on the rate of serious postoperative infection or death observed after high-risk gastrointestinal operations. Betafectin Gastrointestinal Study Group." Arch Surg 1999 Sep;134(9):977-83.

(4) Vetvicka, V; Terayama K, Mandeville R, Brousseau P, Kournikakis B, Ostroff G (2002). "Pilot Study: Orally-Administered Yeast β1,3-glucan Prophylactically Protects Against Anthrax Infection and Cancer in Mice." (PDF). Journal of the American Nutraceutical Association (Birmingham, AL : The Association) 5 (2): 5–9.

(5) Dr. Vaclav Vetvicka, "An Evaluation of the Immunological Activities of Commercially Available Beta 1, 3 Glucans." JANA Vol 10, No 1, 2007

(6) Dr. Vaclav Vetvicka, Jana Vetvickova, "A Comparison of Injected and Orally Administered ß-glucans." JANA Vol 11, No 1, 2008

Biobran MGN-3, BRM4, Noxylane4

This product is an immune system stimulator derived from rice bran. Enzymes of the shiitake mushroom break down rice bran into a variety of bioactive substances which are fractionated and concentrated. The product itself does not contain mushroom extract, the enzymes are removed from the final product, so it can be safely taken by those with mushroom allergies.

Active compounds include arabinoxylan, a short-chain polysaccharide as well as other hemicelluloses and polysaccharides.

History of Biobran

AHCC, mentioned previously, was a predecessor to Biobran MGN-3, and both products were developed by the same Japanese researcher, Hiroaki Maeda.

Biobran was developed in 1992. Maeda was director of research and development of Daiwa Pharmaceutical in Tokyo, a phytonutrient manufacturing company directed by Yasuo Nonomiya. Maeda later tested the product with Mamdooh Ghoneum PhD, professor of immunology at the Charles Drew University of Medicine and Science in Los Angeles. The product is named after the three main developers (Maeda-Ghoneum-Ninomiya), with the '3' symbolizing the fact that it is a third generation product.

However, AHCC is marketed by a different company than BioBran, which was distributed by Lane Labs until the FDA stopped them from selling the product in 2004 due to medical claims. Biobran MGN-3 was subsequently renamed and reintroduced to the market under the name BRM4. It is manufactured in Japan by Daiwa Pharmaceuticals, the same company which made the original MGN-3, and the product has the exact same active ingredients. The company also sells a new product, Noxylane4, which has the added component HAI (heated algal ingredient), a patented amino acid derived from sea algae, which improves absorption.

Maeda and Ghoneum claim that their product is a better immune system modulator than AHCC. It increases the number and activity of NK-cells, T-cells, B-cells and other components of the immune system. Biobran also significantly increases the quality of life of patients undergoing conventional cancer treatment.

Dr. Ghoneum stated, "I have been researching immunomodulators for over 30 years now and Biobran is the most powerful immunomodulator that I have ever tested."

Studies

Multiple studies by Dr. Ghoneum and independent researchers are listed on the company website:

http://www.biobran.org/

According to the studies listed, MGN-3 is indeed a better activator of NK cells, lymphocytes and T-cells than AHCC or other popular supplements containing arabinoxylan. This is true even when low doses of MGN-3 are compared to high doses of AHCC. MGN-3 increases cytokine production, and one of Ghoneum's studies shows it can even affect levels of Tumor Necrosis Factor.

The research includes human studies, not just in-vitro and animal tests. In a human study of 24 subjects who were given various doses of MGN-3, lytic activity of NK cells from peripheral blood increased up to 310% over baseline after 1 week of treatment with MGN-3. Lower doses showed a slower response, but after 2 months of treatment, all doses cause an increase in NK lytic activity of approximately 500%. After 2 months of treatment, NK cells killed 2700% more cancer cells than untreated NK cells.[1]

Other tests have shown an increase in the activity of B-cells by 250% or greater, and increases in T-cell activity by 200%.

MGN-3 enhanced antibody-induced apoptosis of human T cell leukemia cells. [2]

Instructions

Take 2 capsules 3 times daily for 3 weeks. After 3 weeks, reduce dosage to the maintenance level of 2 capsules daily. For best results, take MGN-3 two hours after taking other supplements.

Suppliers

50 capsules of 500mg $130.

http://www.feelgoodnatural.com/

It is known to be a more expensive product than AHCC. However, it may be more effective.

References

(1) M. Ghoneum, "Enhancement of Human Natural Killer Activity By Modified Arabinoxylan From Rice Bran (MGN-3)." Int J. Immunotherapy XIV (2), 89-99, 1998

(2) (2Ghoneum M, "Modified arabinoxylan rice bran (MGN-3/Biobran) sensitizes human T cell leukemia cells to death receptor (CD95)-induced apoptosis." Cancer Letters, vol 201, Issue 1, Pages 41-49, 10 November 2003

Hybridized Mushroom Extract

Discovered in 1989, hybridized mushroom extract (AHCC) is used widely in hospitals throughout Japan and China as an adjunctive therapy for cancer, hepatitis, HIV/AIDs and other diseases involving immunodeficiency. It was developed by Dr. Toshiko Okamoto of the Faculty of Pharmaceutical Sciences, Tokyo University, for Amino Up Chemical Co., Ltd. Other researchers involved in the development of AHCC were Hiroaki Maeda and Mamdooh Ghoneum PhD, who later developed Biobran MGN-3, another immune system modulator.

Since 1994, over 300 medical researchers and physicians have gathered in Sapporo, Japan for the annual **AHCC Research Association** symposiums.

In Japanese hospitals, it is used as a standard preventative regimen for all incoming patients to decrease the risk of hospital-acquired infections. AHCC is also administered to protect the immune system of cancer patients undergoing radiation and chemotherapy. AHCC has been shown in multiple studies to lead to increased longevity, improved quality of life and fewer side effects from conventional cancer therapy. AHCC is compatible with chemo and radiotherapy.

The hybrid is derived from several mushrooms including Shiitake (*Lentinula edodes*), Maitake (*Grifola frondosa*), Reishi (*Ganoderma Lucidum*) , Kawaratake (*Coriolus versicolor*), and Suehirotake mushrooms *(Schizophyllum commune)*, all of which have a long history of medicinal use in Japan. The extract is called AHCC (activated hexose correlate compound), and it is sold in America by BioSciences corporation under the brand name ImmPower.

The proprietary hybrid is grown under laboratory conditions in a liquid medium based on rice bran, rather than in the soil or wood growth medium in which these fungi grow naturally. After being harvested, the mushrooms are enzymatically modified through fermentation. This breaks down the large polysaccharides normally found in medicinal mushrooms, which have a size range of around 100,000 daltons, to a smaller, more bioactive and easily absorbed size of 5,000 daltons. The active component is an oligosaccharide with an alpha, 1- 4 glucan structure.

The alpha-glucan component of AHCC has a mechanism of action similar to that of the beta-glucans mentioned previously. It combats cancer by boosting the immune system.

AHCC stimulates cytokine (IL-2, IL-12, TNF, and INF) production, which increases immune function. It increases NK cell activity up to 300%. It increases the formation of cytotoxic granules within NK cells. The more ammunition each NK cell carries, the more cancer cells or pathogens it can destroy. It increases the number and the activity of lymphocytes, specifically increasing T-cells up to 200 percent. It increases Interferon levels, which stimulates NK cell activity and inhibits the replication of viruses. It increases Tumor Necrosis Factor, which causes apoptosis in cancer cells.

Studies

A 1995 clinical trial showed that ingestion of 3 grams per day of AHCC significantly lowered the level of tumor markers in patients with various types of cancer. 3 ovarian, 3 prostate, 3 breast cancer and 2 multiple myeloma patients had their tumor associated antigen (TAA) markers measured before, during and after taking AHCC. Levels of CA 125 decreased significantly in 2 of the 3 ovarian cancers. All prostate cancers showed significant decreases. 1 of 3 breast cancers showed a reduction of CA 15-3. 1 of 2 myelomas showed a large reduction of BJP, and the other showed a slight decrease.[1]

Researchers at Kansai Medical University in Japan found that AHCC caused a significant increase in postoperative life span in patients who underwent surgery for liver cancer. The study compared the post-operative outcomes of 113 patients taking AHCC with 156 patients who did not take the extract. Rate of tumor recurrence in the two groups was 34% vs. 66% resepectively, and patient survival was 80% vs. 52%.[2]

The Kansai research team also performed a 3-year study of 127 patients with stage III and IV stomach and breast cancers and found that patients taking AHCC showed a 40% increase in mean survival rates compared to a demographically-matched sample of patients of similar age and cancer type.

Animal and human studies have shown that AHCC improves the function of the immune system by increasing the production of cytokines, increasing the activity of natural killer cells by as much as 300-800%, increasing populations of macrophages and T-cells by up to 200%, and increasing the number of dendritic cells.

A study of 17 patients with cancer of the breast, lung, ovary, prostate, and stomach, and myeloma and rhabdomyosarcoma were given 3 gm/day AHCC for 2-6 months. Natural Killer cell binding to tumor target cells was found to be enhanced after 2 weeks of treatment (2-3 fold) and after 1-2 months it was found to be enhanced 2-10 fold. Researchers concluded, "AHCC is a potent immunomodulator and may be useful in immunotherapy of cancer."[3]

Animal studies show that AHCC reduces toxicity and mortality due to toxic chemotherapy. It prevents hair loss and liver toxicity due to chemotherapy.[4]

In another study, researchers dosed healthy mice with several common chemotherapy drugs: paclitaxel, multi-drug chemotherapy with paclitaxel plus cisplatin, 5-fluorouracil (5FU) plus irinotecan, cisplatin plus 5FU, or doxorubicin plus cyclophosphamide. Bone marrow suppression, kidney and liver toxicity, and mortality due to chemotherapy was greatly reduced by AHCC supplements. Researchers concluded, "AHCC can be beneficial for cancer patients receiving chemotherapy."[5]

Instructions

The usual dose given to patients in studies was 3 grams per day.

Suppliers

While there are multiple brands of AHCC for sale, most AHCC products on the market come from common suppliers and then are private labeled.

References

(1) Ghoneum M., Wimbley M., Salem F., McKlain A., Attallah N., Gill G., "Immunomodulatory and AntiCancer Effects of Active HemiCellulose Compound (AHCC)." International Journal of Immunotherapy XI 1995; (1) 23-28.)

(2) 2Matsui Y. et al.;"Improved prognosis of postoperative hepatocellular carcinoma patients when treated with functional foods: a prospective cohort study." J Hepatol, 37, 1:78-86, 2002

(3) Mamdooh Ghoneum, "NK Immunomodulation in 17 Cancer Patients." Paper presented at the 2nd meeting of the Soc. Natural Immunity-Taormina, Italy.

(4) Sun B. et al.; "The effect of active hexose correlated compound in modulating cytosine arabinoside-induced hair loss, and 6-mercaptopurine- and methotrexate-induced liver injury in rodents." Cancer Epidemiology 2009 Oct;33(3-4):293-9

(5) Shigama K. et al.; "Alleviating effect of active hexose correlated compound for anticancer drug-induced side effects in non-tumor-bearing mice."J Exp Ther Oncol 2009; 8(1):43-51

Trametes Versicolor

This multicolored mushroom is also known as *Coriolus versicolor* and *Polyporus versicolor*, and popularly called Turkey Tail due to its resemblance to the tail of the wild turkey. In China it is known as the medicinal mushroom *yun zhi*. It is a common polyphore mushroom which grows throughout the northern forests of the world. In Japan and China it has been widely used for more than 30 years as an adjuvent treatment for cancer. In Japan, it is covered by government health insurance as a standard medication.

Its active ingredient is Polysaccharide-K (PSK), also known as PSP (polysaccharopeptide), marketed as the drug Krestin. It is a protein-bound polysaccharide which boosts the immune system, especially T-helper cells. It also has antioxidant activity.

PSK reduces implanted tumors as well as those induced by radiation and mutagens.[1]

One large study on trametes versicolor involved 8 randomized clinical trials with a total of 8009 patients who had undergone curative surgery for gastric cancer. Patients were randomly assigned chemotherapy alone or chemotherapy with mushroom extract. Patients treated with mushroom extract showed an overall 12% improvement in survival. Researchers concluded, "The results of this meta-analysis suggest that adjuvant immunochemotherapy with PSK improves the survival of patients after curative gastric cancer resection."[2]

PSK has shown to be a useful adjunct in treating breast, colorectal, gastric, and lung cancers. It inhibits cancer by a variety of biochemical mechanisms, from stimulation of the immune system to the induction of differentiation-promoting cytokines.[3]

In his book "Mycelium Running," medicinal mushroom expert Paul Stamets notes special effectiveness of Turkey Tail extract in treating uterine cancer.

Instructions

The usual dose is 2 to 3 grams of dried, powdered turkey tail mushrooms three times daily.

Extracts of Turkey Tail containing higher concentrations of what is purported to be the active ingredient, PSK, also exist, but these exclude other potentially beneficial compounds which may act synergistically. These extracts are taken in the same dose as the whole mushroom. The extracts also cost much more than unrefined mushroom powder, which has been used successfully in Oriental medicine for thousands of years.

Suppliers

http://www.iherb.com

References

(1) Kobayashi H., et al.; "Antimetastatic effects of PSK (Krestin), a protein-bound polysaccharide obtained from basidiomycetes: an overview." Cancer Epidemiol. Biomarkers Prev. 4 (3): 275–81. 1995

(2) Oba K, Teramukai S, Kobayashi M, Matsui T, Kodera Y, Sakamoto J (June 2007), "Efficacy of adjuvant immunochemotherapy with polysaccharide K for patients with curative resections of gastric cancer." Cancer Immunol. Immunother. 56 (6): 905–11

(3) Fisher, M. Y. (May 2002). "Anticancer effects and mechanisms of polysaccharide-K (PSK): implications of cancer immunotherapy." Anticancer research, 22 (3): 1737–1754

Natural Products – Single Ingredient

Aloe Vera

The Aloe vera plant has been used for millenia to heal wounds and illnesses of various kinds, and new studies have shown that this plant also helps fight cancer. It is particularly effective as an adjunct to chemotherapy and radiation by boosting the immune system and preventing damage to healthy tissues caused by conventional cancer treatment.

The FDA has approved the use of Aloe vera derivatives for some veterinary purposes, but it has not approved these same substances for use in fighting human cancer. Substances from the Aloe vera plant are being used in Europe and other parts of the world to fight cancer and are showing great success.

In the United States, one alternative practitioner using Aloe Vera to treat cancer was shut down by the FDA in 2001 due to complaints from local oncologists who were losing business.

The clinic in Tampa, Florida, was run by Ivan Danhof, MD, Ph.D., who had developed a particulary effective Aloe Vera extract called Albarin. Ironically, Dr. Danhof was going through the bureaucratic process at the time to obtain IND (investigational new drug) status for the medication. His Aloe Vera extract was being administered intravenously to 100 terminal cancer patients assigned to hospice care. Dr. Danhof claimed that 94 of them survived with no side effects from Albarin, and the overall recovery rate was 80%.

The FDA raid ended the clinical trial before results could be compiled and submitted for government approval. After the raid, all the patients were denied access to further treatments. Albarin is no longer available, but another product, Serovera, claims to be made under the supervision of Dr. Danhof. However, it is for oral consumption, not IV use.

How Aloe Works

Aloe Vera has multiple therapeutic uses, yet most people only know about the topical applications of Aloe Vera gel for sunburns. In reality, Aloe vera is useful for both external and internal applications. Its internal gel matrix is comprised of a multitude of different phytochemicals with amazing medicinal benefits.

The Aloe Vera plant contains at least 6 antiseptic agents: salicylic acid, lupeol, urea nitrogen, phenols, cinnamonic acid, and sulphur.

All of these substances kill or inhibit bacteria, mold, fungus, and viruses, which is why the plant is effective against many internal and external infections. Lupeol and salicylic acid are also analgesics, or pain-killers.

Aloe Vera contains antioxidants, enzymes, vitamins, minerals, and anti-inflammatory fatty acids such as campersterol and B-sitosterol (plant sterols), which is why it is an effective treatment for trauma and inflammatory conditions. It can be used to treat cuts, burns, abrasions, allergic reactions, rheumatic fever, rheumatoid arthritis, acid indigestion, ulcers, inflammatory conditions of the digestive system and other internal organs. B-sitosterol also lowers cholesterol levels, offering benefits for heart patients.

Aloe contains at least 23 polypeptids which are immune system stimulators, making Aloe juice useful in immune system disorders and infections, including HIV/AIDS. The polypeptids, plus the anti-tumor agents Aloe emodin and Aloe lectins, explains its ability to control cancer.

Aloe Vera enhances the effect of vitamin C, vitamin E and other antioxidants. It is said to improve the ability of blood to transport oxygen and nutrients to the body's cells. It is a widely held belief among herbalists that Aloe vera makes nutritional substances more effective due to its blood-enhancing effects. If this is correct, it means Aloe can influence other anti-cancer treatments, too, helping them more effectively target tumours. Aloe vera acts as a natural drug-delivery system, and unlike artificial chemicals, it is entirely compatible with the human body.

Worldwide, hundreds of studies have proven the anti-inflammatory, anti-bacterial, and anti-viral actions of aloe vera. "The beneficial healing effects of Aloe...are so miraculous as to seem more like a myth than fact," says John P. Heggers, Ph.D., of the University of Texas Medical School.

Aloe vera increases the function of the immune system to allow it to destroy tumors. Studies show strong immuno-modulatory and antitumor properties of polysaccharides found in Aloe Vera.

Aloe vera halts inflammation. Topical application of aloe is well known to ease inflammation of joints, reducing arthritis pain. Aloe can also be used internally, reducing inflammation systemically. Regular consumption of aloe vera for 2 weeks typically results in a significant reduction in symptoms of inflammation.

Aloe juice diminishes digestive tract irritations such as ulcers, colitis, and irritable bowel syndrome. Aloe increases the release of digestive enzyme pepsin by the stomach, helping digestion and helping to heal ulcers, according to a 1963 study from the Journal of the American Osteopathic Society. In a study of asthma patients, six months of oral use of Aloe diminished symptoms in almost half of the participants.

Aloe vera also reduces cholesterol and triglycerides.

Aloe Vera Studies

A 2002 animal study was performed to test whether daily consumption of Aloe would cause any health problems. Instead of showing negative effects, the animals showed a significant decrease in heart and kidney disease as well as a decrease in leukemia. The animals consuming aloe vera actually lived 10% longer than those in the control group. Researchers concluded, "these findings suggest that life-long Aloe vera ingestion does not cause any obvious harmful and deleterious side effects, and could also be beneficial for the prevention of age-related pathology."[1]

In a 1998 human clinical study, Aloe was found to enhance the treatment of various tumors when combined with melatonin. The study included 50 patients suffering conventionally untreatable cancers of the lung, gastrointestinal tract, breast or brain (glioblastomas). They were treated with melatonin alone (20 mg/day orally at bedtime) or melatonin combined with Aloe vera tincture (1 ml twice daily). Partial tumor regression occurred in 2 of 24 patients treated with the combination therapy, compared to none of the patients given melatonin alone. The cancer stabilized 12 of 24 patients given Aloe plus melatonin versus 7 of 26 patients treated with melatonin alone. The percentage of nonprogressing cancers was significantly higher in the group given Aloe, and the 1-year survival was also significantly higher. Both treatments were well tolerated.[2]

Acemannan

While Albarin, which was known to be an effective anti-cancer formula, is no longer available, there is another Aloe extract called Acemannan. Its active constituent is acelated mannan (a polysaccharide, or complex sugar) linked by β-1,4-glycosidic bonds. It is an injectable drug.

Acemannan is manufactured by Carrington Laboratories, Inc. In 1991, based on intitial studies, the USDA granted Carrington Labs conditional approval to market the drug under the name of Acemannan Immunostimulant(TM). In July 2000, conditional status was removed, and an unrestricted license was issued.

It has been used to treat various types of tumors in pet dogs and cats. It causes tumor necrosis and encapsulation, and infiltration of tumors by immunocytes. It extends the life of animals. Researchers concluded, "It is believed that acemannan exerts its antitumor activity through macrophage activation and the release of tumor necrosis factor, interleukin-1, and interferon."[3]

In another experiment, a group of laboratory mice were implanted with sarcoma cells. Without treatment, these tumors would grow rapidly and kill all the test animals in 20-46 days. However, in mice treated with acemannan at the time of tumor cell implantation, the survival rate was approximately 40. Their tumors were invaded by immunocytes, had dead or dying cores, and had regressed.[4]

In 1991, Acemannan was found to be an effective treatment for feline leukemia. This is a retroviral disease that usually kills the majority of affected cats, with 40% of them dying within 4 weeks of disease onset, and 70% within 8 weeks. Injections of acemannan for 6 weeks significantly improved both the quality of life and the survival rate of the infected cats. After 12 weeks of treatment, 71% of treated cats were still alive and in good health.[5]

There are a number of companies selling other concentrated Aloe products, but active ingredients may vary, and it is difficult to tell how much acemannan any of them contain.

How to Grow and Care for Aloe Plants

The best way to get fresh Aloe Vera gel is to grow it yourself. The commercial Aloe Vera products are second rate and comparable to fresh orange juice vs bottled juice. Fresh always wins: Aloe retains its medicinal integrity when picked and used immediately.

It can be used as ingredient in smoothies. Cut a large aloe vera leaf out of a backyard Aloe plant, slice off the thick green skin of the leaf, and drop the large gel piece into a blender.

There are over 250 species of Aloes in the world, mostly native to Africa. They range in size from little one-inch miniatures to massive plant colonies consisting of hundreds of plants, each as large as 2 feet in diameter. Although most Aloes have some medicinal or commercial value, the most commonly cultivated variety is Aloe barbadensis, which is the plant commonly known as Aloe Vera.

Aloe has been widely grown as an ornamental plant for many years. In warm climates, it can grow outside all year. All Aloes are semi-tropical succulents, and will only survive outdoors in areas where there is no chance of freezing (USDA zones 10 or 11). Because Aloe plants consist of 95% water, they are very sensitive to frost. However, they make excellent house plants when they are given sufficient light. In colder climates, Aloes in containers benefit from being placed outdoors in summer. Older specimens may even bloom, producing a high stalk covered with bright coral-colored flowers.

If Aloes are grown or placed outdoors in warm climates, they do best in full sun or light shade. The soil should be moderately fertile, and well-drained.

Established plants will survive a drought quite well, but grow better when watered regularly. Due to their popularity, Aloe vera plants are sold in almost every garden shop or nursery. The nectar from Aloe flowers is a favorite food for hummingbirds.

Instructions

It is not advisable to rely solely on Aloe vera to cure cancer, and it is best used as an adjunct to other treatments, either alternative or conventional.

Suppliers

Aloe plants are available at nurseries.

Pasteurized aloe vera juice is available in health food stores, and sometimes very cheaply in gallon jugs in the vitamin section of Walmart.

Serovera, supposedly much like Albarin:

http://www.serovera.com
The supplier of Acemannan is given below.

**VETERINARY PRODUCTS LABORATORIES
301 W. OSBORN, PHOENIX, AZ, 85013**

Phone : 888-241-9545
Fax : 800-215-5875
Website : www.vpl.com
Email : info@vpl.com

Other Aloe concentrates :

Carrington Lab manufactures a concentrate called *MPS-Gold*, but this product is made up of whatever short-chain polysaccharides are left after the long chains have been extracted to make Acemannan. There is another product called *Mole-Cures A.M.P Aloe Vera*, but they also buy from Carrington.

Alpha-Omega Labs, based in the Bahamas and Equador, manufactures an extract of aloe barbadensis miller, a variety of aloe plant which has a high content of polymannan. The product is unfractionated aloe vera gel powder, 200:1. According to the manufacturer, it contains not less than 25 to 35% extra long chain acemannans. They claim that their low-temperature dehydration technique yields a product with larger polysaccharide molecules than freeze-drying or spray drying.

Freeze dried = up to 500,000 - 800,000 daltons
Dehydrated = up to 1,000,000 - 2,000,000 daltons

Alpha-Omega's product is sold by distributor Al Low & Associates in Texas, phone: (800) 807-4779. No online ordering, just a pdf order form to fax:

http://www.4rhealthproducts.com/mail-or-fax-order.pdf

Here is another company which features a 28:1 whole leaf liquid concentrate, as well as powder:

http://healthy-living.org/html/aloe_7000.html

Serovera:

70 Capsules per Bottle 500mg Each 1-3 Month Supply 375mg High-potency, Freeze-Dried AMP $159 per bottle (or less with discount).

http://www.serovera.com

References

(1) Ikeno Y, Hubbard GB, Lee S, Yu BP, Herlihy JT, "The influence of long-term Aloe vera ingestion on age-related disease in male Fischer 344 rats." Phytother Res 2002 Dec;16(8):712-8.
(2) P. Lissoni, et al., "Biotherapy with the pineal immunomodulating hormone melatonin versus melatonin plus aloe vera in untreatable advanced solid neoplasms." Nat Immun, 1998;16(1):27-33

(3) Harris C, Pierce K, King G, Yates KM, Hall J, Tizard I., "Efficacy of acemannan in treatment of canine and feline spontaneous neoplasms." Mol Biother. 1991 Dec;3(4):207-13

(4) Peng, SY, et al., "Decreased mortality of Norman murine sarcoma in mice treated with the immunomodulator, Acemannan." Mol Biother 1991;3:79-87

(5) Sheets MA, Unger BA, Giggleman GF, et al. "Studies of the effect of acemannan on retrovirus infections: clinical stabilization of feline leukemia virus-infected cats." Mol Biother. 1991;3:41-45

Anamu

Anamu *(Petiveria alliacea)* is a herb which grows in the Amazon rainforest and some tropical areas in South America and the Carribean. Anamu plants can grow as high as a meter and have dark green leaves with tall spikes. White flowers are found in between these spikes.

The plant is widely used as a medicine by traditional healers. Inhalation of crushed anamu roots is said to cure sinusitis, while a tea of the leaves can treat influenza and colds. The leaves are ground into a paste and applied topically as an analgesic for headaches, arthritis, and injuries.

Anamu contains multiple biologically active chemicals, including triterpenes, flavonoids, steroids, and sulfur compounds. The University of Illinois at Chicago conducted a screening study to identify medicinal plants, and evaluated more than 1400 plant extracts as new therapies for the prevention and treatment of cancer. Anamu was one of 34 plants found to display anti-cancer properties. The researchers discovered that dibenzyl trisulfide was one of two of the active phytochemicals in anamu with anti-tumor effects.

In addition, Anamu contains multiple other bioactive compounds which have also been demonstrated to have anticancer properties. These include flavanoids, triterpenes, steroids, lipids and several sulfur-containing amino acids.[1-5]

Clinical experiments have confirmed anti-inflammatory effect of anamu in cases of arthritis. Other studies on anamu show that the plant possesses a wide range of therapeutic properties against many types of cancer. It has also been used to treat leukemia, lymphoma, and cancer of the breast, brain, and liver.

Studies

In an Italian experiment in the 1990s, ethanol and water extracts of whole-herb anamu were discovered to be cytoxic to leukemia and lymphoma cancer cells, and inhibited the growth of breast cancer cells.[6]

Anamu extract had a cytotoxic effect in-vitro against a line of liver cancer cells.[7]

Another in vitro study in 2001 reported that anamu retarded the growth of brain cancer cells. The German study documenting anamu's activity against brain cancer cells related its actions to the sulfur compounds found in the plant.[8]

Apart from its anti-inflammatory and anti-cancerous properties, anamu is also an antimicrobial and immunostimulant. In mice test subjects, anamu extracts were able to induce production of new immune system cells.[9-12]

In an in-vitro study, Anamu was found to exert multiple biological activities against several lines of cancer cells. It induced G2 cell cycle arrest and caused apoptotic cell death in a mitochondria independent way. It down-regulates cytoskeleton, chaperone, and signal transduction proteins, and other proteins involved in metabolic pathways. Also, it up-regulates production of proteins involved in intracellular degradation. Researchers concluded, *"Petiveria alliacea* appears to be a good candidate to be used as an antitumor agent."[13]

Amanu also shows antibacterial traits against common pathogens such as Staphylococcus, E.coli, Shigella and Mycobacterium tuberculosis, and also against some viruses. A study found amanu prevented replication of a bovine viral diarrhea virus, leading researchers to reccommend further testing of anamu as a treatment for hepatitis C infection in humans.[14]

After conventional cancer treatments the immune system is at its weakest, and there is a high risk of infection. Anamu can not only prevent cancer reccurrence, but it also protects and strengthens the body during the recovery process.

Anamu does not interact with conventional chemotherapy, and has few side effects. It may lower blood sugar levels. However, animal tests showed it can cause uterine contractions, which may cause miscarriage and therefore the herb is not recommended for pregnant women.

Apart from this, there have been no other side effects of anamu noted. A few experiments claimed that amanu extracts caused the development of brain tumors in animals, but subsequent studies did not back up these findings.

Due to its many health benefits, the growing worldwide popularity of this ancient rain forest herb is unsurprising.

Instructions

Traditional preparation of anamu is usually an infusion dried anamu in water. Half cup of the infusion should be taken daily.

Anamu now comes in packs of loose herb, as well as capsules and tablets. These capsules or tablets should be taken twice a day or more depending on the advice of your doctor or the product recommendation.

Infusion: 1/4 to 1/2 cup 2-3 times daily
Capsules: 1-3 g daily

Suppliers

Anamu powder 1 pound $28.

http://www.rain-tree.com/anamu-powder.htm

References

(1) De Sousa JR, Demuner AJ, Pinheiro JA, Breitmaier E, Cassels BK. "Dibenzyl trisulphide and trans-N-methyl-4-methoxyproline from Petiveria alliacea." Phytochemistry 1990, 29:3653-3655.

(2) Delle-Monache F, Menichini F, Cuca LE. "Petiveria alliacea: II. Further Flavonoids and Triterpenes." Gazzeta Chimica Italiana 1996, 126:275-278

(3) Delle-Monache F, Cuca LE. "6-C-formyl and 6-C hidroxymethyl flavonones from Petiveria alliacea." Phytochemistry 1992, 31:2481-2482

(4) Kubec R, Musah RA: "Cysteine sulfoxide derivatives in Petiveria alliacea." Phytochemistry 2001, 58:981-5

(5) Kubec R, Kim S, Musah RA. "S-Substituted cysteine derivatives and thiosulfinate formation in Petiveria alliacea-part II. Phytochemistry 2002, 61:675-80.

(6) Rossi, V., et al.,"Antiproliferative effects of Petiveria alliacea on several tumor cell lines." Pharmacol. Res. Suppl. 1990; 22(2): 434.

(7) Ruffa, M. J., et al. "Cytotoxic effect of Argentine medicinal plant extracts on human hepatocellular carcinoma cell line." J. Ethnopharmacol. 2002 ; 79(3): 335-339.

(8) Rosner, H., et al. "Disassembly of microtubules and inhibition of neurite outgrowth, neuroblastoma cell proliferation, and MAP kinase tyrosine dephosphorylation by dibenzyl trisulphide." Biochem. Biophys. Acta, 2001; 1540(2): 166-77.

(9) Queiroz, M. L., et al. "Cytokine profile and natural killer cell activity in Listeria monocytogenes infected mice treated orally with Petiveria alliacea extract." Immunopharmacol. Immunotoxicol. 2000 Aug;22(3):501-18; 5.

(10) Quadros, M. R., et al. "Petiveria alliacea L. extract protects mice against Listeria monocytogenes infection—effects on bone marrow progenitor cells." Immunopharmacol. Immunotoxicol. 1999 Feb; 21(1): 109-24.

(11) Williams, L., et al. Immunomodulatory activities of Petiveria alliaceae L." Phytother. Res. 1997 ; 11(3): 251253; Rossi, V., "Effects of Petiveria alliacea L. on cell immunity." Pharmacol. Res. 1993; 27(1): 111-12

(12) Marini, S., "Effects of Petiveria alliacea L. on cytokine production and natural killer cell activity." Pharmacol. Res. 1993 27 1: 111-112.

(13) Urueña, C., et al. "Petiveria alliacea extracts uses multiple mechanisms to inhibit growth of human and mouse tumoral cells." BMC Complement." Altern. Med. 2008 Nov 18; 8:60.

(14) Ruffa, M. J., et al. "Antiviral activity of Petiveria alliacea against the bovine diarrhea virus." Chemotherapy 2002; 48(3): 144-47.

Arjuna

Arjuna is the common name for the herbal tree known as *Terminalia Arjuna*. It is an evergreen plant native to India that grows up to 100 feet. The white-to-pinkish-gray bark of the arjuna is one of the most frequently used herbs in ayurvedic medicine. Three related species of Terminalia are used for medicinal purposes, Terminalia arjuna, Terminalia bellerica, and Terminalia chebula.

Arjuna has anti-cancer, anti-oxidant, anti-microbial, and cardioprotective properties. It also helps heal wounds and gastric ulcers.

It is known to contain triterpene glycosides, glycosides, flavanoids and other strong antioxidants. Components include triterpenoids such as arjunin, arjunic acid, arjunolic acid, arjungenin, and terminic acid; glycosides such as arjunetin, arjunoside I, arjunoside II, arjunaphthanoloside and terminoside A; sitosterol; flavonoids including arjunolone, arjunone, bicalein, luteolin, gallic acid, ethyl gallate, quercetin, kempferol, pelorgonidin, oligomeric and proanthocyanidins; tannis and minerals.[1]

An in-vitro test of the anti-cancer activity of Arjuna found that one created derivative from the plant performed twice as well as the standard chemotherapy drug vinblastine. The study was performed using oral, ovarian and liver cancer cell lines.

Bioassays have identified the anti-cancer compounds in Arjuna as gallic acid, ethyl gallate and the flavone leutonolin. Ellagic acid is an antimutagenic agent and ellagitanin is a moderately cytotoxic compound.

Researchers concluded, "Luteolin has a well established record of inhibiting various cancer cell lines and may account for most of the rationale underlying the use of T. arjuna in traditional cancer treatments."[2]

The flavanoid luteolin has multiple anti-tumor actions. In-vivo studies show that luteolin is anticarcinogenic, inhibits angiogenesis, causes apoptosis in tumor cells, reduces tumor growth and enhances the effects of chemotherapy. Biochemical mechanisms for these effects include "modulation of ROS levels, inhibition of topoisomerases I and II, reduction of NfkappaB and AP-1 activity, stabilization of p53, and inhibition of PI3K, STAT3, IGF1R and HER2."[3]

Other researchers identified the most cytotoxic compound as arjunic acid; however, it was only 1/5 as cytotoxic as the standard chemo drug vinblastine against liver tumor cells. The researchers then prepared seven derivatives of arjunic acid and cytotoxic activity was reevaluated.

All derivatives displayed anti-tumor effects, but three of the derivatives were highly active, 7-9 times greater than the starting material, arjunic acid. Two derivatives were 4-5 times more active than arjunic acid against oral cancer cells. When the derivatives were compared to vinblastine, the compound 2-0-palmitoylarjunic acid showed twice the activity of the drug against liver cancer cells.[4]

Researchers at the University of Madras Department of Pharmacology and Environmental Toxicology performed a rat study to test the antioxidant properties of ethanolic extract of Terminalia arjuna bark (EETA) on toxin-induced liver cancer. Levels of lipid peroxides, indicators of tissue damage, were found to be significantly lower in rats administered EETA.[5]

In another study, a 70% extract of Terminalia chebula fruit was found to inhibit various tumor cell lines. Tumor lines tested included human and mouse breast cancer, human osteosarcoma, human prostate cancer, and a non-cancerous, immortalized human prostate cell line. In all cell types, the extract decreased cell viability, inhibited cell proliferation, and induced cell death in a dose dependent function. Cell death was due to apoptosis at lower doses, but at higher concentrations, necrosis occurred. Chebulinic acid and ellagic were the most effective tumor growth inhibitors found in the study.[6]

An aqueous extract of Terminalia arjuna was administered to mice with lymphoma. Arjuna contains catalase, superoxide dismutase, S-transferase and glutathione, all strong anti-oxidants. Arjuna extracts greatly increase the concentration of these enzymes in cells.

Antioxidant levels are usually low in mouse lymphoma and the resultant oxidative stress enhances the growth of cancer. Arjuna was also found to downregulate anaerobic metabolism (a basic characteristic of tumors) by blocking the function of lactic dehydrogenase.[7]

Caution

T.arjuna may produce mild gastritis, headache and constipation. It has no known drug interactions. No haematological, metabolic, renal or hepatotoxicity has been reported even with long term consumption of 24 months.

Traditionally contraindicated during pregnancy.

Instructions

Usual dosage of Arjuna is 1-2 g/day.

Dried bark
1-6 g

Liquid extract 1:1 in 45% ethanol
0.7 to 2.0 ml 3 times daily

Supplier

Very inexpensive. You can buy 4 bottles (550 mg X 120) capsules of Arjuna for $8 on Ebay.

References

(1) Dwivedi S. "Terminalia arjuna Wight & Arn.--a useful drug for cardiovascular disorders." J Ethnopharmacol 2007; 114(2):114-129).

(2) Pettit G. R. et al., "Antineoplastic agents 338. The cancer cell growth inhibitory. Constituents of Terminalia arjuna (Combretaceae)." J. Ethnopharmacology, 1996 Aug;53(2):57-63.

(3) Miguel López-Lázaro, "Distribution and Biological Activities of the Flavonoid Luteolin." Mini-Reviews in Medicinal Chemistry, 2009, 9, 31-59 31

(4) Saxena M, Faridi U, Mishra R, Gupta M, Darokar MP et al. 2007. "Cytotoxic agents from Terminalia arjuna." PlantaMed 14:73;1429-1524.

(5) Sivalokanathan S., Ilayaraja M., Balasubramanian M.P., "Antioxidant activity of Terminalia arjuna bark extract on N-nitrosodiethylamine induced hepatocellular carcinoma in rats." Mol Cell Biochem, 2006 Jan;281(1-2):87-93.

(6) Ammar Saleema, et al., "Inhibition of cancer cell growth by crude extract and the phenolics of Terminalia chebula retz. Fruit." Journal of Ethnopharmacology 81 (2002) 327-336.

(7) Verma N., Vinayak M., "Effect of Terminalia arjuna on antioxidant defense system in cancer." Mol Biol Rep 2009 Jan; 36(1):159-64.

Artemisia

The Chinese herb Artemisia has been used since ancient times to combat malaria, and modern medicine is rediscovering its use, as malaria is becoming increasingly more resistant to the conventional treatment, quinine. Artemisinin is an extract of sweet wormwood, *Artemisia annua L.*, known in Chinese traditional medicine as Qing Hao. It is now a major drug for the treatment of malaria in Vietnam, China, and other areas of Asia and Africa. It is usually combined with other anti-malarials.

In 1996, Dr. Henry Lai and Dr. Narendra Singh of the University of Washington patented the use of Artemisinin as a cancer treatment (US Patent 5,578,637). It is used by alternative practitioners to treat a wide range of cancers, and it is currently being investigated as a possible cure for breast cancer and leukemia.

Chemically, artemisinin is a sesquiterpene lactone which contains an unusual peroxide bridge, a rare feature in a natural compound.

Artemisinin works by combining chemically with iron in the body and creating free radicals that attack cancer cells from within. Tumor cells replicate faster than normal cells, and therefore contain a higher concentration of iron. This makes artemisinin selectively toxic to cancer cells.

The same mechanism gives the plant its anti-malarial properties. The parasite that causes malaria cannot eliminate iron from the red blood cells it inhabits, so it eats and stores it. Artemisinin converts these iron stores into a poison that kills the parasite.

Studies

Artemisinin has previously been shown to selectively kill cancer cells, and in one study, it decreased the development of breast cancer by 40% in rats that had been given a cancer-causing agent. In the study, rats were treated with a single 50 mg/kg dose of DMBA, a compound known to cause breast cancer. The rats were randomly divided into two groups, with one group's food supplemented with 0.02% artemisinin.

The rats fed artemisinin showed a 40% decreased incidence of breast cancer compared to controls. In addition, the tumors which did develop in the artemisinin group were smaller and fewer.

"Since artemisinin is a relatively safe compound that causes no known side effects even at high oral doses, the present data indicate that artemisinin may be a potent cancer-chemoprevention agent," said the researchers.[1]

Combining artemisinin with hyperbaric oxygen produced synergistic effects. Leukemia cells treated with either artemisinin alone or hyperbaric oxygen showed cell growth of 85% compared to untreated cells. Combining the two therapies reduced growth by another 22%, or down to 63% of that seen in untreated cells.[2] Artesunate, another artemisia derivative, caused apoptosis in chemotherapy-resistant leukemia cells.[3,4]

In 1999, working with a veterinarian, Drs. Lai and Singh also used artemisin to treat cancer in dogs. Numerous anecdotal reports from pet owners using Artemisinin to treat dogs with lymphoma, osteosarcoma, and metastases from osteosarcoma state that the dogs survived longer than expected.

In addition to the animal studies, Dr. Lai has also received several reports of substantial reductions of PSA levels from prostate cancer patients using various Artemisia compounds.

The plant contains at least 20 known biologically active compounds, as well as hundreds of other chemicals which may function synergistically.[5]

Other compounds extracted from the same plant, aside from artemisinin, have also been used to treat cancer. These include artesunate, dihydroartemisinin, and artemether as oral products and injectibles. Artemether maintains blood levels for a longer time period. Artemether may be more effective than Artemisinin alone in brain cancers, because it crosses the blood-brain barrier more readily.

Wellcare Pharmaceuticals manufactures a product called Artemix, which contains Artesunate, Artemether, and Artemisinin. The combination treatment may be more effective than Artemisinin alone.

There are several alternative practitioners using Artemisa compounds clinically, and patient studies are ongoing. Dr. Singh, Dr. Lai's co-author, is a medical doctor from India working in Washington on studies involving Artemisia compounds.

Dr. Bernard Bihari has combined Artemisia compounds with low dose naltrexone (1.75 to 4.5 mg LDN per day) as part of his protocol in treating cancer patients. Dr. Biharia has also used low-dose naltrexone extensively to treat HIV/AIDS, as it seems to halt progression of that disease by stimulating the immune system.

These practitioners report successful treatments of lung, brain, breast, laryngeal and pancreatic cancers with various Artemisia products.

Artemisia has been the subject of numerous research papers, and has been proven effective against multiple cancer cell lines including breast cancer[6], cholangiocarcinoma[7], glioblastoma[8], hepatoma[9], kaposi's sarcoma[10], leukemia[11], melanoma[12,13,14], myeloma[15], pancreatic[16,17,18], stomach,[19] and uterine[20] cancer, and epithelial cells expressing papilloma virus.[21]

Caution

Artemisinin is usually well-tolerated at the doses used to treat malaria. Side effects from the artemisinin can include nausea, vomiting, anorexia, and dizziness. Mild blood abnormalities have also occurred. One report of liver toxicity has been reported in a patient using relatively high-dose artemisinin for an unstated medical condition (not malaria).

A mouse study using five brands of Artemisinin combination therapies found no major heart, liver or kidney toxicity.[22]

Instructions

Artemisinin is being used as self-treatment by cancer patients at doses of 100 to 600 mg a day. Some patients use both the oral and injectable forms simultaneously, but most are just using one form of the oral compound.

Patient studies are being conducted to find the best combination of derivative form, dosage and timing.

The optimal anti-cancer protocol is still being investigated, but the following recommendations have been made by various alternative practitioners.

Dosage: Initially, Dr Lai recommended a dose of 2.2-4.4 mg of Artemisinin per pound of bodyweight. More recently, he stated that it may be best to use only Artemether, twice daily 12 hours apart, to keep up therapeutic blood levels.

Dr.Singh believes taking all three forms of Artemisinin together once a day at bedtime is the most effective treatment.

Dr Guillermo Couto, a veterinarian conducting an Artemisinin study at Ohio State University, believes a dose of 6.6-8.8mg Artemisinin per pound of body weight is most effective.

Holley Pharmaceuticals recommends doses as high as 11-16 mg Artemisinin per pound. (For kilogram dosages, multiply the dose per pound by 2.2)

If using whole Artemisia powder, Hans-Martin Hirt at the German Cancer Research Centre in Heidelberg, Germany, recommends 5 grams dried plant per day for 7 days, either made into a tea or consumed with food. If no positive results are seen after that time period, stop using it.

Timing: Again, opinions differ. Some patients split the dose, taking some in the morning and some before bed. Some take the entire dose at bedtime.

There is agreement that Artemisinin should **not** be taken within 3 hours of iron-rich food, such as meat. It should also not be combined with anti-oxidants since the substance works by creating free radicals that destroy tumor cells, and anti-oxidants block production of free radicals.

Giving it with some form of dietary fat is recommended by some. The substance is quite bitter-tasting, and may be mixed with cream cheese or peanut butter to hide the taste.

Cycling: Herbal remedies are often more effective if they are "cycled" or "pulsed", that is, taken for a certain time period, and then not taken for a time. The belief is based on the theory that if the body rests between doses, it will be less likely to build up resistance to the effects of the drug. Artemisinin may be cycled or pulsed by days or weeks.

Suppliers

Artemisinin and its derivatives are available from various suppliers. Iherb has products from several manufacturers.

http://www.iherb.com/Artemisinin

References

(1) Henry Lai and Narendra Singh, "Oral artemisinin prevents and delays the development of 7, 12-dimethylbenz(a)anthracene (DMBA)-induced breast cancer in the rat." Cancer Letter, 2006 Volume 231, Issue 1, Pages 43-48, 8.

(2) Yusuke Ohgami, Catherine Elstad, Eunhee Chung, Donald Shirachi, Raymond Quock, Henry Lai,"Effect of Hyperbaric Oxygen on the Anticancer Effect of Artemisinin on Molt-4 Human Leukemia Cells." Anticancer Research November 2010 vol. 30 no. 11 4467-4470

(3) Efferth, T., Giaisi, M., Merling, A., Krammer Peter, H. & Li-Weber, M. "Artesunate Induces ROS-Mediated Apoptosis in Doxorubicin-Resistant T Leukemia Cells." International Journal of Oncology 18, 767-773 2001.

(4) Efferth, T. et al. "Activity of drugs from traditional Chinese medicine toward sensitive and MDR1- or MRP1-overexpressing multidrug-resistant human CCRF-CEM leukemia cells." Blood cells, Molecules & Diseases 28, 160-168 (2002).

(5) Ferreira JF, Luthria DL, Sasaki T, Heyerick A. "Flavonoids from Artemisia annua L. as Antioxidants and Their Potential Synergism with Artemisinin against Malaria and Cancer." Molecules. 15(5):3135-3170 (2010).

(6) Shafi G, et al., "Artemisia absinthium (AA): a novel potential complementary and alternative medicine for breast cancer." Mol Biol Rep 2012 Jul;39(7):7373-9. Epub 2012 Feb 5.

(7) Chaijaroenkul W, et al., "Cytotoxic Activity of Artemisinin Derivatives Against Cholangiocarcinoma (CL-6) and Hepatocarcinoma (Hep-G2) Cell Lines." Asian Pac J Cancer Prev. 12(1):55-59 (2011).

(8) Efferth, T., Ramirez, T., Gebhart, E. & Halatsch, M.-E. "Combination treatment of glioblastoma multiforme cell lines with the anti-malarial

artesunate and the epidermal growth factor receptor tyrosine kinase inhibitor OSI-774." Biochemical Pharmacology 67, 1689-1700 (2004).

(9) Deng, X.-R., Yu, H.-P., Wang, K.-Q. & Li, X.-M. "Inhibitory effect of artemisinin on hepatoma H22 cells." Shiyong Linchuang Yixue 8, 1-3, 7 (2007).

(10) Dell'Eva, R. et al. "Inhibition of angiogenesis in vivo and growth of Kaposi's sarcoma xenograft tumors by the anti-malarial artesunate." Biochemical Pharmacology 68, 2359-2366 (2004).

(11) Deng, D.A., Xu, C.H. & Cai, J.C. "Derivatives of arteannuin B with antileukemia activity." Acta Pharmacetica Sinica 27(4): 317-320 (1992)

(12) Berger, T.G. et al. "Artesunate in the treatment of metastatic uveal melanoma - first experiences." Oncology Reports 14, 1599-1603 (2005).

(13) Buommino E, Baroni A, Canozo N, Petrazzuolo M, Nicoletti R, Vozza A, Tufano MA. "Artemisinin reduces human melanoma cell migration by down-regulating alphaVbeta3 integrin and reducing metalloproteinase 2 production." Invest New Drugs 27, 412-418 (2009)

(14) Cabello CM, et al., "The redox antimalarial dihydroartemisinin targets human metastatic melanoma cells but not primary melanocytes with induction of NOXA-dependent apoptosis." Invest New Drugs. 2011 May 6. [Epub ahead of print]

(15) Chen H, et al., "Artesunate inhibiting angiogenesis induced by human myeloma RPMI8226 cells." Int J Hematol. 2010 Oct 14. [Epub ahead of print]

(16) Du, J.-H., Ma, Z.-J., Li, J.-X. & Zhang, H.-D. "An oncosis-like cell death of pancreatic cancer Panc-1 cells induced by artesunate is related to generation of reactive oxygen species." Zhongguo Aizheng Zazhi 18, 410-414 (2008).

(17) Chen, H., Sun, B., Pan, S., Jiang, H. & Sun, X. "Dihydroartemisinin inhibits growth of pancreatic cancer cells in vitro and in vivo." Anti-Cancer Drugs 20, 131-140 (2009).

(18) Du JH, et al., "Artesunate induces oncosis-like cell death in vitro and has antitumor activity against pancreatic cancer xenografts in vivo." Cancer Chemother Pharmacol. 65(5): 895-902 (2010).

(19) Alcântara DD, et al., "In vitro evaluation of the cytotoxic and genotoxic effects of artemether, an antimalarial drug, in a gastric cancer cell line (PG100)." 2011 Sep 23. doi: 10.1002/jat.1734. [Epub ahead of print]

(20) Chung, S.Y. et al. "Effect of natural compounds on P-glycoprotein activity in human uterine sarcoma cells." Yakche Hakhoechi 35, 249-254 (2005).

(21) Disbrow, G.L. et al. "Dihydroartemisinin is cytotoxic to papillomavirus-expressing epithelial cells in vitro and in vivo." Cancer Research 65, 10854-10861 (2005).

(22) U. Georgewill , O. Ebong : Artemisinin Combination Therapies; Safe Or Not Safe ?. The Internet Journal of Pharmacology. 2012 Volume 10 Number 1. DOI: 10.5580/2b58

Avemar

Avemar, sometimes referred to by the generic name MSC, is made from wheat germ fermented by baker's yeast through a patented process (US patent# 6355474), standardized to yield 0.4 mg/kg of the naturally occurring flavone 2,6-dimethoxy-p-benzoquinone (2,6-DMBQ) present in wheat germ.

While it is made from fermented wheat germ, it is considered to be a semi-synthetic product and comes as a granule or in capsule form.

History of Avemar

Pioneering work on this compound was done at the Semmelweis Medical University in Budapest, Hungary by Dr.Albert Szent-Györgyi, a Nobel Prize recipient in 1937 for his discovery of vitamin C and his studies on the process of cellular metabolism. Szent-Györgyi was determined to find a non-toxic alternative to chemotherapy, which was just being developed in this era and was initially based on experiments with mustard gas, a chemical weapon used in WWI. He theorized that supplements of the chemical DMBQ, found naturally in wheat germ, could help regulate cellular metabolism, allowing normal cells to grow while preventing cancerous cells from spreading. The theory was confirmed with experiments in the 1960s, using natural and synthetic DMBQ against various cancer cell lines. His studies were published in the Proceedings of the National Academy of Sciences USA.

However, as aggressive chemotherapy increasingly became the medical establishment's treatment of choice against cancer, Szent-Györgyi's research was forgotten, and he died in 1986.

After the fall of communism in Hungary in 1989, scientists were freed to pursue independent interests, and at this time Szent-Györgyi's discovery was picked up by Dr. Mate Hidvegi. However, before he could complete his research, funding ran out. For lack of any other option, Hidvegi, a devout man, prayed to the Virgin Mary for guidance and an investor. The very next day, a stranger gave Hidvegi a check in the range of $100,000.00. Hidvegi continued his work, and by 1998, he patented a process to ferment wheat germ with baker's yeast, producing a concentrated extract called FWGE (Fermented Wheat Germ Extract). In honor of the help he felt he had received through prayer, he called his product Avemar, from Ave Maria (Ave meaning hail and Mar meaning Mary).

Avemar is one of the world's most well-researched natural substances, reviewed in more than 100 studies in over 20 medical journals. In the United States, Avemar has been scientifically proven to balance glucose metabolism at the celular level. It has immunomodulating as well as direct cytotoxic effects on cancer cells.

Cancer cells use glucose as energy, which is why many anti-cancer diets are low in sugar and carbohydrates. Tumor cells use up to 20-30 times more glucose than normal cells. Glucose is used for the production of energy as well as to make more nucleic acids for cell division. Avemar blocks the uptake of glucose by cancer cells and therefore blocks the production of RNA and DNA so that replication of the cells is limited. It also inhibits the primary enzymes that the tumor cells need to function and replicate.
Avemar also enhances tumor necrosis factor-alpha or TNFalpha. This blocks angiogenesis or blood vessel formation necessary for tumor growth. Without an increased blood supply, the tumor will not be able to continue growing past a certain point.

In research on Avemar and cancer, it has been found that Avemar stimulates the immune system, allowing it to kill cancer cells. It selectively inhibits MHC-1, which is the main histocompatibility complex expressed on cancer cell surfaces, allowing them to hide from the immune system. When the expression of this protein is low, suggesting abnormal cell function, Natural Killer cells prompt apoptosis of the affected cell.

It is also known to cause the process of apoptosis or programmed cell death in tumor cells. This seems to be effective within the first day of use.

Avemar supports detoxification of the body, and helps the body get rid of any toxins made by the tumor and rids the body of the dead cells created by apoptosis. It has anti-inflammatory properties.

In breast cancer, Avemar has been shown to block estrogen binding to cells so that breast cancer cell growth is not stimulated.

Interestingly, Avemar has been studied as an alternative treatment for pets with cancer.

Avemar restores the individual's immune system to its precancerous state. Because it acts on antibodies formed against the body's own cells, it is helpful in the treatment of autoimmune disease in addition to its effect on cancer. In Europe, it is a popular therapy for auto-immune diseases, including rheumatoid arthritis, Sjogren's disease, scleroderma and type I diabetes. People with a variety of autoimmune conditions can experience relief of pain and other symptoms of their disease by taking oral capsules of Avemar.

Avemar can be used together with chemotherapy and prolongs survival time in even the most severe cases of cancer. It is considered an adjunct to be used along with regular chemotherapy, radiation and surgery to treat cancer. It is not considered to be a primary treatment. In Hungary, where it originated, it is classified as a "medical nutriment for cancer patients." Nevertheless, research seems to indicate that it has significant anti-cancer properties on its own. It is especially effective when it comes to the prevention of cancer recurrences and metastases.

Avemar Studies

The bioactivity of Avemar seems to be unique in its effectiveness against cancer. It has a generic name of MSC. More than a hundred studies have been published showing it has immunomodulating and anti-metastatic effects.

One non-randomized, non-blinded clinical trial investigated the effects of Avemar on colorectal cancer. The study group included 66 patients already undergoing conventional treatment who agreed to take Avemar for 6 months in addition to their other treatments. The control group consisted of 104 patients who received standard care alone.

The rate of progression-related events was significantly lower in the Avemar group versus the control group (3.0% vs 17.3%, respectively), as was the incidence of new metastases (7.6% vs 23.1%) and mortality (12.1% vs 31.7%). A lower incidence of cancer progression was seen in the Avemar group. However, the authors noted that because the study subjects were not randomly allocated to each treatment there were significant differences in the characteristics of the two groups at the start of the study. The non-Avemar control group was older (66.1 vs. 61.7 years), had a greater proportion of patients undergoing radiotherapy (53.8% vs. 27.3%) and a much shorter time interval from diagnosis to study entry (1.1 months vs. 11.2 months).[1]

In an open-label, non-randomized, non-blinded pilot trial in pediatric cancer patients with various solid tumors, the incidence of chemotherapy-related febrile neutropenia was lower in patients given Avemar (24.8% vs 43.4%).[2]

In a randomized clinical trial on melanoma patients the effectiveness of dacarbazine (DTIC)-based chemotherapy was compared to that of the same treatment supplemented for one year with Avemar. After a

7-year follow-up period significant differences were seen in both progression-free interval and overall survival in favor of the Avemar group. Mean progression-free interval was 55.8 months versus 29.9 months, and survival time was 66.2 months versus 44.7 months. The study concluded, "The inclusion of Avemar into the adjuvant protocols of high-risk skin melanoma patients is highly recommended."[3]

The Hungarian Association of Oral and Maxillofacial Surgeons (Magyar Arc-, Állcsont- és Szájsebészeti Társaság) reviewed Avemar research and issued the following conclusion: "For patients suffering from head- and neck tumors - primarily malignant tumorous diseases of the oral cavity, the progression of the disease can be slowed significantly, the five-year survival rate increased considerably, the quality of life improved, and the oxidative stress on the patients reduced by the long-term application of the supplementary formula Avemar. The Association considers the supportive treatment with the formula Avemar as an important part of the complex therapeutic protocols applied in stages II, III and IV of malignant tumorous diseases of the oral cavity."[4]

Instructions

Avemar has been described as having a peculiar taste, but it has been found that removing the taste lessens the effectiveness of the product.

Avemar cannot be taken at the same time as Vitamin C or other substances which enhance cellular energy such as CoQ10.

It is recommended that Avemar be taken when the stomach is empty, which means before meals or two hours or more after a meal. For long term complementary therapy, it should be taken for at least 6 months.
Recommended dosage 17gm (1 sachet) per day, dissolved in 200-250 ml cold water.

Suppliers

Avemar is available on ebay for $90 to $135.

References

(1) Jakab F, Shoenfeld Y, Balogh A, et al, "A medical nutriment has supportive value in the treatment of colorectal cancer." Br. J. Cancer, August 2003; 4;89(3):465-9.

(2) Garami M, Schuler D, Babosa M, et al., "Fermented wheat germ extract reduces chemotherapy-induced febrile neutropenia in pediatric cancer patients." J. Pediatr. Hematol. Oncol, October 2004; 26(10):631-5.

(3) Demidov LV, Manziuk LV, Kharkevitch GY, Pirogova NA, Artamonova EV, "Adjuvant fermented wheat germ extract (Avemar) nutraceutical improves survival of high-risk skin melanoma patients: a randomized, pilot, phase II clinical study with a 7-year follow-up." Cancer Biother Radiopharm. 2008 Aug; 23(4):477-82.

(4) Barabás J, Németh Z., "Recommendation of the Hungarian Society for Face, Mandible and Oral Surgery in the indication of supportive therapy with Avemar." Orv Hetil. 2006 Sept 3; 147(35):1709-11.

BEC 5, Egg Plant Extract – Skin Cancer

BEC5 / Curaderm is a skin cream which contains a purified plant extract from the Devil's apple (*Solanum linnaeanum*, also known *as Solanum Sodomaeum* and *Solanum hermannii*), which grows in the Australasia region. Devil'sApple is a member of the same family as eggplant, potatoes and tomatoes. The standardized extract contains 0.005% Solasodine Glycosides, chemicals also found in smaller quantities in the eggplant or aubergine.

This product was developed in 1979, after Australian biochemist Dr. Bill Cham heard an anecdotal report about a cow which had stopped the growth of a skin cancer on its eye by rubbing the lesion against the fruit of the Devil's Apple plant. Dr. Cham isolated the active compounds in the plant, solasodine rhamnosyl glycosides (solasonine and solamargine and di- and mono-glycosides). Great care was taken to obtain these purified glycoalkaloids without traces of their inhibitors, known as "Free Sugars." The Curaderm-BEC5 cream was first released on the Australian market in 1990. To date, it is estimated that BEC5 has been used by more than 80,000 patients.

The topical cream can eradicate non-melanoma skin cancers, specifically basal and squamous cell carcinomas. It is also effective against benign skin lesions, including keratoses, keratoacanthomas, sun spots, and age spots caused by skin damage due to UV light (sunlight).

Non-melanoma skin cancers rarely spread beyond their immediate location, but they erode normal tissue and surgical excision often causes great disfigurement, especially in cases of head and neck cancer. BEC5 eliminates the need for surgery and often results in a cure with minimal scarring.

Australia, the World Skin Cancer Continent, Suppresses BEC5 Skin Cancer Cure

Australia has its own version of the FDA, the Therapeutic Goods Administration (TGA), which regulates health products. Initially, this government agency allowed BEC5 to be sold over the counter in Australia. However, after a television program on skin cancer was aired which showed very satisfied patients who had cured themselves with BEC5, dermatologists lost many patients who decided to use the skin cream instead of submitting to surgery. Subsequently, Australian dermatologists lobbied heavily to restrict access to the product, on the spurious grounds that it was toxic, having been derived from a poisonous plant, the Devil's Apple. Visibility and subsequent sales of BEC5 dropped sharply, as prescription products are not allowed to be advertised in Australia.

Dr. Cham protested, stating the amount of BEC in one tube of Curaderm BEC5 is the equivalent to approximately 5 grams of eggplant (roughly 1 tablespoon), and that numerous clinical studies showed no toxicity.

For 8 years, Dr. Cham attempted to have BEC5 reclassified as an OTC product once again, but the TGA refused to reconsider its decision to restrict consumer access to the product.

Finally, Dr. Cham gave up dealing with Australian authorities and successfully applied to have his product registered as an OTC medication in the Republic of Vanuatu, an island nation in the South Pacific. Dr. Cham claims Australia sent healthcare workers to Vanuatu, where they attempted to raid the premises of a BEC5 distributor and threatened prosecution. However, authorities in Vanuatu refused to cooperate, and BEC5 continues to be sold as an OTC product. It is allowed to be sold directly to the end-user worldwide in a three month supply.

In addition to numerous research papers, Dr. Cham has also written a book about his experiences, *The Eggplant Cancer Cure.*[1]

How BEC5 Works

BEC5 contains a plant sugar called rhamnose bound to a glycoalkaloid. Receptors for the sugar portion of the glycoalkaloids exist on the membranes of susceptible cancer cells, but not on the surface of normal cells. The glycoalkaloid-rhamnose compound binds to the receptors on cancer cells, and subsequently enters the cancer cell and causes cell death by apoptosis or necrosis. Since normal cells lack the receptor for the compound, they are completely unaffected. This is contrasted with conventional skin cancer treatments such as surgical excision, radiation and topical chemotherapy treatments such as 5-FU (Adrucil®, Fluorouracil®, Efudex®, Fluoroplex®), which also destroy healthy cells surrounding the lesion.[2,3]

These compounds also affect the immune system, causing mice with sarcoma once effectively treated with solasodine compounds to be resistant to re-inoculation with cancer.[4]

Studies

Curaderm was used in a clinical trial to treat 56 keratoses, 39 basal cell cancers and 29 squamous cell cancers. All lesions regressed, and no adverse effects were seen on the liver, kidneys or haematopoietic system. A placebo formulation used as a control had no effect on a smaller number of treated lesions.[5]

Numerous clinical trials in Australia and Great Britain have confirmed BEC5's ability to cure non-melanoma skin cancers with no harm to normal tissues. In one open study with 72 patients, treatment with BEC5 cream resulted in the regression of all treated lesions (56 actinic keratoses, 39 BCCs and 29 SCCs), with 100% healing after 1-13 weeks of treatment.

Recent trials in 10 UK hospitals found that a twice daily topical application of BEC5 cream to cancerous skin lesions caused complete remission in 78% of patients within 2 months. The remaining 22% of patients also showed improvement but needed longer treatment times. They did not require standard skin cancer treatments such as chemotherapy, radiotherapy or surgery.

The dermatologists at the Royal London Hospital concluded, "BEC5 is a topical preparation which is safe and effective, an ideal therapy for outpatient treatment... It is a cost effective treatment for both primary and secondary skin cancer care."

The only side effects were minor skin irritation and redness. Ulceration of the lesion site occurred during treatment, but after treatment the wound healed with minimal scarring. Histological analyses of biopsies over the course of treatment and during 5- and 10-year follow-up show no tumor recurrence.

Twice daily application of Curaderm-BEC5 under occlusive dressing for 2 months resulted in a 78% success rate. Three months of treatment resulted in virtually 100% success rate.[6,7,8,9]

Intralesional injection of solasodine glycosides into large tumors is highly effective, more than intravenous administration.[10] According to Dr. Cham, the glycoside compounds in BEC5 completely eliminated terminal cancer in animals such as horses, leaving the animals cancer-free for the remainder of their normal life span.[11]

BEC5 - Not Just For Skin Cancer

BEC5 is effective against Kaposi's sarcoma and has also been used to treat herpes infections. Currently, clinical trials are being performed using internal administration of the glycoalkaloids in BEC5 in patients with terminal internal cancers.

In-vivo and in-vitro studies show solasodine compounds are effective against multiple tumor lines, including cell cultures of lung Ehrlich carcinoma, K562 leukaemia, colon (HI29) cancer, liver (Hep G2) cancer cells, promyelocytic leukaemia (HL-50) ovarian and lung cancer.[12,13,14]

They also sensitize cells to the effects of chemotherapy.[15]

Intravenous Use

In 2000, Solbec Pharmaceuticals Ltd. licensed the intellectual property rights to BEC5 from Dr. Cham after it was found to be effective in treating mesothelioma in mice.[16]

Solbec Pharmaceuticals developed a formulation called Coramsine (also referred to as experimental drug SBP002), a 1:1 combination of solasonine and solamargine, which showed positive results in FDA clinical trials. In 2005 and 2006 Cormasine was given Orphan Drug status by the FDA for the treatment of melanoma and renal cell carcinoma. The Orphan Drug program is an FDA incentive program for the development of drugs targeting conditions affecting fewer than 200,000 patients, or affecting more than 200,000 patients but being unlikely to make a profit.

The FDA approval process was never completed due to the company's inability in 2008 to raise the capital needed to fund the completion of all the required tests. The last tests of this drug were performed in 2008, after which Solbec returned the rights to the drug to Dr. Cham.

In a Phase I clinical trial, Coramsine was administered intravenously to patients with a varienty of cancers. Minor responses occurred in 2/19 of the patients, but liver toxicity occurred at doses above 1 mg/kg/day.[17]

Muliple studies on solasodine compounds:

http://curaderm.net/

Caution

Side effects are minor, usually limited to skin reddening, although during the curative phase, erosion, ulceration and shedding of unwanted skin cells can also occur. It can create a burning sensation on contact. If a severe reaction occurs, decrease or discontinue use.

It is advisable to consult a dermatologist for a biopsy to insure the lesion to be treated is basal or squamous cell cancer, and not melanoma. Not all melanomas are dark, they can have mixed colors or even no pigmentation at all. Melanoma is a serious, quickly progressing and metastasizing cancer for which a topical treatment such as BEC5 is NOT an appropriate cure.

Used with caution if allergic to eggplant or aspirin.

Instructions

Clean the area to be treated with a mild antiseptic (to remove old skin cells). BEC5 should be applied relatively thickly to the area at least twice a day, then covered with a micro pore dressing.

Avoid contact with eyes. If any excess remains on the skin, wipe away with cold water. Treatment should continue for a minimum of 1 week and a maximum of 3 months, depending on the size of the lesion and regularity of application.

Store your BEC5 in the fridge. It is an emulsion of multiple ingredients which enhance absorption. It tends to separate if stored at high temperatures, making it difficult to apply and less absorbable by skin. If you shake a container of BEC5 and hear a sloshing sound, it has separated. To reconstitute it, place tube in hot water (at least 60 degrees celsius) for a few minutes. Then shake vigorously, place it in the freezer for 10 minutes, then subsequently store in the fridge.

Suppliers

A 20 ml. bottle of BEC5 can treat one large skin cancer, two medium sized ones, six small ones or twelve sun spots.

Widely available on the internet for approximately $125.00.

http://www.amazon.com/Curaderm-Bec5-20-ml-Cream

Home-made Egglant Extract

The commercial formula has the great advantage of having been clinically tested on humans and found to be effective. It contains fractionated, standardized compounds. However, many people have made their own version and anecdotal reports exist that it also works. The homemade remedy uses a vinegar solution to extract from eggplant the same glycocides and glycoalkaloids found in BEC5.

Recipe For Homemade Eggplant Remedy

Some people have made the recipe using white vinegar, while others recommend raw organic apple cider vinegar. Finely grind up a medium sized eggplant, put it into a glass jar and fill up the jar with the vinegar. Store the jar in the refrigerator for 3 days. After this, the vinegar will have darkened, indicating that it is ready to use.

Apply the vinegar directly to skin lesions with a cotton ball, or secure the soaked cotton onto the skin with tape. Treatment may take several weeks. Both commercial BEC5 cream and the homemade remedy also heal non-cancerous skin conditions.

References

(1) The Eggplant Cancer Cure: A Treatment for Skin Cancer and New Hope for Other Cancers from Nature's Pharmacy by Bill E. Cham (Jan 1 2008)

(2) Cham B.E., "Saloasodine glycosides as anti-cancer agents: Pre-clinical and clinical studies." Asia Pacif. J. Pharmacol., 1994, 9:113-118.

(3) Cham B.E. "Solasodine Rhamnosyl Glycosides Specifically Bind Cancer Cell Receptors and Induce Apoptosis and Necrosis. Treatment for Skin Cancer and Hope for Internal Cancers." Research Journal of Biological Sciences 2007 Volume: 2 Issue: 4 Page No.: 503-514

(4) B. E. Cham and T. R. Chase, "Solasodine Rhamnosyl Glycosides Cause Apoptosis in Cancer Cells, Do They Also Prime the Immune System Resulting in Long Term Protection Against Cancer?" Planta Medica, in Press.

(5) Cham, B. E., B. Daunter and R. Evans, 1992. Topical treatment of malignant and premalignant skin cancers by very low concentrations of a standard mixture of salasodine glycosides. Clin. Digest Series Dermatol., 1992.

(6) Punjabi, S., I. Cook, P. Kersey, R. Marks, A. Finlay, G. Sharpe, et al. "A double blind, multi-centre parallel group study of BEC-5 cream in basal cell carcinoma." Eur. Acad. Dermatol. Venereol. 2000. 14:47-60.

(7) Cerio, R. and S. Punjabi, 2002. "Clinical appraisal of BEC5." Barts and the London NHS.

(8) Cham, B. E., B. Daunter and R. Evans, "Topical treatment of malignant and premalignant skin cancers by very low concentrations of a standard mixture of salasodine glycosides." Clin. Digest Series Dermatol., 1992.

(9) Cham, B.E., 1994. "Solasodine glycosides as anti-cancer agents: Pre-clinical and clinical studies." Asia Pacif. J. Pharmacol., 9:113-118

(10) B. E. Cham, "Cancer Intralesion Chemotherapy with Solasodine Rhamnosyl Glycosides," Research Journal Biological Sciences, Vol. 3, 2008, pp. 1008-1017.

(11) Cham, B.E., 2007. Solasodine rhamnosyl glycosides specifically bind cancer cell receptors and induce apoptosis and necrosis. Treatment for skin cancer and hope for internal cancers." Res. J. Biol. Sci., 2007, 2 (4): 503-514.

(12) Cham, B.E., "Saloasodine glycosides as anti-cancer agents: Pre-clinical and clinical studies." Asia Pacif. J. Pharmacol., 1994 9:113-118.

(13) L. Sun, Y. Zhao, H. Yuan, X. Li, A. Cheng and H. Lou,"Solamargine, a Steroidal Alkaloid Glycoside, Induces Oncosis in Human K562 Leukemia and Squamous Cell Carcinoma KB Cells," Cancer Chemotherapy and Pharmacology, Vol. 65, No. 4, 2010, pp. 1125-1130.

(14) Tania Robyn Chase, "CuradermBEC5 for Skin Cancers, Is It? An Overview." Journal of Cancer Therapy, 2011, 2, 728-745 Published Online December 2011

(15) L. Y. Shiu, L. C. Chang, C. H. Liang, Y. S. Huang, H. M.Sheu and K. W. Kuo, "Solamargine Induces Apoptosis and Sensitizes Breast Cancer Cells to Cisplatin," Food Chemistry Toxicology, Vol. 45, No. 11, 2007, pp. 2155-2164

(16) Van der Most RG, "Antitumor efficacy of the novel chemotherapeutic agent coramsine is potentiated by cotreatment with CpG-containing oligodeoxynucleotides." J Immunother 2006 Mar-Apr;29(2):134-42.

(17) Millward M, Powell A, Tyson S, Daly P, Ferguson R, Carter S. "Phase I trial of coramsine SBP002 in patients with advanced solid tumors. Abstract of presentation at 2005 ASCO Annual Meeting." J. Clin. Oncol. 23

Berries

Cranberries

History of cranberries

Cranberries are red, glossy, tart berries related to the blueberry. They belong to the genus *Vaccinium*. Cranberries are found in North America, northern Europe and northern Asia., growing in low trailing vines that sit atop large sandy bogs.

The cultivated berry is larger than the wild species. The most commonly cultivated species of cranberry is Vaccinium oxycoccos. Another cultivated variety is bigger and is called Vaccinium macrocarpon.

Cranberries were cooked and eaten at celebrations, including Thanksgiving, by the American Indians. Cranberry consumption was picked up as a tradition in the beginning of the 18th century by the New Englanders. Commercial cultivation and export began in this era as well. Popular places for cultivating cranberries include Wisconsin, Oregon, the New England states, Washington, Great Britain and Scandinavia.

Peak season for cranberries runs from October through December.

Due to the tart taste of cranberries, commercial cranberry juice is usually diluted and sweetened, or mixed with apple juice or other berry juices.

Medicinal use of cranberrries

The link between Cranberry juice and cancer protection has recently been found. Before that, however, cranberries were widely used to treat other medical conditions. Cranberry juice and cranberries have been found to prevent and treat bladder infections. They have also been found to lower the LDL or "bad" cholesterol and raise HDL or "good" cholesterol. Stroke recovery is enhanced with cranberry juice as well. Cranberries were traditionally used as an astringent and to stop bleeding. Their antibiotic effect was known by the end of the 18th century.

Cranberries are best known as a natural treatment for infections, particularly bladder infections. The active ingredient seems to be hippuric acid, which acidifies the urine and prevents bacteria from sticking to the wall of the bladder. The bacteria are flushed out through the urinary tract. The berry also contains proanthocyanidins, which are antioxidants that lessen the adherence of bacteria to the wall of the bladder. Cranberries are also used to treat bacterial respiratory infections. They also act against a common organism that causes stomach ulcers and stomach cancer: Helicobacter pylori or H. pylori.

Cranberries Against Cancer

Cranberry juice and cranberries contain proanthocyanidins that prevent cancers from getting a blood supply. Without a blood supply, small cancers remain small and cannot grow because they receive no nourishment.

Cranberries, in vitro, have been found to kill ovarian, prostate and brain cancer, as well as breast cancer. This is thought to be related to the cranberry's high concentration of proanthocyanidin-A compounds. These chemicals are unique to cranberries, and so far have not been found in other types of foods. The exact chemical mechanism of their action is unknown.

One study showed that a preparation made from 27% cranberry juice and platinum-based chemotherapy made the chemotherapy six times more effective against ovarian cancer. The amount of juice used in this in-vitro study would be equivalent of 1 cup of juice consumed by a patient.[1]

It has not been tested as extensively in other types of cancers but there is every reason to believe that the combination of cranberries and platinum-based chemotherapy will work on many different types of cancer.

In the US, ovarian cancer is the fifth leading cause of cancer death in women and is the leading cause of death due to gynecological malignancies.

It should be noted that cranberry juice does not represent a cure in and of itself for cancer. It is an adjunctive therapy that makes the chemotherapy more effective.

Instructions

Data indicate that whole, fresh cranberries work better than extracts made from cranberries. This is true of both the anti-cancer and antibiotic properties.

Ideally you should drink unsweetened, freshly-made cranberry juice, but it is very bitter. When using cranberry juice for medicinal purposes, take 2 ounces of cranberry juice (unsweetened) and mix it with 8 ounces of water for best overall taste and effectiveness.

Suppliers

If you must purchase a prepared product, R.W.Knudsen cranberry juice is very high in polyphenols.

References

(1) Singh Ajay, et al., "Cranberry proanthocyanidins are cytotoxic to human cancer cells and sensitize platinum-resistant ovarian cancer cells to paraplatin." Phytotherapy Research, 26 Jan 2009, 23: 1066–1074)

Raspberries

Two "berry" Good Solutions To Cancer

One promising and totally risk-free breakthrough comes from ordinary red raspberries. A researcher at the Medical University of South Carolina (MUSC) has found a nutrient in this delicious fruit that prevents the division of tumor cells. It is not necessary to eat raspberries every day to get the benefit, as fruit concentrate was used in the study.

The active ingredient seems to be ellagic acid, a polyphenol antioxidant found in numerous fruits and vegetables such as raspberries, strawberries, cranberries, pomegranates, walnuts, and pecans. The compound occurs naturally in plants in the form of ellagitannin. It inhibits DNA mutation through its antioxidant action, prevents the destruction of the P53 gene by cancer cells, and prevents mutagenic and carcinogenic compounds from binding with DNA by masking the binding sites.

Dr. Daniel Nixon of MUSC began his research on ellagic acid in 1993. His study used raspberry extract, which contains the entire ellagitannin complex.

Dr. Nixon's in-vitro study demonstrated that ellagic acid causes cervival cancer cells to undergo apoptosis. He wrote, "DNA synthesis basically stops for a period of time, and in our study, a very profound apoptotic cell death occurred among human cervical cancer cells approximately 36 hours after being exposed to ellagic acid."[1]

Dr. Nixon followed a number of patients, some with normal colons, others with precancerous lesions, each of whom ate 1 cup of raspberries once a day, providing 40 mg ellagitannin complex. The patients had colonic biopsies every 3 months. The study is yet unpublished, but Dr. Nixon stated that he noted a decrease in abnormal cell proliferation in the group fed raspberry puree.

Dr. Nixon studied cervical cancer cells, but tests by other reearchers reveal similar results for colon, prostate, breast, skin, pancreatic, and other cancers.

While Dr. Nixon used raspberry extract, other labs have used pure ellagic acid, either naturally-derived or synthetic, with similar results.

The amount of ellagic acid used in the Dr. Nixon's in-vitro tests would be equivalent to eating one cup of raspberries per day.

Black Raspberries

Black raspberries have anti-inflammatory, antioxidant, anti-cancer, and anti-neurodegenerative properties.

Black raspberries are extremely effective in preventing colorectal tumors, according to a 2010 University of Illinois study published in *Cancer Prevention Research*. Colorectal cancer is the third most common cancer and the second leading cause of cancer-related death in America, according to the National Cancer Institute.

Dr. Wancai Yang fed freeze-dried black raspberries to two strains of mice bred to develop intestinal tumors. He found reduced tumor incidence of 45% and reduced number of tumors of 60% in *Apc1638+/−* mice, and reduced tumor incidence and numbers of 50% in *Muc2−/−* mice. Black raspberries inhibit tumor development through suppression of a protein, known as beta-catenin, which binds to the APC gene.

The two strains of mice used in the study, Apc1638 and Muc2, each have a specific genetic defect, causing the mice to develop either intestinal tumors (the Apc1638 strain) or colitis (Muc2). Colitis is an inflammation of the large intestine, which can be a precursor to colorectal cancer.

Both mouse strains were randomly placed in one of two groups. For 12 weeks, both groups were fed a high-risk Western diet high in fat and low in calcium and vitamin D. One group received a supplement of 10% freeze-dried black raspberry powder for 12 weeks.

The researchers found that in both mouse strains the black raspberry supplements had a wide range of protective effects in the intestine, colon and rectum and decreased tumor formation.

"We saw the black raspberry as a natural product, very powerful, and easy to access," said Yang.[2]

References

(1) Daniel Nixon, "Alternative and Complementary Therapies in Oncology Care." Journal of Clinical Oncology, Vol 17, No 11s (November Supplement), 1999: pp 35-37

(2) Xiuli Bi, Wenfeng Fang, Li-Shu Wang, Gary D Stoner, Wancai Yang, "Black raspberries inhibit intestinal tumorigenesis in apc1638+/- and Muc2-/- mouse models of colorectal cancer." Cancer Prevention Research, 2010, Volume: 3, Issue: 11, Pages: 1443-1450.

Brazilian Peppertree

The Brazilian Peppertree is native to Argentina, Brazil and Paraguay. In both North and South America, three different species, *Schinus aroeira, Schinus molle,* and *Schinus terebinthifolius* are all interchangeably referred to as "peppertrees." All 3 varieties species have traditional medical uses. The Peppertree is a member of the family Anacardiaceae, which also contains poison ivy, poison oak, and poison sumac. Those with sensitivities to these plants should use Peppertree with caution.

The Peppertree was introduced into Florida in the mid-1800s as an ornamental plant, and is known there as the Christmas Berry or Florida Holly. Its bright red berries and brilliant green foliage are frequently incorporated into Christmas wreaths. It also grows in California, and is considered an invasive species in Hawaii.

Peppertree contains triterpenes and sesquiterpenes, known to have anti-tumor properties. Some of these compounds are unique to the Peppertree. Many of the Peppertree's medicinal effects are attributed to its essential oil. The berries can contain up to 5% essential oil, and the leaves up to 2%.

Traditionally, Peppertree bark and leaves are typically used as antiseptic wound cleansers, and as treatment for nasopharyngeal bacterial infections. They have also been used to treat infections throughout the body, including bronchitis, eye infections, gingivitis, tuberculosis, urogenital infections such as gonorrhea, and warts; and also non-infectious conditions such as depression, hypertension, menstrual disorders, and rheumatism.

All parts of Peppertree, including its leaves, bark, fruit, seeds, resin, and oleoresin (also called "balsam") have been used by traditional healers in South America. The plant has an ancient history of use and is shown in ancient religious artifacts and on idols of the Chilean Amerindians.

In the 1990s a patent was awarded to a medicine containing Peppertree oil to be used against *Pseudomonas* and *Staphylococcus* infection in humans and animals.

In the 1970's the plant showed effectiveness against tumors in a study conducted with patients who suffered from various types of cancer. The testing and research monitored cell activity as well as bacterial activity of several strains.

In 1976, it was found in a medicinal plant screening study to have anti-tumor effects.[1]

One research team identified 42 compounds in Peppertree essential oil, accounting for 97.2% of the total oil. The major constituents were alpha and beta-pinene. The essential oil was cytotoxic to several tumor cell lines, especially against breast cancer and leukemia. The oil also displayed weak antioxidant effects. The main mechanism of cancer cell death was apoptosis.[2]

The antitumor effects of polyphenols purified from the Peppertree (Schinus terebinthifolius) were tested on the androgen-insensitive DU145 human prostate cancer cell line. An F3 fraction purified from leaf extract inhibited cancer cell proliferation more than 30 times compared to the crude essential oil.

The F3 polyphenol fraction induced G0/G1 cell growth arrest and cell apoptosis by activating lysosomes, intracellular organelles that can autodigest the cell.[3]

Schinus Molle extract inhibited the growth of human liver cancer cells in-vitro.[4]

Caution

Peppertree has an anti-hypertensive effect, and patients using blood-pressure medication should use Peppertree with caution.

Not to be used during pregnancy.

Long-term, chronic use of Peppertree is not advised, as it has strong antibacterial effects and may lead to die-off of friendly bacteria in the digestive tract. Supplements of probiotics and digestive enzymes are advisable if this plant is used for longer than one month.

Instructions

For Brazilian Peppertree (Schinus molle) bark extracted in distilled water and 40% alcohol, dosage is:

60 drops (2 ml) 2-3 times daily.

Supplier

$23 for the 2 Oz extract on Ebay

References

(1) Bhakuni, D., et al. "Screening of Chilean plants for anticancer activity. I." Lloydia 1976; 39(4): 225–43.

(2) Diaz, C., et al. "Chemical composition of Schinus molle essential oil and its cytotoxic activity on tumour cell lines." Nat. Prod. Res. 2008; 22(17): 1521-34.

(3) Queires, L., et al. "Polyphenols purified from the Brazilian aroeira plant (Schinus terebinthifolius, Raddi) induce apoptotic and autophagic cell death of DU145 cells." Anticancer Res. 2006 Jan-Feb; 26(1A): 379-87.

(4) Ruffa, M. J., et al. "Cytotoxic effect of Argentine medicinal plant extracts on human hepatocellular carcinoma cell line." J. Ethnopharmacol. 2002; 79(3): 335–39

Cartilage (Shark & Bovine)

Cartilage has been widely used since the 1950s to treat both osteoarthritis, inflammatory conditions and cancer. It was popularized in the 1992 book "Sharks Don't Get Cancer: How Shark Cartilage Could Save Your Life," written by Dr. I William Lane, Ph.D, who was subsequently interviewed on the news program 60 Minutes.

Dr. Lane founded Lane Labs, which sells shark cartilage even today. However, in 2000, the Federal Trade Commission fined Dr. Lane $1 million for making health claims for his supplement. He was barred from promoting his product, or any other shark cartilage supplement, as a preventative or cure cancer.

Cartilage from a variety of species has documented anti-inflammatory, anti-allergenic and anti-angiogenesis properties.[1]

It is usually taken orally, but may also be administered intravenously.

Sharks

Sharks have skeletons composed entirely of cartilage, and they have no bone marrow. The function of the bone marrow, which produces immunocytes in other species, is provided by two completely unique immune organs, the Leydig's and Epigonal organs, that are poorly understood by biologists. Sharks are thought to be the earliest species to have developed a sophisticated immune system complete with immunoglobin, T-cell receptors, MHCs and RAG proteins.[2]

Sharks have an average lifespan of 25 years, but scientists believe they can live to be 100 years old or more.

Actually, just to set the record straight, sharks do ocassionally develop cancer, though at an impressively low rate. This may be because they have an innate resistance to the disease, and also because they are pelagic fish which live in clean, deep sea water which is relatively free of pollutants.

Substances such as aflatoxin, which reliably produce tumors in other animal test subjects, do not have this effect on nurse sharks.[3]

However, in 2004, biologist Dr. Gary Ostrander and his colleagues at the University of Hawaii, published a survey of the Registry for Tumors in Lower Animals, stating that his team had found 42 tumors in Chondrichthyes species (the class of cartilaginous fish that includes sharks, rays and skates). Findings included 12 malignant cancers as well as metastatic cancer. Two sharks had multiple tumors, suggesting individual susceptability or exposure to high levels of carcinogens. There were even tumors found in the shark's cartilage itself.[4]

The cartilaginous skeleton of the shark makes up approximately 6% of the shark's body weight, compared to animals with bony skeletons, in which cartilage makes up approximately .5-.6% of total body weight. This makes sharks an inviting target for supplement producers seeking to obtain cartilage.

Marine biologists and enviromentalists are appalled at the ongoing slaughter of sharks, both as a food item and for shark fin soup. Sharks reproduce slowly, and are being harvested at the unsustainable rate of at least 100 million per year. It is difficult to say how much of this situation can be blamed on the supplement industry, as a great deal of shark cartilage is derived from sharks caught as part of the food fishery, which would otherwise go to waste.

Though shark cartilage shows superior biological activity compared to cartilage from other species, the diminishing number of sharks may someday force manufacturers to source their supplements from more sustainable sources, such as bovine cartilage. It is possible that fractionization and concentration of the active ingredients would allow a comparable product to be made from the cartilage of other species.

Studies

Cartilage itself is devoid of blood vessels.

In the 1970s, Henry Brem and Judah Folkman at the Johns Hopkins School of Medicine first deduced that since cartilage lacks blood vessels, it must contain some biological factor inhibiting their formation.

This development of a blood supply, called angiogenesis, is vital to the growth of malignant tumors, and any substance that can prevent this process is of interest to medical researchers.

Brem and Folkman discovered that inserting cartilage from baby rabbits alongside tumors in animal subjects completely prevented tumor growth. Further research showed calf cartilage had similar anti-angiogenic effects.[5]

Subsequently, these researchers isolated the protein fraction in cartilage responsible for the anti-angiogenesis effects. This fraction contained several different proteins, the major one having a molecular weight of about 16,000 daltons.[6]

Another researcher, Robert Langer, repeated Brem and Folkman's experiment using shark cartilage. Since shark skeletons are entirely composed of cartilage, Langer felt they would be a more abundant source of therapeutic material. As expected, the shark cartilage, like calf and rabbit cartilage, inhibited tumor angiogenesis.

Animal studies of tumor neovascularization show that in a weight-for-weight comparison, shark cartilage has approximately 1,000 times more antiangiogenic activity than bovine cartilage. Protein composition of cartilage from different species varies greatly. In addition, the method of extraction is extremely important in the quality of the resulting product. Yield of bioactive proteins was substantially greater after a 41-day extraction period, compared to a 1-day extraction process for calf cartilage.

It was initially postulated that the anti-angiogenesis action of cartilage was correlated with its inhibition of proteolytic enzymes, as these would be needed by the tumor in order to remodel tissue to accommodate new blood vessels; however, this turned out not to be the case.[7]

Bioactive molecules extracted from shark cartilage range in size from 1000 to 35,000 daltons or more. The intestinal membrane is permeable to macromolecules of up to about 50,000 daltons, so these molecules are likely to be absorbed easily through the intestinal tract.

Human Studies

Clinical studies have produced mixed results.

Dr. Lane, who initially introduced shark cartilage, oversaw a Cuban study involving 29 Stage III and Stage IV terminal patients with various forms of cancer, all diagnosed by 2 physicians as having a life expectancy of less than 6 months.[8]

This study, which ran from late 1992 to early 1993, was covered by 60 Minutes, which spent $350,000 on this segment of their show, and thoroughly vetted the research to be sure they were not observing a fraud. The documentary team made 4 visits to Cuba, documenting the health improvements of the patients. 2-1/2 years later, 50% of the patients were still alive, including all 9 brain tumor patients.

Some criticized the methodology of the study, and claimed the response rate of the Cuban study was only 20%, not 50%.[9] However, to have any level of response at all from terminal cancer patients is quite remarkable.

In further patient studies, Dr. Lane found different response rate for different types of cancer. Best results were achieved against tumors of the prostate, breast, brain and central nervous system, with an almost 90% response rate. Ovarian cancer had a response rate of 70%. Liver cancer had a good response. Lung cancer responded in 50% of cases. Pancreatic cancer responded at high doses, up to 140 gms of cartilage per day. Treatment of other tumors had less dramatic results.

An interview with Dr. Lane:

http://www.consumerhealth.org/articles/

However, some FDA-approved American studies produced no positive results.

Mice implanted with SCCVII carcinoma were fed water solutions of two commercially available shark cartilage extracts, Sharkilage and MIA Shark Powder, at doses ranging from 5-100 mg daily for 25 days. Compared to a control group of non-treated animals, the test subjects did not show any inhibition of tumor growth.[10]

In one human study, 60 patients with advanced, previously treated cancer were given oral supplements of shark cartilage (Cartilade) at a dose of 1 g/kg daily in three divided doses. Of the 60 patients, 47 were available to be evaluated at the end of the study. No complete or partial positive responses to the treatment were noted, and the trajectory of disease was similar to that of comparable patients given only palliative care. Researchers concluded that shark cartilage was "inactive in patients with advanced-stage cancer and had no salutary effect on quality of life."[11]

Another human study was a two-group, randomized, placebo-controlled, double-blind, clinical trial. 83 patients with terminal breast or colorectal carcinoma were randomly assigned to receive either a shark cartilage supplement or an identical-appearing and smelling placebo 3 to 4 times each day. The Benefin brand of shark cartilage from Lane Labs was used, at the manufacturer's recommended dosage level, starting at 24 grams per day and increasing to 96 grams per day as tolerated by the patients. No difference in outcome was observed between the two groups.[12]

AE-941 (Neovastat), a standardized shark cartilage extract manufactured by the pharmaceutical company Aeterna Zentaris of Quebec City, was recently tested in a Phase III trial on patients with inoperable stage III non-small cell lung cancer. The study, a randomized, double-blinded, placebo-controlled trial, involved 379 subjects who were treated with chemoradiotherapy and either AE-941 or a placebo, given during and after chemoradiotherapy. AE-941 did not improve overall patient survival.[13]

Dr. Lane himself states that there is a great difference in quality between different brands of supplements, which may explain some of the discrepancies in research results. According to Dr. Lane, processing cartilage with heat destroys the active factors, and unfortunately many supplement manufacturers use the cheapest manufacturing techniques possible. However, one of the unsuccessful studies used Dr. Lane's own product.

Instructions

The recommended dose is 1 gram per kg of body weight, or 1 gram per 2.2 lbs of body weight.

If using shark cartilage powder rather than capsules, it is advised that it be mixed in a blender with pulpy juice such as tomato or fruit nectar. Up to 20 grams (4 level teaspoons) should be mixed with 6-8 ounces of juice. This amount should be consumed 3-4 times daily.

It can also be mixed with 3-4 oz of fluid and used in a retention enema.

According to Dr. Lane, treatment must be continued for at least 6-8 weeks to produce results, though ocassionally improvement will occur after 1 month. One course of treatment can last up to 20 weeks, and after that, the patient must stay on a maintenance dose of 10-15 grams per day. If the cancer recurs, the higher dose must be resumed.

Other chronic illnesses, such as arthritis or psoriasis, may also improve from shark cartilage.

Caution

Do not use during pregnancy or during initial wound healing, as these processes require angiogenesis. In patients who have had a recent heart attack, it will prevent the formation of new collateral circulation.

It may stop menstruation in women, as the monthly buildup of uterine endometrium involves angiogenesis.

Side effects are limited to gastric upset.

Supplier

Anyone interested in using shark cartilage should probably buy the Lane Labs brand, as it is the original product and has documented positive results associated with it.

http://www.compassionet.com/c-140-shark-cartilage.aspx

References

(1) Prudden, John and Balessa, "The biological activity of bovine cartilage preparations." Seminars in Arthritis and Rheumatism, 1974 Vol 3 (4):287-320)

(2) Flajnik MF, Rumfelt LL., "The immune system of cartilaginous fish." Curr Top Microbiol Immunol 248, 249–270, 2000

(3) Luer CA&Luer WH., "Acute and chronic exposure of nurse sharks to aflatoxin." Fed Proc 41, 925, 1982.

(4) Ostrander GK et al, "Shark cartilage, cancer and the growing threat of pseudoscience." Cancer Res 64, 8485-8491 (2004)

(5) Brem H, Folkman J., "Inhibition of tumor angiogenesis mediated by cartilage." J Exp Med. 141, 427–439, 1975.

(6) Langer R, Brem H, Falterman K, Folkman J., "Isolations of a cartilage factor that inhibits tumor neovascularization." Science 193, 70-72,1976.

(7) Lee A, Langer R, "Shark cartilage contains inhibitors of tumor angiogenesis." Science 221 (4616): 1185-7, 1983

(8) Jose R. Menendez Lopez, M.D.,Ph.D., Jose E. Femandez-Britto Rodriguez, M.D., Ph.D, D. Sc, I.W. Lane Ph.D, "Shark Cartilage Administration in Human Advanced Cancer Diseases." Alternative Research Data Vault, 6941 58th Way,Pinellas Park, Florida 33780

(9) Mathews J, "Media feeds frenzy over shark cartilage as cancer treatment." J Natl Cancer Inst. 1993;85:1190–1191).

(10) Horsman MR, Alsner J, Overgaard J, "The Effect of shark cartilage extracts on the growth and metastatic spread of the SCCVII carcinoma." Acta Oncologica 37, 441-445 ,1998

(11) Miller DR et al. "Phase I/II trial of the safety and efficacy of shark cartilage in the treatment of advanced cancer." J. Clin. Oncol 16, 3649-3655,1998.

(12) Loprinzi, C.L. et al., "Evaluation of shark cartilage in patients with advanced cancer: a North Central Cancer Treatment Group trial." Cancer 104, 176-182, 2005

(13) Charles Lu, et al., "Chemoradiotherapy With or Without AE-941 in Stage III Non–Small Cell Lung Cancer: A Randomized Phase III Trial." J Natl Cancer Inst (2010) 102 (12): 859-865

Cat's Claw

Cat's Claw, a plant which derives its popular name from its claw-shaped thorns, is a woody vine native to the Amazon rainforest of South and Central America. Traditionally, medicines have been made from the inner bark and root, taken in the form of capsules, tea and extracts. It contains several biologically active alkaloids, tannins, and phytochemicals. It has been used to treat cancer, arthritis, gastrointestinal disease, and as a contraceptive. Uncaria tomentosa has also been used as an adjunct to standard AIDS treatment.

Cancer patients who take Cat's Claw in combination with standard cancer therapies report a lessening of side effects of chemotherapy and radiation, such as hair loss, anorexia, nausea, and secondary infections due to immune system suppression.

There are two species of Cat's Claw, *Uncaria tomentosa* and *Uncaria guianensis*. Each subtype has a different chemical profile and unique medicinal properties, a fact often ignored by supplement manufacturers. Uncaria tomentosa has been heavily researched for its anti-cancer and immunological effects, while Uncaria guianensis is used to treat osteoarthritis.

Some supplement manufacturers state that Uncaria tomentosa is further divided into 2 subtypes. One subtype of Uncaria tomentosa has roots containing mostly pentacyclic (5-carbon-ring) oxindole alkaloids, including pteropodine, speciophylline, and mitraphylline. These have been shown in in-vivo studies to have desirable immune-strengthening effects.

The second chemotype contains tetracyclic oxindole alkaloids which supposedly counteract the immune-strengthening effects of the pentacyclic alkaloids, suppress cardiac function, and produce neurological effects such as loss of coordination and sedation.

Without chemical testing, it is impossible to tell the proportion of alkaloids in a given plant. Wild-harvested plants vary widely due to natural genetic variation and environmental factors. One researcher, noting the variable quality of many Cat's Claw products, went so far as to state, "those wishing to use cat's claw are best advised to restrict consumption to products certified to be free (or at least not containing more than 0.02%) of tetracyclic oxindole alkaloids as determined by suitable analytical methods."[1]

However, other herbalists have noted that plants of the same species can show wide variations in biochemistry, and the theory that there are two varieties of Uncaria tomentosa has not been proven. Another confounding factor is the unscrupulous sale of the more readily available lowland Uncaria guianensis as Uncaria tomentosa.

Multiple studies of Cat's Claw have shown therapeutic effect with whole bark extract, without using elaborate methods to fractionate the product.

Studies

Klaus Keplinger did the first research on Cat's Claw in the 1970s and 1980s, and his studies were the basis for the approval of Cat's Claw as a herbal medicine in Austria and Germany. Numerous further studies in Europe and Peru found that oxindole alkaloids can increase the function of the immune system by up to 50%. The oxindole alkaloids display this action either as whole-bark extract or as individual fractionated compounds. Keplinger obtained a patent for his extraction method of oxindole compounds (US patent 5,723,625 March 3, 1998).

The compounds found in Cat's Claw act as anti-inflammatory, antioxidant and anticancer agents.[2]

One research paper, a meta-analysis of 19 existing in-vivo and in-vitro studies, found Cat's Claw induced apoptosis by activation of caspase-3 in some tumor cell lines, and also inhibited the growth of normal T and B lymphocytes by non-toxic and non-apoptotic means. It has immune-stimulating, anti-inflammatory, and cancer preventative actions. SAOS osteosarcoma, MCF7 breast cancer and HeLa cervical cancer cells were treated with a 120 mg/ml and a 240 mg/ml water extract of Cat's Claw. After 96 hours of exposure, 84-96% of all 3 tumor cell lines were killed by the 240 mg/ml extract, compared to 23% (SAOS), 51% (MCF7) and 83% (HeLa) by the 120 mg/ml extract.[3]

 Recent studies indicate that at least six of the Cat's Claw vine's alkaloids can increase the functioning of the immune system by up to 50%.

Caution

Do not take while pregnant.

Instructions

Cat's Claw taken orally in capsule form is very poorly absorbed. It is best taken as a double-extracted water/alcohol tincture or as a strong tea.

If you plan to make your own preparation, add ½ tsp of lemon juice per cup of water to your tea while extracting it. This will produce a tea with more alkaloids and fewer tannins.

Supplier

Cat's claw powder is widely available.

Whole World botanicals sells tincture which has been documented to be effective in clinical studies.

References

(1) Tyler, Varro E., "An herb to forget – cat's claw – Uncaria tomentosa." Nutrition Forum, Sept-Oct, 1997

(2) Heitzman ME, Neto CC, Winiarz E, Vaisberg AJ, Hammond GB, "Ethnobotany, phytochemistry and pharmacology of Uncaria (Rubiaceae)." Phytochemistry, Volume 66, Issue 1, January 2005, Pages 5-29

(3) Laura De Martino, et al., "Proapoptotic effect of Uncaria tomentosa extracts." J Ethnopharmacol, 2006 Aug 11;107(1):91-4

Chaparral

Chaparral (*Larrea tridentata*) is commonly referred to as the creosote bush. It is a common shrub with waxy leaves found in the American South-West, and it is usually prepared in the form of a tea.

Traditonally, it has been used by Native Americans to treat gastrointestinal diseases such as stomach ulcers and bowel disorders, cancers, and respiratory illnesses such as bronchitis, colds and flu. It is said to be beneficial to the walls of capillaries throughout the body. It has been made into poultices for sore joints, and charraral tea or lotion is applied topically for skin diseases such as ringworm and athletes' foot. Chaparral will also relieve skin dryness, brittle hair and nails and cracks in the hands or feet. It is also used to treat diabetes.

The plant was listed as a bronchial antiseptic and expectorant in the U.S. Pharmacopoeia for approximately a century. For many years, NDGA was used by the food industry as an antioxidant to prevent rancidity in foods, until a scare over possible renal and hepatic toxicity caused the FDA to remove it from the GRAS (generally regarded as safe) list in in the late 1990s.

Thousands of patient testimonials credit chaparral for tumor remissions and complete cures.

The pharmaceutical industry is currently trying to out-do nature by investigating the anti-cancer activity of what they believe is chaparral's "active ingredient," Nordihydroguaiaretic acid (NDGA). A derivative of NDGA, called terameprocol (EM-1421), is still in the early stages of laboratory testing as an anti-cancer drug.

NDGA inhibits several enzyme reactions, such as lipo-oxygenase, which cause unhealthy inflammatory and immune-system responses. It also reduces inflammatory histamine responses in the lung, which helps asthma symptoms. NDGA is one of the strongest antioxidants known.

Chapparal can improve liver function, increasing metabolism of toxins, increasing the synthesis of fatty acids into high density lipids (HDL, the so-called "good cholesterol"), while decreasing LDL (the type of cholesterol linked to heart disease). The strong antioxidant effects repair free radical damage caused by drugs such as amphetamines and cocaine.

Chapparel contains flavonoids and ligans, which in addition to their anti-oxidant properties also act as antibiotics, anti-fungals, and anti-virals. Chapparal's anti-viral action has led to research about its ability to inhibit HIV and Herpes simplex-1 and 2 in cell cultures. It has been used to reduce symptoms of shingles and herpes, and also helps treat sores from Kaposi's sarcoma in AIDS patients.

Studies

A study published in the *Journal of Dental Research* found that dental cavities were reduced by 75% with the use of chaparral mouthwash.

A water-soluble derivative of NDGA blocks the AIDS virus from binding to cells and initiating infection.[1]

Further NDGA derivatives are being tested as possible therapy for AIDS.[2]

Researchers at the University of Nevada investigated the activity of NDGA and discovered it to be a powerful inhibitor of mitochondrial enzymes, which in turn inhibits cancer growth.

NDGA was shown to reduce the occurrence of colon cancer in rats fed a carcinogenic chemical.[3]

NDGA prevents genetic damage caused by carcinogens.[4]

NDGA prevents the development of breast cancer in animals.[5]

Leukemia cell cultures were inhibited by NDGA.[6]

Human brain cancer cell growth was also inhibited by NDGA.[7] Cancer cell inhibition was exhaustively studied in the doctoral thesis of J. Zemora.[8]

NDGA caused documented regression of deadly melanoma in one patient.[9]

A 1970 study at the University of Utah sponsored by the NCI produced negative results. 45 patients with terminal cancer drank chaparral tea or ingested doses of pure NDGA orally. Only 4 experienced a minor decrease in tumor size, with regressions lasting from 10 days to 20 months. However, tumors grew larger in some patients treated with chaparral, leading the researchers to conclude that chaparral tea was an ineffective anti-cancer treatment.[10]

Further studies to clarify these contradictory results found that low levels of NDGA actually stimulated growth of some types of cancer cells, while higher concentrations suppressed growth.

NDGA has multiple effects on cell proliferation, apoptosis, differentiation, and chemotaxis.[11]

NDGA belongs to a class of compounds that stabilize microtubules in NRK (normal rat kidney) cells, preventing their function in the mitotic process and thus stopping cell division. However, this action protects microtubules from depolymerization by drugs such as vinblastine, nocodazole, ilimaquinone, and colchicine.[12] As such, the compound may interfere with some forms of chemotherapy.

Caution

There are more than a dozen reported instances in which signs of liver damage showed up after several months of taking chaparral leaf, including 4 cases of cirrhosis, and 2 cases of liver failure neccesitating a liver transplant.

The time required for the development of liver problems is usually within 3-12 weeks after beginning the chaparral, but it may also occur after years of chronic consumption.

The toxicity presents clinically with an illness resembling viral hepatitis, with laboratory findings of extreme elevations in serum aminotransferase levels (AST and ALT), but minimal increase in alkaline phosphatase (liver enzymes which tend to be raised in cases of liver damage). Autoimmune and allergic reactions are uncommon. Even in cases where patients do not complain of symptoms, liver enzymes may be raised.[13,14]

A researcher commenting on one of these cases warned that "the public and the medical profession must be wary of all 'harmless' non-prescription medications, whether purchased in pharmacies or elsewhere."[15]

Some of the patients studied were also taking other substances such as alcohol and prescription drugs at the same time, complicating any investigation of toxicity.[16]

It is unknown whether chaparral is toxic to anyone at sufficiently high doses, or only to patients with some genetic inability to metabolize it.

It has also been reported that chaparral can cause kidney damage, including renal cysts and renal failure.

In 1992 manufacturers voluntarily restricted sales until the reports of hepatotoxicity were investigated. Following a lengthy review, a government-appointed research panel concluded, "no clinical data was found... to indicate chaparral is inherently a hepatic toxin." After reviewing this report in 1994, the FDA concluded chaparral did not pose a significant threat to consumer safety. The American Herbal Products Association (AHPA), recommends the following warning be printed on all chaparral product labels: *Seek advice from a health practitioner before use if you have had, or may have had liver disease. Discontinue use if nausea, fever, fatigue, or jaundice occurs.*

However, few of the toxicity reports involved the use of chaparral in its traditional form, as a tea, and a 2001 study by Heron and Yarnell, even prolonged ingestion of a 10% extract was not found to be toxic. Preparation method may be the key to avoiding toxicity. Only approximately 40% of the NDGA contained in the chaparral leaf dissolves into water used to make chaparral tea. Dried tablets of ground leaf swallowed whole deliver a much larger dose.[17]

Traditional healers used chaparral only as weak infusions to be consumed for 2 weeks or less.

The dosages found to create toxicity were capsules of 100 mg to 480 mg, or tablets of 65 mg to 100 mg, consumed at the rate of 4-15 per day for more than a month.[18,19,20]

Instructions

Use this substance with caution, preferably under medical supervision. Use as a tea, and not in capsule form. It should be avoided by patients with any form of liver disease. Do not combine with other drugs.

Suppliers

Dried chaparral in leaf or powder form can be found on Ebay for approximately $10-$12 per pound.

References

(1) Huang RC, Li Y, Giza PE. et al. "Novel antiviral agent tetraglycylated nordihydroguaiaretic acid hydrochloride as a host-dependent viral inhibitor". Antiviral Res. 2003 Mar;58(1):57-64

(2) Gnabre JN, Ito Y, Ma Y, Huang RC. "Isolation of anti-HIV-1 lignans from Larrea tridentata by counter-current chromatography." J Chromatogr A. 1996 Jan 8;719(2):353-64

(3) S. Birkenfeld et al, "Antitumor effects of inhibitors of arachidonic acid cascade on experimentally induced intestinal tumors", Dis Colon Rectum 1987; 30:43–6

(4) Shalini V.K.,"Fuel smoke condensate induced DNA damage in human lymphocytes and protection by turmeric (Curcuma longa)", Molecular Cell Biochemistry, 1990 Jun 1;95(1):21-30.

(5) McCormick D.L., Spicer A.M., "Nordihydroguaiaretic acid suppression of rat mammary carcinogenesis induced by N- methyl-/V-nitrosourea", Cancer Lett., 1987, 37, 139146.

(6) Miller A.M., Cullen M.K., Kobb S. M., Weiner R.S., "Effects of lipoxygenase and glutathione pathway inhibitors on leukemic cell line growth", Journal of Laboratory Clinical Medicine, 1989 Volume: 113, Issue: 3, Pages: 355-361

(7) Wilson D.E., "Effect of nordihydroguaiaretic acid on cultured rat and human glioma cell proliferation", Journal of Neurosurgery, 1989 Oct;71(4):551-7

(8) Zamora JM. 1984. Cytotoxic, Antimicrobial and Phytochemical Properties of Larrea tridentata Cav. Auburn, AL: Auburn University. Dissertation; Zamora JM, Mora EC, Parish EJ. 1992. "A comparison of the cytotoxicity of nordihydroguaiaretic acid and its derivatives". J Tenn Acad Sci 67:77–80

(9) Smart, C.R., et. al. "An interesting observation on nordihydroquaiaretic acid (nsc-4291; NDGA) and a patient with malignant melanoma--a preliminary

report". Cancer Chemotherapy Reports, Part 1, 5392), 147-151, 1969

(10) C.R. Smart et al, "Clinical experience with nordihydroguaiaretic acid— "chapparel tea" [sic] in the treatment of cancer", Rocky Mtn Med Journal, 1970 Nov; 39-43

(11) Arasaki K., et al., "Nordihydroguaiaretic Acid Affects Multiple Dynein-Dynactin Functions in Interphase and Mitotic Cells Molecular Pharmacology February 2007 vol. 71 no. 2 454-460

(12) Nakamura M,et al., "Nordihydroguaiaretic acid, of a new family of microtubule-stabilizing agents, shows effects differentiated from paclitaxel". Biosci Biotechnol Biochem 2003; 67: 151-157.).

(13) Sheikh NM, Philen RM, Love LA. "Chaparral-associated hepatotoxicity." Arch Intern Med 1997; 157: 913-9.

(14) Liu LU, Schiano TD. "Hepatotoxicity of herbal medicines, vitamins and natural hepatotoxins." In, Kaplowitz N, DeLeve LD, eds. Drug-induced liver disease. 2nd ed. New York: Informa Healthcare USA, 2007, pp. 733-54.

(15) Katz M, Saibil F. "Herbal hepatitis: subacute hepatic necrosis secondary to chaparral leaf." J Clin Gastroenterol 1990;12:203-6.

(16) Fleiss PM. "Chaparral and liver toxicity." JAMA 1995; 274: 871; author reply 871-2.

(17) Heron S, Yarnell E, "The safety of low-dose Larrea tridentata (DC) Coville (creosote bush or chaparral): a retrospective clinical study." J Altern Complement Med 2001 Apr;7(2):175-85.

(18) Bruneton J, Pharmacognosy, Phytochemistry, and Medicinal Plants, William Morrow and Co., New York, 1999

(19) Melgarejo and Cupp, Toxicology and Clinical Pharmacology of Herbal Products, 2000, pp 177-190 Humana Press, New Jersey, USA

(20) Alderman et al., "Cholestatic hepatitis after ingestion of chaparral leaf: confirmation by endoscopic retrograde cholangiopancreatography and liver biopsy." J Clin Gastroenterol 1994 Oct;19(3):242-7.

Crinum

Crinum Latifolium is a Vietnamese plant treasured for contributing to prostate and ovarian health. It is grown in Vietnamese family gardens and harvested as needed for medicinal use. If not used as a medicine, it is steamed or boiled and served as a vegetable dish, flavored with soy sauce.

In Vietnam, crinum is the standard first line of treatment for ovarian and prostate diseases. Phan Tung Chae, Ph.D., an internationally known herbalist, claims to have treated prostate cancer using only crinum.

Crinum was used in ancient times by Vietnamese royalty to enhance longevity. It is also known as "The Medicine for the King's Palace" and "Royal Female Herb."

The King of Cambodia treated his prostate cancer with crinum, and has experienced good health for a decade.

Traditional Chinese herbal medicine is well known in the West, but Vietnamese medicine has not been widely publicized.

Vietnamese research

Although much of the research on crinum focuses on its use for prostate diseases, it is increasingly being used to treat ovarian diseases as well.

The use of crinum for ovarian health began with studies by the Hoang family. Dr. Kha Hoang was the Chief Teacher and medical doctor for the Vietnamese royal family. In 1984, his daughter had multiple cysts on her ovary, and surgery was planned to remove it. Dr. Hoang gave her a tea made of crinum leaves, and the cysts disappeared within 6 weeks.

Today, three generations of the Hoang family practice integrated medicine. The family has used crinum in combination with other herbal medicines to treat a variety of prostate and ovarian conditions.

Biopsies have confirmed complete cures in 16 cases of advanced prostate cancer.

Many crinum studies have used a proprietary extract called CriLa, developed over 21 years by Dr. Nguyen Thi Ngoc Tram, an award-winning Pharmacologist. She produces the crinum on an organic plantation using a strain of crinum plants specially bred to contain high levels of active phytochemicals.

After 15 years of research reviews and clinical trials, the Ministry of Health in Vietnam approved CriLa for use in all hospitals and pharmacies in that country. Approximately 8,000 people in Vietnam take CriLa every month.

https://www.crilahealth.com/research

Studies

Most crinum patient studies deal with prostate disease; however, there are also documented individual case reports of female patients who used crinum to treat benign (non-cancerous) conditions such as fibroids and polycystic ovary syndrome. It is recommended in cases of gynecological cancer as well.

Phytochemical analysis of *Crinum* species has found more than 170 different compounds, mostly alkaloids of the *Amaryllidaceae* group, with a wide range of biological activity such as analgesic, anti-tumor, central nervous system, and antiviral effects.[1]

In 2001, the Vietnam Pharmaceutical Corporation published a report showing that aqueous extracts of Crinum leaves caused in-vitro and in-vivo activation of T-lymphocytes and slowed the growth of chemically induced sarcomas in rats.[2]

A 2009 in-vivo study on hamsters inoculated with myeloid (Graffi) tumors showed that CriLa crinum extract decreased tumor size and proliferation, and increased longevity of the test animals. 30 days into the study, all control (untreated) hamsters had died, whereas all in the group treated with crinum were still alive. The last of the crinum group died after 45 days.[3]

A recent in-vitro study found that crinum (CriLa) displays strong antioxidant and anti-inflammatory effects. It causes apoptosis in highly metastatic human prostate carcinoma cells, androgen-sensitive prostate adenocarcinoma cells, and benign prostate hyperplasia cells.[4]

92.6% Success In Treatment Of BPH Symptoms

Crinum is not only useful in treating prostate cancer. It also alleviates the symptoms of one of the most common male problems, enlarged prostate, or benign prostatic hyperplasia (BPH).

The usual symptom of BPH is frequent and sometimes painful urination.

The International Hospital in Vietnam conducted a 7-year study involving more than 500 BPH patients who were treated with crinum. 92.6% of patients had positive results, confirmed by measurements of prostate size and clinical evaluation by urologists.[5] In another Vietnamese study, 158 BPH patients consumed a Crinum-based herbal medication twice daily. The patients were evaluated by clinical and ultrasound examinations after 64 days. In 154 patients, or 97% of the study group, prostate size had returned to normal. A follow-up study 3 years later confirmed the high longterm success rate for those patients who completed therapy.[6]

In a 2005, researchers reported that "Crinum latifolium extract has a very good therapeutic effect on benign hyperthrophy of prostate (BHP)" based on tests performed by the National Institute of Traditional Medicine of Ho Chi Minh City, and the Institute of Aging Disorders of Hanoi. Crinum was administered to 627 patients with BHP. The patients had a 33-93% reduction in urinary symptoms, and 90% of patients tested showed a reduction in prostate size. A significant number of patients achieved normalization of prostate size and urinary health after three months of crinum therapy. No significant adverse reactions were noted.[7]

Instructions

CriLa for cancer treatment: take 5 tablets twice a day after meals for 9 weeks. Benign conditions : 3 tablets twice a day.

Supplier

Generic Crinum Latifolium tea is available for a very low price on Ebay. However, as with many plant products (Paw-paw and graviola come to mind), quality varies widely. Many varieties of Crinum plants look alike, but have huge variations in active phytochemicals.

CriLa tablets are a patented product derived from a known strain of crinum plants, standardized and guaranteed to contain active ingredients. These are sold on Ebay for $8 for 40 tablets, though volume discounts are available.

References

(1) Fennell CW, van Staden J. "Crinum species in traditional and modern medicine." Ethnopharmacol. 2001;78:15–26.; Tram NTN, Titorenkova TV, St Bankova V, Handjieva NV, Popov SS. Crinum L. (Amaryllidaceae)", Fitoterapia. 2002;73:183–208.

(2) Nguyen Thi Ngoc Trama, Maya Mitovab. "GC-MS of Crinum latifolium L. Alkaloids." Zeitschrift für Naturforschung B. (A Journal of Chemical Sciences). 57c, 239D242 (2002); received October 2/November 29, 2001

(3) Ilia Bankov, Elissaveta Zvetkova, "Influence of CriLa Medicine, Alkaloid- and Flavanoid Extracts (fractions) from Vietnamese Crinum latifolium (L.) on cancer disease in experimental animal models as well as on stimulation of the immune system against cancer : to use as raw materials producing Vietnamese drug which treat cancer." Bulgarian Academy of Sciences, 2009

(4) Marcel Jenny, Angela Wondrak, Elissaveta Zvetkova, Nguyen Thi Ngoc Tram, Phan Thi Phi Phi, Harald Schennach, Zoran Culig, Florian Ueberall, and Dietmar Fuchs, "Crinum Latifolium Leave Extracts Suppress Immune Activation Cascades in Peripheral Blood Mononuclear Cells and Proliferation of Prostate Tumor Cells." Sci Pharm. 2011 June; 79(2): 323–335)

(5) "Crinum latifolium, a promising and highly effective treatment for BPH, health and life". The Journal of Health Ministry of Vietnam, December 20, 2002, N 207.

(6) Doan Thu Nhu. "Crinum Latifolium in treatment of Benign Hypertrophy of prostate and cancers." Journal of Health and Life of Vietnamese Health Ministry, December 10, 2002, N 148

(7) Nguyen Thi Ngoc Trama, Maya Mitovab. GC-MS of Crinum latifolium L. Alkaloids, Zeitschrift für Naturforschung B. (A Journal of Chemical Sciences). 57c, 239D242 (2002); received October 2/November 29, 2001 "Crinum latifolium extract has a very good therapeutic effect on benign hyperthrophy of prostate (BHP)". Vietnamese central state news agency September 22, 2005.

Enzymes

Enzymes are biological *catalysts* or assistants. Enzymes consist of various types of proteins that work to drive the chemical reaction required for a specific action or nutrient. Enzymes can either begin a reaction or speed it up.

Cancer cells are protected by a protein-based coating, called "fibrin", that makes it difficult for the immune system to identify and destroy them. This sticky coating can be up to 15 times thicker than the membrane of normal cells. This is where metabolic enzymes are needed. The bulk of these enzymes are proteases, which means they speed up the breakdown of proteins. In sufficient quantities, they digest the protective fibrin membrane and expose the cancer cells to the immune system.

Pancreatic enzymes also activate macrophages and NK cells, modulate cellular adhesion molecules, cytokines and immune complexes. According to a 2001 study, three specific pancreatic enzymes (elastase, carboxypeptidase A, and lipase) caused macrophages to dramatically increase production of tumor necrosis factor-alpha (TNF-alpha) protein.[1]

Dr. Beard, who pioneered the theory that cancer is derived from stem cells, used enzymes successfully against tumors in both animal and human subjects.

Laetrile treatments frequently include the injection of protease enzymes directly into the tumor.

The most well-known enzymes are bromelain and papayin, which are also taken as digestive aids.

Take the enzymes on an empty stomach if possible, since if they are taken with food they will be used in the digestive process rather than being absorbed. However, if stomach irritation occurs, it is better to take them with food rather than discontinuing them altogether.

Wobenzyme is a reputable brand made of a proprietary combination of several different enzymes. It contains pancreatic as well as proteolytic enzymes. Proteolytic enzymes by themselves can be obtained cheaply through bulk vitamin suppliers such as vitamins.com.

References

(1) Jaffray C., "Specific pancreatic enzymes activate macrophages to produce tumor necrosis factor-alpha: role of nuclear factor kappa B and inhibitory kappa B proteins." Journal of Gastrointestinal Surgery, Aug 2000, vol 4 issue 4, 370-378

Fucoidan

In the pursuit of an effective cancer cure, Japanese researchers discovered a highly potent polysaccharide in brown seaweed. This polysaccharide, later named Fucoidan, makes up around 4 % of the total dry weight of numerous types of brown seaweed. It is found in kombu and other varieties of brown seaweed (wakame, mozuku, and hijiki).

Fucoidan is a sulfated polysaccharide with a very complex structure. This compound consists of xylose, galactose, glucuronic acid and sulfuric esterified L-fucose amongst other components. Fucoidan exists in two different molecules, as discovered at the Research Institute for Glycotechnology Advancement and Takara Shuzo's Biomedical Research Laboratories.

The researchers named these two different types U-Fucoidan and F-Fucoidan. The former possesses traces of glucuronic acid that makes up about 20% of the molecule. F-Fucoidan on the other hand is made up mainly of sulfated fucose.

Scientists have been performing research on fucoidan since around 1970, and subsequently, fucoidan has been the subject of approximately 700 papers published in the database of the National Library of Medicine.

Fucoidan-rich seaweeds have been used historically as a food in regions such as Hawaii, Korea, Japan, Polynesia and Tonga.

Sources of Fucoidan

It is best to procure the product from a reputable manufacturer and known source, as Fucoidan is derived from seaweed, and in many places, sea water is highly polluted. This is particularly important as studies have found that some kelp supplements are contaminated with heavy metals such as arsenic. The Fukushima accident has contaminated a large area along the Japanese coast with radiation.

Brown seaweed grows in every ocean, and it is harvested all around the world.

It grows luxuriantly in a 7,200 km stretch along the Indian coast. Brown sea weed, urchins and cucumbers also perform exceptionally well in the Gulf of Mannar, which lies between the southeastern tip of India and the west coast of Sri Lanka. This is a 10,500 square kilometer water body that supports over 3600 different species of fin fishes, crustaceans, mollusks, corals, seaweeds and a variety of marine animals.

It is also harvested in the south pacific, notably in Tonga, along the coasts of Asian countries such as Korea and Japan, and also off the coast of Nova Scotia, Canada.

Studies

Fucoidin causes apoptosis in various cancer cell lines, inhibits angiogenesis, and boosts the immune system. It has health benefits in addition to its anti-cancer effects. Fucoidan is anti-oxidant, anti-viral, cardioprotective, lowers cholesterol, acts as an anti-coagulant, and helps in ridding the body of heavy metals.

Fucoidan stimulates production of granzyme A (GzmA), which in turn causes the production of cytokines, immune-regulating proteins.

It is usually used as an adjunct to other cancer therapies rather than as a cure in itself. It has no side effects on healthy tissues.

Nutraceutical products containing higher concentrations of fucoidan than those found in dried seaweed are available from a range of manufacturers.

Fucoidan has shown effects in-vitro on cancer of the breast, colon, lung, and stomach as well as leukemia, lymphoma and melanoma.

Fucoidan caused apoptosis in colon cancer cells through a variety of biochemical effects.[1]

In patients with advanced colorectal cancer, Fucoidan lessened fatigue due to chemotherapy, allowing chemotherapy to be continued longer. It did not, however, provide a significant increase in patient lifespan in these advanced cases.[2]

Instructions

Take one capsule daily

Supplier

Brand name "Doctor's Best Fucoidan" 70% - 30mg - 150 capsules and costs approximately $28.00.

http://www.vitacost.com/Doctors-Best-Fucoidan

References

(1) Hyun, J.H., et al.,"Apoptosis inducing activity of fucoidan in HCT-15 colon carcinoma cells." Biol Pharm Bull 32,1760-1764.

(2) Masahide Ikeguchi, Manabu Yamamoto, Yosuke Arai, Yoshihiko Maeta, Keigo Ashida, Kuniyuki Katano, Yasunari Miki, Takayuki Kimura, "Fucoidan reduces the toxicities of chemotherapy for patients with unresectable advanced or recurrent colorectal cancer." Oncology Letters, March-April 2011, Volume 2 Number 2, 319-322

Habanero Peppers, Garlic, Ginger & Cod Liver Oil

Kelley Eidem is the inventor of an unconventional cure which he entitled descriptively, "How I Cured Stage 4 Cancer In Two Weeks

For Less Than The Cost Of A Night At The Movies." Eidem is also the author of *The Doctor Who Cures Cancer*, a biography of cancer researcher Dr. Emanuel Revici.

http://hubpages.com/hub/How-I-Cured-Stage-4-Cancer-in-Two-Weeks-For-Less-Than-The-Cost-Of-A-Night-At-The-Movies

Eidem claims to have cured his own stage 4 prostate cancer in a few weeks, and collects anecdotal reports of others' success with his recipe at his website.

http://kelleyeidem.hubpages.com/hub/Cancers-reversed-with-my-simple-recipe-so-far.

One caveat: Eidem's cancer was never diagnosed clinically, only symptomatically and with the help of a self-administered HCG test. However, despite the anecdotal nature of Eidem's story, there are scientific studies that confirm the anti-cancer activity of the substances in this simple cure.

The recipe is as follows:

Grate one habanero pepper each day, putting it on bread. If you cannot tolerate peppers, use freshly ground ginger root. The potent active ingredients from the spices disperse quickly, so they must be grated as closely as possible to the time of consumption.

Grate two cloves of garlic each day, putting them on bread.

Ezekial sprouted bread is highly recommended. Have one piece of bread for the pepper and garlic mixture, and another half piece to eat afterwards.

Smother the grated garlic and habaneros peppers with real butter and eat it. *Do not use margarine!*

Place the peppers and the garlic on one side of the bread, then fold over the bread and eat it. Let yourself breathe deeply for a minute or two to stimulate the lymphatic system, then eat the extra half slice of bread.

Eidem recommends that this be combined with 1-2 tablespoons of Emulsified cod liver oil each day. (Carlson's is probably the highest quality cod liver oil available, and TwinLabs features flavored cod liver oil for those who object to the fishy taste). In some cases, evening primrose oil is used instead.

Clinical Research

Peppers

Capsaicin is the active ingredient in peppers. It is so hot that it can numb the mouth or make it feel as if it is on fire. Capsaicin is a phytochemical that keeps animals from eating the plants which contain the chemical.

Approximately 80% of the capsaicin within a chili pepper is found in its pith and seeds. The outer shell contains much less capsaicin.

Capsaicin was initially extracted in an impure form by Christian Bucholz in 1816. It was then extracted in its crystalline form in 1873. It was initially called capsicin because it was extracted from Capsicum species. By 1873, it was called "capsaicin", a name that stuck.

Its chemical structure was defined in 1919 and synthesized first in 1930. Related chemicals to capsaicin were called capsaicinoids. Capsaicin and dihydrocapsaicin are about twice as potent in terms of a strong taste when compared to multiple other capsaicinoids. There are six natural capsaicinoids and one synthetic form of capsaicinoid.

High concentrations of the substance can burn the skin and mucus membranes. The best treatment for capsaicin burning is cold milk or cold sugar solutions. Even without treatment, the burning sensation diminishes after 6-8 hours.

Capsaicin is a popular component of plant-based arthritis and pain remedies due to its biochemical activation of TRPV1 receptors. TRPV1 is a heat-activated calcium channel which opens at much lower body temperatures when capsaicin is bound to it. This is why we feel heat when we come in contact with capsaicin. The chemical mimics the burning sensation while the nerves are overwhelmed by the sensation. Capsaicin so overstimulates neurons that they become depleted of neurotransmitters. At this point, the nerves are unable to transmit signals such as pain for a long period of time.

The main ingredient of the drug Adlea is capsaicin. This drug, made by drug manufacturer Anisiva, is currently in phase 2 trials for use as a long acting pain reliever in post operative and osteoarthritic pain. It is injected into the site of pain and its effects last as long as 12 weeks. It has also been found to be helpful in treating joint and muscle pain in patients who have fibromyalgia or rheumatoid arthritis.

Capsaicin causes apoptosis in cancer cells, and capsaicin pills have been used experimentally to treat prostate cancer.

A team of researchers at UCLA led by Dr. Soren Lehmann shrank tumors by 80% with capsaicin treatment.[1]

The researchers injected prostate cancer cells into mice and treated one group with a dose of capsaicin equivalent to giving 400 milligrams of capsaicin three times a week to a 170-pound human, or about eight fresh habanero peppers, the hottest on the market. The control group of mice were left untreated. After one to two months of treatment, the tumours in the treated mice were only one-fifth the size of the tumours in the untreated rodents.

The pepper extract caused apoptosis in prostate tumor cells while leaving normal cells unharmed.

It should be noted that low doses of capsaicin can actually boost tumor growth, so if you plan to use this remedy, use the substantial dose that was employed in the study. Capsaicin seems to be the active ingredient in habaneros peppers.

Caution

Do not over-consume peppers, as they can cause severe stomach and intestinal irritation, and potentially stomach cancer.

Garlic

Multiple population studies from around the world prove an epidemiological link between garlic consumption and lowered risk of cancer. Even the staid NCI has published a fact sheet featuring dozens of articles on garlic's role in cancer prevention.

http://www.cancer.gov/cancertopics/factsheet/prevention/garlic-and-cancer-prevention

A 2003 study found that an organosulfur component of garlic called ajoene caused apoptosis in basal cell skin tumors. In this case, the ajoene was applied directly to the tumor, not ingested.[2]

A 2001 study suggested that garlic's effect against various cancers in cell cultures and animal test subjects was due to stimulation of the immune system.[3]

Dr Richard Schulze, a noted herbalist and naturopath, recommends consumption of seven garlic cloves per day as treatment for cancer. For colon cancer he recommends a garlic enema once a day. Crush the cloves and let them sit for ten minutes before use.

Garlic and Breast cancer

Garlic contains a number of biologically active compounds, including the water-soluble chemicals S-allylmercaptocysteine (SAMC) and the S-allylcysteine.

S-allylmercaptocysteine (SAMC), but not S-allylcysteine, was found by researchers to inhibit the growth of colon cancer cells in doses similar to that of sulindac sulfide (SS), a known colon cancer chemopreventive agent. SAMC caused apoptosis, associated with an increase in caspase3-like activity, and stopped cell division at the G2-M stages of mitosis. Sodium sulindac stopped mitosis at G1-S. Together, the two agents stopped tumor cell division in a synergistic action. Researchers concluded, "These findings suggest that SAMC may be useful in colon cancer prevention when used alone or in combination with SS or other chemopreventive agents."[4]

S-allylcysteine (SAC) and *S*-allylmercaptocysteine (SAMC) suppressed proliferation and tissue invasion in a variety of tumor cells lines. Both *in vivo* and *in vitro* studies show that these compounds suppress the growth of breast, colon, esophageal, leukemia, lung and skin cancer.[5]

Another study identified the mechanism by which a garlic compound, diallyl trisulfide, can suppress breast cancer cell invasion and metastasis. A process called epithelial-mesenchymal transition is a crucial event in the invasion of normal tissue by tumors, and the garlic compound prevents this process.[6]

Use of Garlic

Raw parsley or raw parsley juice can help with bad breath due to garlic.

Cautions about garlic consumption relate to its anti-coagulant effects, and the possibility of gastric upset.

Garlic supplements come in many strengths, some pure herb, others extracts, also some are said to be "deodorized".

A common sense caution in regards to the use of peppers, ginger or garlic would be to decrease consumption if stomach upset occurs.

Ginger

Ginger (Zingiber officinale Roscoe) is an excellent source of several bioactive phenolics, such as gingerols, paradols, shogaols and gingerones. It has anticancer and antioxidant properties, and is also an effective remedy for nausea and inflammation.

Ginger has been shown to inhibit the growth of breast, colon, ovarian, prostate, skin and colon cancer cells in-vitro.

Researchers at the University of Minnesota's Hormel Institute found that gingerol prevented mice from developing colorectal tumors, and that ginger caused apoptosis in cancer cells. The study concluded, "These results strongly suggest that ginger compounds may be effective chemo-preventive and/or chemotherapeutic agents for colorectal carcinomas."[7]

Dr. Rebecca Liu and colleagues found that powdered ginger caused autophagy and apoptosis (the cells digested themselves and died) in-vitro in cultures of multiple lines of ovarian cancer cells. The cells were treated with pharmaceutical grade whole ginger extract standardized to 5% [6]-gingerol, solubilized in DMSO.

Researchers found that ginger killed cancer cells at a similar or better rate than the platinum-based chemotherapy drugs commonly used in the treatment of ovarian cancer. Also, researchers said, "The majority of conventional chemotherapeutic agents induce apoptotic cell death. Because ginger can circumvent chemoresistance due to alterations in apoptotic signaling, it has the potential to be effective against chemoresistant disease. Our preliminary results indicate that ginger is a nutraceutical that may have significant therapeutic benefit for ovarian cancer patients."

The findings were presented in 2006 at the annual meeting of the American Association for Cancer Research in Washington, DC.[8]

According to researchers at the Industrial Toxicology and Research Center in India, the anti-tumor action of ginger is attributed to anti-inflammatory compounds known as vallinoids, such as [6]-gingerol and [6]-paradol, as well as some other constituents like shogaols, and zingerone. These compounds have a number of anti-cancer mechanisms.[9]

Mice implanted with human prostate cancer were treated with 100 mg/kg whole ginger extract. Tumor volume in treated mice was reduced by 56% compared to untreated controls. According to the researchers, the ginger extract, "perturbed cell-cycle progression, impaired reproductive capacity, modulated cell-cycle and apoptosis regulatory molecules and induced a caspase-driven, mitochondrially mediated apoptosis in human prostate cancer cells." Normal tissue was unharmed.[10]

Caution

Large amounts of ginger should be taken with caution by diabetics and patients on anticoagulants, as it lowers blood sugar and has a blood-thinning effect.

References

(1) Akio Mori, Soren Lehmann et al.;"Capsaicin, a Component of Red Peppers, Inhibits the Growth of Androgen-Independent, p53 Mutant Prostate Cancer Cells." Cancer Research March 15, 2006 66; 3222.

(2) Tilli, CM, Stavast-Kooy, AJ, Vuerstaek, JD, et al. (2003). "The garlic-derived organosulfur component ajoene decreases basal cell carcinoma tumor size by inducing apoptosis." Archives of Dermatological Research, 295, 117–123

(3) Donald L. Lamm and Dale R. Riggs, "Enhanced Immunocompetence by Garlic: Role in Bladder Cancer and Other Malignancies," Journal of Nutrition. 2001;131:1067S-1070S

(4) Haim Shirin, et al., "Antiproliferative Effects of S-Allylmercaptocysteine on Colon Cancer Cells When Tested Alone or in Combination with Sulindac Sulfide." Cancer Res January 1, 2001 61; 725

(5) Qingjun Chu, "A novel anticancer effect of garlic derivatives: inhibition of cancer cell invasion through restoration of E-cadherin expression." Carcinogenesis, (2006) 27 (11): 2180-2189.

(6) Ahmed S. Sultan and Zaki Sherif, "New suppression strategy for human breast cancer invasion and metastasis." Association for Cancer Research (AACR) Meeting, April 2010

(7) Ann Bode, Ph.D. and Zigang Dong,"Ginger is an Effective Inhibitor of HCT116 Human Colorectal Carcinoma." (Abstract 1345), 2003 American Association for Cancer research conference, Phoenix, Arizona.

(8) Jennifer M. Rhode, Jennifer Huang, Sarah Fogoros, Lijun Tan, Suzanna Zick and J. Rebecca Liu, "Ginger induces apoptosis and autophagocytosis in ovarian cancer cells." Proc Amer Assoc Cancer Res, Volume 47, 2006 Abstract# 4510

(9) Shukla Y, Singh M, "Non-volatile pungent components of ginger." Food and Chemical Toxicology 45 (2007) 683–690.

(10) Karna P., et al., "Benefits of whole ginger extract in prostate cancer." Br J Nutr, 2012 Feb;107(4):473-84

IP_6 & Inositol (Rice Bran Extract)

IP_6 is usually combined with Inositol.

Inositol hexaphosphate (IP_6), also referred to as phytic acid, is a polyphosphorylated carbohydrate naturally found in almost all plant and animal cells, and the commercial product is usually derived from rice bran. It has multiple biological functions, including a strong antitumor effect.

Inositol is a naturally-occurring carbohydrate showing moderate antitumor activity. It is an isomer of glucose, and exists in nine possible configurations, of which the most prominent form is myo-inositol. Myo-Inositol was initially classified as a B vitamin complex (B8), but because the human body can synthesize it to some extent, it is no longer classified as such.

Best laboratory anticancer results have been obtained by combining IP_6 with inositol.

Iron Chelation To Treat Cancer

IP_6 is a very effective mineral chelator, and can remove excess cadmium, calcium, copper, iron, lead, mercury, zinc, and even uranium[1] from the body. It will not remove calcium from bones, or iron in red blood cells. It is an extremely powerful iron chelator, and this may be part of its anti-tumor action, as growing tumors need iron,[2] and iron is a well known pro-oxidant.

IP_6 suppresses iron-caused oxygen generation, and almost completely inhibits iron-caused lipid (fat) peroxidation, the process where lipids become rancid and pro-inflammatory.[3]

In addition, iron and other minerals are important in gene regulation. Excess iron correlates with an increased cancer rate in humans and animals, especially colon cancer.[4]

There have been concerns that IP_6 might have the effect of depleting the body's mineral stores, but experiments on rats have found no significant differences in the serum or bone levels of minerals, even after lengthy treatment with IP_6 and inositol.[5]

Pharmaceutical drugs used as iron chelators are either ineffective or have toxic side effects. The usual iron chelator employed in anti-cancer studies, Desferal (desferrioxamine), does exhibit modest inhibition of tumor growth,[6] an effect limited by its poor ability to enter tumor cells to remove iron.[7]

Adriamycin (doxorubicin), an antibiotic also used as a chemotherapy drug, also binds iron. Its main drawback is that it is extremely cardiotoxic. Under certain conditions it can release iron from its storage protein (ferritin), causing heart damage.[8] The contraction force of the heart can be reduced by up to 50% by the use of Adriamycin.[9] Even if Adriamycin cures cancer, it can produce fatal heart damage.

In 1995 one researcher bemoaned, "There is therefore an urgent need for an orally active, inexpensive iron-chelating drug, because the only currently available iron chelator cannot be administered orally, is expensive and side effects have raised doubts about its safety."[10]

In 1987, researcher Ernst Graf found that only 4 of 22 chelating agents tested, including IP_6, block hydroxyl radical formation. Only IP_6 was found to be economical, safe, and effective.[11]

In 2001, FDA scientists found that 8 out of 12 chelating agents they tested caused DNA mutations. Among the four non-toxic chelators was IP_6.[12]

Recently, an oral iron chelator was introduced, called Ferriprox (deferiprone). It has toxicity problems similar to other pharmaceutical chelating drugs.[13]

Cancer researchers, aware of the multitude of roles played by iron in the development of tumors, have stated the need for a safe and effective iron chelator.[41] It is ironic that pharmaceutical companies are going through so much trouble to develop new iron chelators, and getting such poor results, when an extremely effective and completely non-toxic iron chelator already exists. However, it is natural, cheap, and unpatentable, and so the drug companies will keep trying to find substitutes.

Other Mechanisms of Action

Much of the research on IP_6 has been done by Dr. AbulKalam Shamsuddin, from the University of Maryland, who has been investigating this substance since the 1980s.[14]

IP_6 is rapidly absorbed by cells and undergoes dephosphorylation to lower-phosphate inositol phosphates, which block the internal signals used by the cancer cell to divide and reproduce.[15] As well as reducing tumor cell division, IP_6 increases differentiation of malignant cells, often resulting in a reversion back to their normal phenotype.[14,16] IP_6 and inositol also enhances the body's immune system and displays antioxidant properties, which also contributes to the destruction of tumor cells. It prevents angiogenesis,[17] and inhibits metastasis.[18] This supplement can be combined with chemotherapy, and acts synergistically to boost its effect.[14]

IP6 is a very well-documented supplement, as it has been shown to suppress tumor growth in numerous in-vitro and in-vivo studies. These studies include cancer of the breast,[19,20,21] colon,[22,23,24] liver,[25,26,27] prostate,[28,29,30] and skin,[31] as well as leukemia,[32] rhabdomyosarcoma,[33] fibrosarcoma[34] and asbestos-induced fibrosis.[35]

Human Studies

In a study of breast cancer patients the drop in platelets and leukocytes usually seen after chemotherapy was prevented by IP_6 and Inositol, but tumor marker CEA was unchanged compared to a control group. Quality of life was improved in the IP_6 group.[36]

Other human studies exist, and have been quoted by various researchers, but the texts are difficult to find online.[37,38,39,40]

Instructions

Start with 500 grams twice daily on an empty stomach, then slowly increase to at least three grams twice daily. If gastric upset occurs, decrease the dose. Some studies have used higher amounts, 12-30 grams per day.

Suppliers

This economical supplement is widely available for approximately $70.00 - $80.00 per kilogram from Ebay and large vitamin websites such as Vitamins.com. It comes in either powder or capsule form.

References

(1) Cebrian D, Tapia A, Real A, Morcillo MA (2007). "Inositol hexaphosphate: a potential chelating agent for uranium." Radiation Protection Dosimetry 127 (1–4): 477–9

(2) Buss JL, et al., "Iron Chelators In Cancer Chemotherapy." Current Topics Medical Chemistry 4: 1623-35, 2004

(3) Porres JM, Stahl CH, Cheng WH, et al., "Dietary intrinsic phytate protects colon from lipid peroxidation in pigs with a moderately high dietary iron intake." Proc Soc Exp Biol Med 1999, 221(1):80-6.

(4) Graf E, Eaton JW, "Suppression of colonic cancer by dietary phytic acid." Nutr Cancer 1993, 19(1):11-9.

(5) Vucenik I, Yang GY, Shamsuddin AM, "Inositol hexaphosphate and inositol inhibit DMBA-induced rat mammary cancer." Carcinogenesis 1995, 16:1055-58.

(6) Buss JL, et al., "The Role of Iron Chelation In Cancer Therapy." Current Medicinal Chemistry 10: 1021-34, 2003

(7) Richardson DR, "Iron chelators as therapeutic agents for the treatment of cancer." Critical Review Oncology Hematology 42: 267-81, 2002

(8) Thomas CE, "Release of iron from ferritin by cardiotoxic anthracycline antibiotics." Arch Biochem Biophysics 248: 684-89, 1986

(9) Husken BC, et al., "Modulation of the in vitro cardiotoxicity of doxorubicin by flavonoids." Cancer Chemotherapy Pharmacology 37: 55-62, 1995

(10) Hoffbrand AV, "Iron Chelating Therapy." Current Opinion Hematology 2: 153–58, 1995

(11) Graf E, Empson KL, Eaton JW. 1987, "Phytic acid. A natural antioxidant." Journal of Biological Chemistry 262, 11647–11650.

(12) Whittaker P, et al., "Genotoxicity of iron chelators in L5178Y mouse lymphoma cells." Environmental and Molecular Mutagenesis 38: 347–56, 2001

(13) Kontoghiorghes GJ, "Quantum chemical analysis of the deferiprone–iron binding reaction." Current Med Chemistry 11: 2161-83, 2004

(14) Ivana Vucenik, Shamsuddin AbulKalam, "Cancer Inhibition by Inositol Hexaphosphate (IP6) and Inositol: From Laboratory to Clinic." J. Nutr. November 1, 2003 vol. 133 no. 11 3778S-3784S

(15) Huang, C., Ma, W.-Y., Hecht, S. S. & Dong, Z., "Inositol hexaphosphate inhibits cell transformation and activator protein 1 activation by targeting phosphatidylinositol-3' kinase." Cancer Res. 1997 57: 2873–2878.

(16) El-Sherbiny, Y., Cox, M. C., Ismail, Z. A., Shamsuddin, A. M. & Vucenik, I., "G0/G1 arrest and S phase inhibition of human cancer cell lines by inositol hexaphosphate (IP6)." Anticancer Res. 2001 21: 2393–2404.

(17) Vucenik, I., Passaniti, A., Tantivejkul, K., Eggleton, P., Vitolo, M. & Shamsuddin, A. M., "Anti-angiogenic potential of inositol hexaphophate (IP6)." Rev. Oncologia 2002 4 (Suppl 1): 79.

(18) Tantivejkul, K., Vucenik, I. & Shamsuddin, A. M., "Inositol hexaphosphate (IP6) inhibits key events of cancer metastases: II. Effects on integrins and focal adhesions." Anticancer Res. 2003 23: 5

(19) Tantivejkul, K., Vucenik, I. & Shamsuddin, A. M., "Inositol hexaphosphate (IP6) inhibits key events of cancer metastases: I. In vitro studies of adhesion, migration and invasion of MDA-MB 231 human breast cancer cells." Anticancer Res, 2003 23: 5 (in press).

(20) Shamsuddin AM, Yang GY, Vucenik I. Novel anti-cancer functions of IP6: Growth inhibition and differentiation of human mammary cancer cell lines in vitro." Anticancer Res 1996, 16:3287-92.

(21) Tantivejkul K, Vucenik I, Eiseman J, Shamsuddin AM, "Inositol hexaphosphate (IP6) enhances the anti-proliferative effects of adriamycin and tamoxifen in breast cancer." Breast Cancer Res Treat 2003, Jun;79(3):301-12.

(22) Shamsuddin, A. M., Elsayed, A. & Ullah, A., "Suppression of large intestinal cancer in F344 rats by inositol hexaphosphate." 1989. Carcinogenesis 9: 577–580.

(23) Shamsuddin, A. M. & Ullah, A. "Inositol hexaphosphate inhibits large intestinal cancer in F344 rats 5 months after induction by azoxymethane." Carcinogenesis 1989 10: 625–626.

(24) Shamsuddin, A. M., Ullah, A. & Chakravarthy, A., "Inositol and inositol hexaphosphate suppress cell proliferation and tumor formation in CD-1 mice." Carcinogenesis 1989 10: 1461–1463.

(25) Lee HJ, Lee SA, Choi H, "Dietary administration of inositol and/or inositol-6-phosphate prevents chemically-induced rat hepatocarcinogenesis." Asian

Pac J Cancer Prev 2005, Jan-Mar;6(1):41-7.

(26) Vucenik I, Tantivejkul K, Zhang ZS, Cole KE, Saied I, Shamsuddin AM, "IP6 in treatment of liver cancer. (I). IP6 inhibits growth and reverses transformed phenotype in HepG2 human liver cancer cell line." Anticancer Res 1998, 18(16A):4083-90.

(27) Vucenik I, Zhang ZS, Shamsuddin AM, "IP6 treatment of liver cancer. (II). Intra-yumoral injection of IP6 regresses pre-existing human liver cancer xenotransplanted in nude mice." Anticancer Res 1998, 18(6A):4091-96.

(28) Singh, R. P., Agarwal, C. & Agarwal, R., "Inositol hexaphosphate inhibits growth, and induces G1 arrest and apoptotic death of prostate carcinoma DU145: modulation of CDKI-CDK-cyclin and pRb-related protein-E2F complexes." Carcinogenesis 2003 24: 555–563.

(29) Agarwal C, Dhanalakshmi S, Singh RP, Agarwal R, "Inositol hexaphosphate inhibits growth and induces G1 arrest and apoptotic death of androgen-dependent human prostate carcinoma LNCaP cells." Neoplasia 2004, Sep-Oct;6(5):646-59.

(30) Agarwal C, Dhanalakshmi S, Singh RP, Agarwal R, "Inositol hexaphosphate inhibits constitutive activation of NF- kappa B in androgen-independent human prostate carcinoma DU145 cells." Anticancer Res 2003, Sep-Oct;23(5A):3855-61.

(31) Gupta KP, Singh J, Bharathi R, "Suppression of DMBA-induced mouse skin tumor development by inositol hexaphosphate and its mode of action." Nutr Cancer 2003, 46(1):66-72.

(32) Deliliers GL, Servida F, Fracchiolla NS, Ricci C, Borsotti C, Colombo G, Soligo D, "Effect of inositol hexaphosphate (IP(6)) on human normal and leukaemic haematopoietic cells." Br J Haematol 2002, Jun;117(3):577-87.

(33) Vucenik, I., Kalebic, T., Tantivejkul, K. & Shamsuddin, A. M., "Novel anticancer function of inositol hexaphosphate (IP6): inhibition of human rhabdomyosarcoma in vitro and in vivo." Anticancer Res. 1998 18: 1377–1384.

(34) Vucenik, I., Tomazic, V. J., Fabian, D. & Shamsuddin, A. M., "Antitumor activity of phytic acid (inositol hexaphosphate) in murine transplanted and metastatic fibrosarcoma, a pilot study." Cancer Lett. 1992 65: 9–13.

(35) Shamsuddin AM, "IP6: Nature's Revolutionary Cancer-Fighter." Kensington Books. New York, NY. 1998. Page 80.

(36) Ivan Bačić, Nikica Družijanić, Robert Karlo, Ivan Škifić and Stjepan Jagić, "Efficacy of IP6 + inositol in the treatment of breast cancer patients receiving chemotherapy: prospective, randomized, pilot clinical study." Journal of Experimental & Clinical Cancer Research 2010, 29:12

(37) Juricic J, Druzijanic N, Perko Z, Kraljevic D, Ilic N, "IP6 + Inositol in treatment of ductal invasive breast carcinoma: our clinical experience." Anticancer Res 2004, 24:3475

(38) Sakamoto K, Suzuki Y, "IP6 plus Inositol treatment after surgery and post-operative radiotherapy: report of a case: breast cancer." Anticancer Res 2004, 24:3617.

(39) Druzijanic N, Juricic J, Perko Z, Kraljevic D, "IP6 + Inositol as adjuvant to chemotherapy of colon cancer: our clinical experience." Anticancer Res 2004, 24:3474

(40) Druzijanic, N., Juricic, J., Perko, Z. & Kraljevic, D., "IP-6 & inositol: adjuvant to chemotherapy of colon cancer. A pilot clinical trial." Rev. Oncologia 2002 4: 171.

(41) Weinberg ED, "The role of iron in cancer." European J Cancer Prev 5; 19-36, 1996.

Graviola

Graviola is derived from the South American plant *Annona muricata.* The herbal preparation for cancer comes from the seeds, leaves, bark and stem of the plant. There are many other plants in this genus, which yield various potent cytotoxic substances. These are especially effective against prostate and pancreatic cancers and work well even against lung cancer.

Researchers are focusing the antitumor and pesticidal properties of a group of phytochemicals called annonaceous acetogenins (annonaceous means that these substances are derived from Graviola plants). Acetogenins can be derived from several plants, including paw-paw, graviola, mountain graviola and others.

Scientists are continually finding new compounds in Graviola, so the number of acetogenins in each type of Graviola is still under revision. However, Graviola (*Annona muricata*) is currently said to contain 82 different acetogenin chemicals, in 10 distinct subgroups. Mountain graviola (*Annona montana*) contains the main annonacin chemical found in graviola (*Annona muricata*), along with 26 more acetogenins not found in graviola (in 6 distinct subgroups). American paw paw contains 28 acetogenins.

There is some overlap in the contents of each plant, but each holds some unique compounds and has a slightly different mechanism of action.

Purdue University has conducted a great deal of animal research on annonaceaous acetogenins, with funding from The National Cancer Institute and/or the National Institute of Health. So far, Purdue University and its staff have filed at least nine U.S. and or international patents on the results of their studies. After 10 years of research they succeeded in isolating and synthesizing annonacin, a major anti-cancer component of graviola.

In 1997, Purdue University concluded that several of the Annonaceous acetogenins are not only effective in killing cancer cells, but also seem to have a special toxicity to chemotherapy-resistant cells. This research is detailed in the paw-paw chapter.

The dose required to kill cancer cells is far below that which will injure healthy human cells. Graviola has few side effects. Given its low toxicity, scientific research supporting its effectiveness, and reasonable market price, it is potentially useful for all cancer patients.

It is said to be particulary effective against prostate, pancreatic, and lung cancer.

Studies

Six acetogenins (four previously known and two newly discovered) exhibited significant cytotoxic activity against two human hepatoma cell lines.[1]

A 2002 animal study compared the effects of the main graviola acetogenin annonacin and chemotherapy drug adriamycin. Eighteen mice were inoculated with lung cancer cells, then divided into 3 groups. One group (the control group) received no treatment, the second group was treated with adriamycin, and the third group was given annonacin at a dose of 10mg/kg.

After 2 weeks, the tumor sizes in all the groups were compared. 5 out of 6 in the control group were still alive, 3 out of 6 in the adriamycin group, and all 6 of the annonacin group. The adriamycin group showed a 54.6% reduction in tumor size compared to the control group, but despite this, half of the mice had died due to adriamycin toxicity. However, the annonacin group, all still alive, showed a reduction in tumor size of 57.9%. This result was better than that of adriamycin, with no toxicity.

This led the researchers to conclude, "On considering the antitumor activity and toxicity, annonacin might be used as a lead to develop a potential anticancer agent."[2]

Another review in the Skaggs Scientific Report 1997-1998 states, "Annonaceous acetogenins, particularly those with adjacent bis-tetrahydrofuran (THF) rings, have remarkable cytotoxic, antitumor, antimalarial, immunosuppressive, pesticidal, and antifeedant activities."

Related Compounds

A. bullata, a cuban tree in the same botanical family, also contains acetogenins in its leaves and bark.[3] One of them, bullatacin, was isolated and tested on multidrug-resistant human breast adenocarcinoma cells (MCF-7/Adr) and the original non-drug-resistant wild type cells (MCF-7/wt). Bullatacin was more cytotoxic to the MCF-7/Adr (MDR) cells while it was more cytostatic to the MCF-7/wt cells. That is, it killed the MDR cells while only inhibiting the growth of non-drug-resistant cells.[4] It also caused apoptosis in human hepatocarcinoma cells in-vitro.[5] The compound can be artificially synthesized.[6]

One 1999 Purdue study by Dr. X.X. Liu and colleagues was done on annoglacins, chemical compounds related to acetogenins, but derived from a different tree altogether, *Annona glabra*, a Polynesian tree called the pond or alligator apple. Tests showed that the annoglacins were selectively cytotoxic to colon adenocarcinoma cells, showing 10,000 times the potency of adriamycin, a commonly used chemotherapy drug. Researchers stated, "Annoglacins A and B were selectively 1000 and 10,000 times, respectively, more potent than Adriamycin against the human breast carcinoma (MCF-7) and pancreatic carcinoma (PACA-2) cell lines in our panel of six human solid tumor cell lines."[7]

Caution

Graviola has significant antimicrobial properties. Uninterrrupted long-term use may lead to a decrease in friendly bacteria in the digestive tract, with subsequent overgrowth of candida. Supplementing the diet with probiotics and digestive enzymes is advisable if this product is used for more than 30 days.

Large single dosages may cause nausea or vomiting. Reduce the dose or take with food if nausea occurs. Drinking plenty of water (at least 8 glasses a day) is helpful to reduce Herxheimer reactions.

Graviola should not to be used during pregnancy or breast-feeding. Do not use Graviola in combination with vitamin C, CoQ10 or other supplements which increase cellular ATP. ATP inhibition is the main mechanism of action of graviola, and taking CoQ10 will counteract this effect.

Graviola has demonstrated hypotensive, vasodilator, and cardiodepressant activities in animal studies. People should check with their doctors before taking graviola and monitor their blood pressure accordingly.

Instructions

The recommended dosage is 2 grams three times daily in capsules or tablets. An infusion (tea) can be substituted, one cup 3 times daily, or a 4:1 standard tincture (2–4 ml three times daily).

Suppliers

Graviola 600 mg (Annona Muricata) $12.99

http://www.herbspro.com/3345/Graviola.htm

Iherb.com has a wide variety of graviola products.

http://www.iherb.com/Search?kw=graviola&x=0&y=0

References

(1) Chang, F. R., et al. "Novel cytotoxic annonaceous acetogenins from Annona Muricata," J Nat Prod; 2002 Apr;65(4):470-5.

(2) Wang, L.Q et al, "Annonaceous acetogenins from the leaves of Annona montana", Biorg Med Chem 2002; 10(3):561-5

(3) Y.-H. Hui, J. K. Rupprecht, Y. M. Liu, J. E. Anderson, D. L. Smith, C.-J. Chang, J. L. McLaughlin (1989). "Bullatacin and Bullatacinone: Two Highly Potent Bioactive Acetogenins from Annona bullata". J. Nat. Prod. 52 (3): 463–47

(4) Nicholas H. Oberlies, Vicki L. Croy, Marietta L. Harrison, Jerry L. McLaughlin. "The Annonaceous acetogenin bullatacin is cytotoxic against multidrug-resistant human mammary adenocarcinoma cells." Cancer Letters 115 (1997) 73-79

(5) Hwa-Woei Chiha, Hui-Fen Chiub, Kung-Sung Tanga, Fang-Rong Changc, Yang-Chang Wu (2001). "Bullatacin, a potent antitumor annonaceous acetogenin, inhibits proliferation of human hepatocarcinoma cell line 2.2.15 by apoptosis induction". Life Sciences 69 (11): 1321–1331.

(6) H. Naito, E. Kawahara, K. Maruta, M. Maeda, S. Sasaki (1995). "The First Total Synthesis of (+)-Bullatacin, a Potent Antitumor Annonaceous

Acetogenin, and (+)-(15,24)-bis-epi-Bullatacin". J. Org. Chem. 60 (14): 4419–4427.

(7) Liu XX, Alali FQ, Pilarinou E, McLaughlin JL. "Two bioactive mono-tetrahydrofuran acetogenins, annoglacins A and B, from Annona glabra." Phytochemistry 1999 Mar;50(5):815-21.

Mountain Graviola

Mountain graviola (*Annona montana*), commonly known as mountain soursop, is a tree belonging to the Annona family. The tree is a traditional medicinal plant which grows in Central America and the Caribbean islands.

It closely resembles the graviola tree and the two plants are often mistakenly considered the same. Despite the similarity in appearance, they are different trees with different chemical compositions.

Annona montana or mountain graviola has leaves which are glossier and wider than those of Annona muritica or graviola. Also, Annona montana bears fruits faster. These fruits have fibrous pulps and grow to about 15 centimeters long. It is said that Montana fruits are sourer than those of Muritica.

Mountain graviola has similar ATP-inhibiting effects as the muricata.

Anecdotal reports state that liver and ovarian cancer patients using mountain graviola herbal medicines have been healed within a year, with no recurrences reported.

Extracts of the muricata and montanta are often combined by supplement manufacturers to boost effectiveness.

One good Graviola supplement is Graviola Max, manufactured by Raintree Nutrition, which combines both graviolas in one capsule. Also on their website is an interesting table showing the different acetogenins in graviola, mountain graviola, and paw-paw.

http://www.rain-tree.com/graviola-max-capsules.htm

A 120 capsule bottle is $29.95.

Suggested Use: Take 3 capsules 3-4 times or as directed by a healthcare professional.

Graviola versus Paw Paw as a Cancer-Fighting Supplement

As detailed in the paw-paw article, graviola products are inconsistent in quality, as they have not been standardized and the concentration of active compounds in raw material is extremely variable. Buyer beware.

For many years the components of Graviola and Pawpaw have been used in the creation of formulas for medical and health purposes. Many independent studies have been performed on the properties of Graviola and Pawpaw, with data being compared and reviewed to gain a better understanding of the effectiveness of the plant products.

Through the collection of data from independent studies there is evidence that Graviola may not be as powerful as Pawpaw when it comes to cancer fighting supplements, for several reasons:

- Natural variation in potency and concentration of chemical compounds between plants
- When the plants are harvested
- What happens during and after the harvesting process and its effects on the final product
- Variation in production and manufacturing process by distributors.

There have been positive outcomes reported with the use of Graviola, but its potency has shown to be much less compared to Pawpaw. To gain a better understanding of Graviola and Pawpaw it helps to review the history, background, and origin of the plants.

Variation In Potency & Concentration Of Chemical Compounds.

Each acetogenin is a slightly different chemical, with slightly different cellular effects. Each type of plant has a synergistic combination of these chemicals in different proportions, in the case of graviola at least 128 different compounds. Scientists have isolated many and tested their individual actions, but how they work as individual chemicals may be different from how they work all together in a whole plant extract.

There have been over 100 pages of research content published in scientific and medical related publications describing the findings and the effects of Pawpaw. Because Pawpaw has had such good testimonials regarding its effectiveness, some believe that companies manufacturing Graviola try to take advantage of the good name of Pawpaw, with some referring to Graviola as "Brazilian paw paw."

Independent studies performed on Graviola products showed possible discrepancies within the product formulas. The Graviola products are inconsistent, with great variation in the amount of active ingredients from one bottle to another.

One finding that stood out during the studies included the fact that potency levels of Graviola products were much lower, with Pawpaw being 50 times more potent than certain Graviola products.

One recommended paw-paw product, Nature's Sunshine, has a standardized acetogenin content. The quality is monitored and consistent, and the manufacturing process was created by a scientist who studied the plant.

Time of Harvest

If a plant is harvested too soon, not only will it be unripe, but it may not have developed all its potential chemical compounds. Also, pawpaw and graviola have varying concentrations of acetogenins depending on the season and time of day they are picked.

What Happens During And After The Harvesting Process Affects The Final Product

Some manufacturers use only the fruit, while others use twigs and leaves as well.

Variation In production & Manufacturing Process By Distributors

Formulas used to mix the components with Graviola seemed to affect the potency of the overall product.

Some of the various acetogenins found in Graviola and Pawpaw have different interactions with other compounds, which can affect the potency of the product.

Manufacturing of the products plays another important role in helping the product reach it maximum potency potential. Many people realize that companies often look for ways to save on production costs but this process may affect how well the product works. Quickly processed, freeze-dried fruit will have more active compounds than plants stored for weeks and then heat-dried.

Understanding the manufacturing process can give a better insight in the condition of the ingredients as well as how the ingredients are combined to create therapeutic formulas. Manufacturers would do well to test each batch and review potency levels. Due to the number of acetogenins in graviola, this is an expensive process and many manufacturers avoid doing it. Not all products are created equal, and in some cases the customer may not be getting the required amount of active ingredients.

Instructions

Capsules are usually easier to digest than tablets.

Like paw-paw, graviola works by starving cancer cells. Take it regularly without breaks for the entire treatment period, at least 2-3 months. Any drug holidays allow the tumor to recover.

Suppliers

Use a standardized product, such as Nature's Sunshine paw-paw, or buy a reputable brand of graviola. Bargain hunting for the cheapest brand of graviola may leave you with an inferior product.

Laetrile, Apricot Pits, Vitamin B17

This is a controversial substance in the treatment of cancer; however, it has been used as a treatment for more than 150 years worldwide. The terms amygdalin, vitamin B17 and Laetrile are often used interchangeably, compounding the confusion. While they are all related compounds that release cyanide, there are some differences in their chemistry.

Amygdalin is a nitriloside found in the pits of certain fruits. The standardized extract form is referred to as Laetrile or vitamin B17.

Nitrilosides are actually a group of sugary, water-soluble compounds found in up to eight hundred plants, most of which are edible. The molecules contain a component of sugar, benzene, an acetone component and a hydrogen cyanide component.

As a whole molecule, it is not dangerous at all but if hydrolyzed by the enzyme beta-glycosidase, it turns into free hydrogen cyanide, sugar, and acetone or benzaldehyde.

Amygdalin is the most common nitriloside. Apricot pits contain a high concentration of amygdalin and plant seeds have been found to contain as much as two percent nitriloside. It is found in most fruit seeds, although in lesser concentrations. These include peach, cherry, apple, nectarine, and orange seeds. Flax, millet, wheatgrass and some beans (such as lima beans) also contain these compounds. Cassava (tapioca) is also a rich source.

The highest concentrations of amygdalin are found in the pit of the bitter almond tree, which was banned in America in 1995 after an unprecendented decades-long campaign by the FDA to restrict public access to any source of this substance.

The seed is the soft component of the seed inside the hard outer shell of the pit. If you break open the hard shell of an apricot pit, you will find the seed within it.

Apricot pits are said to prevent cancer and to cure existing cancer. Some cultures routinely eat the seeds of these types of fruits. These include the Hunzas, the Abkhasians and the Navajos. Of note is that these tribes have an extremely low incidence of cancer.

The seed should not be the main course of your meal, but in order to keep cancer away, it is estimated that an average size adult should eat seven apricot seeds daily.

When eating a fruit, eat the seeds too. If you are eating apricot seeds from a package, eat about as many seeds as you would consume if you ate the fruits. Don't throw away the fruit and just eat the seed. You need to eat the fruit for its benefits for your health. It just takes a few apples or apricots a day to get the benefit of both the fruit and the seeds. Apricot seeds are particularly bitter so you may need to sprinkle them in regular food or take them with a bit of applesauce or honey.

The nutritional benefits of apricot seeds don't just extend to the seed. The apricot itself is rich in vitamin A, vitamin C, vitamin B2 (riboflavin), easily digestible sugars and niacin (vitamin B3). It contains healthful minerals, including sulfur, manganese, sodium, cobalt and bromine.

Multiple studies using Laetrile have yielded mixed results, with some researchers complaining that their tests were deliberately sabotaged and positive results suppressed.

Laetrile is not approved by the FDA for the treatment of cancer, and was banned for use in the US after a vigorous campaign by the FDA. However, patients can still obtain it from the Internet and at foreign clinics. In the years since Laetrile was banned by the FDA, cancer patients have been travelling to Mexico to receive Laetrile treatments in Mexican clinics and hospitals.

History of Laetrile

Laetrile is a trade name that stands for levo-mandelonitrile-beta-glucoronoside. It is a nitrile related to vitamin B17, and was initially synthesized by Ernst T. Krebs Jr.

It is chemically similar to amygdalin, found in apricot pits and other fruit seeds. In some settings, the name Laetrile is used interchangeably with amygdalin because of the similarity of the two compounds. The American patent for Laetrile is for mandelonitrile-beta-glucuronide, a semi-synthetic derivative of amygdalin, while the formula produced in Mexico, mandelonitrile beta-D-gentiobioside, is made from pulverized apricot pits.

Amygdalin is not a newly-discovered compound. It was initially isolated by French chemists around 1830, and was used to treat cancer in Russia as early as 1845, and in America in the 1920s. However, it was found to be unacceptably toxic. It breaks down enzymatically to benzaldehyde, hydrogen cyanide, glucose and prunasin.

In 1952, Ernst T. Krebs Sr. and Ernst T. Krebs Jr. attempted to modify the compound to reduce its toxicity in cancer treatment. They called their amygdalin derivative Laetrile. In amygdalin, two glucose molecules are linked to mandelonitrile. In Laetrile, one sugar molecule is linked to mandelonitrile, and the bond has a different configuration. The chemical properties of the two compounds are almost indistinguishable.

Krebs Sr. was a pharmacist by trade before he obtained his medical degree in 1903. He and his son purportedly developed several compounds for different diseases, but these substances were not helpful and were subsequently banned.

The son, Krebs Jr, was not a medical doctor, having been expelled by his medical college for failing classes. Nevertheless, he worked hard with his father to create Laetrile.

Krebs Sr. wrote a book on Laetrile stating that cancer proteins could be broken down by enzymes he had obtained from his work in pharmacy. He recommended the use of proteolytic enzymes to break down tumors, combined with Laetrile treatment.

Those who believe in the ability of Laetrile to control cancer have studied the similarity between cancer cells and placental trophoblasts that invade the uterine wall and help create the placenta. Krebs supported the view, first introduced by John Beard in 1902, that all forms of cancer arise from these undifferentiated cells.

These cells are now referred to as stem cells. The theory that they are linked to cancer development has been revived in recent years, as researchers have found that both cancer cells and trophoblasts secrete a distinctive hormone, HCG (human chorionic gonadotropin), which can be used to test for both pregnancy and the presence of malignancy.

Krebs found that trophoblasts were killed by amygdalin. According to Krebs, cells metabolized amygdalin, and its related compound Laetrile, back to its constituent compounds through the enzyme beta-glucosidase, releasing cyanide in the process.

According to Kreb's initial theory, cancer cells contained higher amounts of beta-glucosidase, so they produce more cyanide than normal cells. Also, cancer cells supposedly lack a mitochondrial enzyme, rhodanese, which detoxifies the cyanide by converting it to thiocyanate, a relatively non-toxic chemical. Cancer cells are killed by a buildup of cyanide.

Some researchers found beta-glucosidase present in only trace amounts in animal cells, and equivalent amounts of rhodenase in both normal and cancerous tissue.

In response to these objections, in 1955 Krebs revised his theory of how Laetrile works by postulating that the enzyme involved in the release of cyanide within cancer cells was beta-glucuronidase, not beta-glucosidase. However, this enzyme is also present equally within cancerous and non-cancerous tissue, so this still provided no definitive explanation for the action of Laetrile.

In 1970, Krebs Jr. proposed that Laetrile acted as a vitamin, and he referred to it as vitamin B17.

In 1981, a researcher found beta-glucosidase present in human and rat intestinal mucosa, and completely absent in all tumor cell samples studied.[1]

Modern theories are still not entirely clear in explaining the exact mechanism of action of Laetrile, but some researchers speculate that it is due to a synergistic effect of benzaldehyde, cyanide and prunasin in suppressing tumor metabolism.[1-4]

Clinical Use

Some people believe that Laetrile is purely a cure for cancer, while others believe that cancer can also be prevented by consuming vitamin B17 or amygdalin.

Much of the controversy over the use of laetrile occurred from 1960 to 1980. Peak interest in Laetrile occurred in the 1970s, and it is no longer in the headlines. It is still used by a number of alternative clinics in Mexico.

One California cancer specialist, Dr. John Richardson, treated many terminally ill patients with Laetrile—up to 6000 patients by 1976. He also treated patients who were felt to be pre-cancerous, although what was considered to be pre-cancerous was unclear and included people with ill-defined symptoms. Most of the patients treated with Laetrile alone died, while those who took Laetrile, a special diet and vitamins did better.

During the 1980s, Dr. Harold W. Manner (PhD), used Laetrile in conjunction with what he termed "metabolic therapy" that included the use of vitamins and proteolytic enzymes. In fact, he injected tumors directly with proteolytic enzymes, causing lysis and destruction of the tumors. The role of Laetrile in the tumor destruction was unclear. Though he claimed a succes rate of 68-74%, he never provided patient histories to prove his case.

The issue of access to Laetrile was extensively litigated in the 1970s in *U.S v. Rutherford*, a class action lawsuit by Glen Rutherford and several other patients. Glen Rutherford was a fifty-five year old man who had polypoid colon cancer. He refused surgery and was treated instead with cautery of the polyp and administration of Laetrile and vitamins, and was subsequently found to be free from cancer.

He launched the lawsuit after officials confiscated a supply of Laetrile he was attempting to transport from Oklahoma to Kansas for his own personal use. He claimed that lay people with terminal cancer should be given access to Laetrile in the US.

At that time, people labeled terminally ill were allowed to import Laetrile from foreign countries if a formal request was made by their physician. This law was in place from the early 1970s to 1987, when the affidavit program was finally dissolved.

Currently, Laetrile is being legally sold on the Internet, and widely used at alternative clinics in foreign countries.

Clinical Tests

Animal Studies

Multiple tests of Laetrile have been done by Sloan-Kettering and the NCI. According to Dr. Ralph Moss, in many cases, results showed clear benefits from Laetrile, but authorities ignored the findings and stated that Laetrile failed to cure cancer.

One example of this is an animal study done in 1973 by the Southern Research Institute in Birmingham, Alabama. The study was passed on to the National Cancer Institute, which then announced that it proved Laetrile ineffective in treating cancer.
Four groups of mice with tumors were used in the experiment. One group received no treatment. Another group received too small a dose of Laetrile. A third group received the proper dose of Laetrile. The last group received too high a dose of Laetrile.

The mice that received too little Laetrile died just as quickly as those in the control group which received no Laetrile at all. Those that received too much died sooner than those in the control group. However, the group that received the proper dose had a survival time significantly longer than the group that received none at all.

In view of such results, one may wonder how the National Cancer Institute could conclude that Laetrile was useless. Here is how it was done: all three groups of animal test subjects given the Laetrile were lumped into the same statistical set. This included the group which received too little to be effective, as well as the group given a deliberate overdose.

When these two groups were added to the properly-treated group that survived significantly longer, they brought down the average survival time to the point where it could be said "honestly" that the treated mice, as a total group, had not survived significantly longer than those which had received no Laetrile at all.

However, the most egregious case of research suppression involved the work of Dr. Kanematsu Sugiura, a scientist employed by Sloan-Kettering.

From 1972 to 1977, Laetrile was meticulously tested on mice at Sloan-Kettering under the supervision of Dr. Sugiura, a prominent and respected researcher. Dr. Sugiura reported five results in his mouse test subjects: (1) Laetrile prevented metastases; (2) it improved general health; (3) it inhibited the growth of small tumors; (4) it provided pain relief; and (5) it acted as a cancer preventative agent. He felt it was not a complete cure for cancer, but a good palliative drug.

Dr. Sugiura's laboratory issued a formal statement which said, "The results clearly show that Amygdalin significantly inhibits the appearance of lung metastases in mice bearing spontaneous mammary tumors and increases significantly the inhibition of the growth of the primary tumors….Laetrile also seemed to prevent slightly the appearance of new tumors….The improvement of health and appearance of the treated animals in comparison to controls is always a common observation…. Dr. Sugiura has never observed complete regression of these tumors in all his cosmic experience with other chemotherapeutic agents."

Dr. Elizabeth Stockert and Dr. Lloyd Schloen, also biochemists at Sloan-Kettering, conducted other tests with positive results. Dr. Schloen added proteolytic enzymes to the Laetrile injections, as is commonly done in clinical use of Laetrile, and noted a 100% cure rate among mice with tumors.

However, a cheap, easily-synthesized cancer cure made from a plant extract did not have the exclusive profit-making potential desired by the heads of Sloan-Kettering.
Subsequently, public attempts were made by Dr. Sugiura's own employers to discredit his work. Other scientists at Sloan-Kettering, outraged over the cover-up, began to circulate a series of anonymous news releases to the public under the name *Second Opinion*. Copies of important internal company memos, as well as copies of Sugiura's laboratory reports, were leaked to the media and Laetrile advocates.

In response to the furor, Sloan-Kettering announced another round of tests, which produced negative results. Their opponents claimed that animal test subjects and medication had been mixed up. Despite pressure, Dr. Sugiura refused to renounce his own work.

Dr. Ralph Moss (Ph.D), the Assistant Director of Public Affairs at the Sloan-Kettering during these events, was the spokesman in charge of writing the official press releases claiming that Laetrile was ineffective. Secretly, Moss was one of the leaders of the *Second Opinion* whistleblowers group, who had tried to publicize the internal practices of Sloan-Kettering. Finally, in November of 1977, he decided to reveal his identity to the public. He called his own press conference, and before an audience of reporters and cameramen, claimed that his employers had falsified evidence. He provided supporting documents and names of the purported malefactors.

Sloan-Kettering fired Ralph Moss the next day.[5]

Time passed, the scandal subsided, and the short memory of the public once more allows Sloan-Kettering to be known as a "reputable" scientific institution.

In the end, the attempt by the cancer establishment to discredit Laetrile completely was unsuccessful, because too many positive experiments were known to the public, and news about Laetrile was spread by word of mouth within the community of cancer patients. However, the lack of success was obviously not due to lack of trying.

Many people still believe that Laetrile was tested and found to be unsuccessful because they have not personally examined the experimental data, only heard the official pronouncements. Given the behavior of Sloan-Kettering and the NCI, the public would be well advised to be skeptical of their statements.

Human Studies

Tests in Israel (Rubin, 1977) found laetrile to be most effective against adenocarcinoma and Hodgkin's disease, less effective against melanomas and sarcomas, and least effective against leukemia.

Other alternative practitioners have found the best results against cancers of the brain, breast, lung, and prostate, and lymphomas.

The quality of laetrile used (there are multiple manufacturers) also influences the results.
A 1962 clinical trial of 10 terminal patients used intravenous Laetrile in doses of 9-133 gms over a treatment period ranging from 4-43 weeks. The researchers concluded, "The use of Laetrile... in 10 cases of inoperable cancer, all with metastases, provided dramatic relief of pain, discontinuance of narcotics, control of fetor [stench from a tumor], improved appetite, and reduction of adenopathy [swollen lymph nodes]. The results suggest regression of the malignant lesion.... No other side effects [other than transient episodes of low blood pressure] were noted except slight itching and a sensation of heat in the affected areas, which was transitory in all cases."[6]

Unfortunately no followup was done to determine how long the improvement in patient condition lasted, or whether survival was extended.

In 1978, the NCI performed a retrospective study of American clinical experience with Laetrile. They surveyed more than 385,000 doctors, 70,000 other health practitioners, and even contracted pro-Laetrile patient support organizations. Though it was estimated that roughly 70,000 Americans had undergone Laetrile treatment at the time of the study, only 93 cases were finally produced for evaluation, and 26 of those were disqualified due to inadequate documentation, leaving 57 cases.

Of the 57 cases examined, 2 patients showed complete response (total disappearance of cancer), 4 had partial regression (tumor size reduction greater than 50%), 9 were "stabilized" (tumors stopped growing), and 3 showed "increased disease-free intervals."

In summary, 18 out of 57, or approximately one third, displayed some beneficial response to Laetrile treatment, a response rate unmatched by any conventional FDA-approved chemotherapeutic agent. Despite these results, the official NCI report stated, "These results allow no definite conclusion supporting the anti-cancer activity of Laetrile."[7]

A 1982 clinical trial of Laetrile treatment in 178 patients with various cancers produced no observable benefit, and some patients developed high blood levels of cyanide. Researchers concluded, "Amygdalin (Laetrile) is a toxic drug that is not effective as a cancer treatment."[8]

Caution

In Turkey and the Balkans, where apricot seeds are commonly eaten as a snack, rare deaths have occurred due to cyanide poisoning. One death may have occurred in America.

Do not consume large quantities of apricot seeds or B17 capsules without slowly building up from a low starting dose.

Instructions

Chew 7 pits a day, starting with one pit and gradually increasing your consumption.

Some people with cancer take up to 35 pits a day. Do not exceed this dose. Do not give more than 10 pits to a child. If shortness of breath or fatigue develop, discontinue use of seeds IMMEDIATELY until symptoms subside, then restart at a lower dose.

Apricot seeds and laetrile can be used together in the management of cancer. Some manufacturers have encapsulated B17 into 100 mg capsules or tablets that are much easier to take than just eating apricot seeds.

In a clinical setting, high levels of Laetrile can be administered intravenously. This is said to be safer, as much more conversion of Laetrile to cyanide occurs after oral administration.[9]

Suppliers

1 pound of apricot seeds costs as little as $20 on ebay.

There are many brands of Laetrile available, and not all are of equally good quality. Be sure to buy from a reputable company with good references.

Be sure to take proteolytic enzymes (also known as pancreatic enzymes) along with the Laetrile. Brands such as Megazyme Forte contain trypsin, chymotrypsin, bromalin and zinc nutrients. Take 2 pills three times daily. Other good brands are: Vitalzym, 10Zymes (also from Essense of Life), and Wobenzym N.

Laetrile is administered intravenously at some Mexican clinics.

References

(1) Newmark J, et al., "Amygdalin (Laetrile) and prunasin beta-glucosidases: distribution in germ-free rat and in human tumor tissue." PNAS October 1, 1981 vol. 78 no. 10 6513-6516

(2) Rauws AG, Olling M, Timmerman A, "The pharmacokinetics of prunasin, a metabolite of amygdalin." J Clin Toxicol 19 (8): 851-6, 1982.

(3) Kochi M, Takeuchi S, Mizutani T, et al., "Antitumor activity of benzaldehyde." Cancer Treat Rep 64 (1): 21-3, 1980.

(4) Kochi M, Isono N, Niwayama M, et al., "Antitumor activity of a benzaldehyde derivative." Cancer Treat Rep 69 (5): 533-7, 1985.

(5) Moss RW, "The laetrile controversy." The Cancer Industry: The Classic Expose on the Cancer Establishment. Brooklyn, NY: First Equinox Press, 1996.

(6) Morrone JA, "Chemotherapy of inoperable cancer: preliminary report of 10 cases treated with laetrile." Exp Med Surg 20: 299-308, 1962.

331

(7) Ellison NM, Byar DP, Newell GR, "Special report on Laetrile: the NCI Laetrile Review. Results of the National Cancer Institute's retrospective Laetrile analysis." N Engl J Med 299 (10): 549-52, 1978.

(8) Charles G. Moertel, M.D., Thomas R. Fleming, Ph.D., Joseph Rubin, M.D., Larry K. Kvols, M.D., Gregory Sarna, M.D., Robert Koch, M.D., Violante E. Currie, M.D., Charles W. Young, M.D., Stephen E. Jones, M.D., and J. Paul Davignon, Ph.D. "A Clinical Trial of Amygdalin (Laetrile) in the Treatment of Human Cancer." N Engl J Med 1982; 306:201-206

(9) Gostomski FE: The effects of amygdalin on the Krebs-2 carcinoma and adult and fetal DUB(ICR) mice. [Abstract] Diss Abstr Int B 39 (5): 2075-B, 1978.

Limonene (D-Limonene)

Limonene is a colorless hydrocarbon with a strong orange fragrance. It is largely used in cleaning products and as a coolant, as it is insoluble in water and therefore can be used in water separating units. It eliminates the need for products such as mineral spirits, acetone, glycol ethers and chlorinate solvents. It is used to impart an orange fragrance in solvents. Limonene is a versatile compound and very safe to use.

It is chemically classified as a monoterpene, a family of substances found in the essential oils of citrus fruits and other plants. D-Limonene is the chemical substance found in oil extracted from citrus rind.

Two extraction methods are used.

In the first method, at the time of juicing whole citrus fruits, oil is extracted by separating the oil from the juice before distilling it. The residue oil that is left behind after recovery of the fragrances and flavors is collected, and is further processed to extract d-Limonene. The oil can also be used to make flavored and fragranced substances.

In the second method, peels are removed before the fruit pulp is juiced. These peels are passed through a steam extractor to remove the oil. The steam is condensed, the oil collected from the surface of the cooled water, and d-Limonene is then extracted. However, this latter product is termed technical grade d-Limonene, while the Limonene collected through distillation is known as food grade d-limonene.

D-Limonene can also be extracted from orange or lemon peel using liquid Carbon dioxide.

The limonene is distilled from the oil without breaking down due to its stable structure. Limonene is then converted into various other forms prior to use. Most of the limonene is converted to carvone, which is a compound used in many cosmetics to impart the citrus fragrance. It is also used in food manufacturing and for medicinal purposes.

People are exposed to low levels of d-limonene on a widespread scale, due to consumption of citrus fruits and juice. A glass of pure orange juice contains approximately 20 mg d-limonene.

D-Limonene Skin Cancer Cure

Increased consumption of d-limonene correlates with a lower incidence of squamous cell skin cancer.

There are anecdotal reports of topically applied d-limonene or orange peel essential oil to treat non-melanoma skin cancer. It can be combined with surfactants (detergents) or pretreatment of skin with household ammonia for better absorption. Though the results are not immediate, it is a natural method with very minimal if any side effects.

Studies

D-limonene, which comprises >90% of orange peel essential oil, prevents the development of cancer by activating carcinogen-destroying enzymes. It also stimulates cancerous cell differentiation, prevents tumor growth by inhibition of proteins which regulate cell growth, and causes apoptosis in tumor cells.

D-limonene prevents against the induction of mammary, skin, liver, lung and forestomach cancers in-vivo if administered during the initiation phase of cancer. Combined with its metabolite perillyl alcohol, it has chemotherapeutic effects against liver and pancreatic cancer in test animals. More human trials are being planned.[1]

Evidence from one Phase I human trial shows a partial response from a patient with breast cancer given 15 gm/day of d-limonene and disease stabilization of more than 6 months in 3 patients with colorectal cancer.[2]

In addition to treating cancer, d-limonene has also been used successfully to dissolve cholesterol-based gallstones.[3]

It is also used to relieve heartburn and indigestion.

Caution

While it is classified as a GRAS (generally recognized as safe) compound when used in small quantities as a flavoring agent, it can be fatal in high doses. LD50 (the dose needed to kill 50% of test animals) was 5.6 and 6.6 grams/kg in male and female mice respectively, and 4.4 and 5.1 mg/kg in male and female rats.

It concentrates in fatty tissues such as the breast.

D-limonene is almost completely absorbed through the gastrointestinal tract, and 52-83% is cleared from the body within 48 hours.
20 healthy males given a single dose of 20 gm of d-limone complained of diarrhea and intestinal cramping, but tests showed no abnormalities of pancreatic, liver or kidney function.
D-limonene is a skin and eye irritant. It also makes the skin photosensitive and can cause skin rash and sunburns.

In a study of 32 patients with treatment-resistant solid tumors, maximum tolerated oral dose was 15 gm/day. One breast cancer patient consumed this dose for 11 month. Only gastrointestrinal side effects were noted.[4]

Instructions

There is no established treatment protocol for the use of this substance in treating cancer, but studies suggest up to 15 grams per day is safe.

Supplier

1000 mg 60 softgels under $8 from http://www.iherb.com/D-limonene-Orange-Peel-Extract

References

(1) Pamela L. Crowell, "Prevention and Therapy of Cancer by Dietary Monoterpenes." J. Nutr. March 1, 1999 vol. 129 no. 3 775

(2) Sun J, "D-Limonene: Safety and Clinical Applications." Altern Med Rev 2007 12(3):259-264

(3) Igimi H. Et al., "Medical dissolution of gallstones. Clinical experience of d-limonene as a simple, safe and effective solvent." Dig Dis Sci 1991; 36; 200-208

(4) Jidong Sun, "D-limonene : Safety and Clinical Applications." Alt Med Review, Volume 12, Number 3 2007

Marijuana (Cannabis Sativa)

Who would have thought that marijuana would be capable of killing cancer cells? Marijuana, or cannabis, contains 483 known compounds. At least 80 of them are cannabinoids, which include THC or tetrahydrocannabinol, the best-known psychoactive compound. The five most important cannabinoids found in cannabis are tetrahydrocannabinol, cannabidiol, cannabinol, beta-caryophyllene, and cannabigerol. THC is the best known, but it acts synergistically with the other chemicals in the plant.

Marijuana and its components have a long history of use for medical purposes. In ancient Greece it was used for veterinary medicine, helping animal wounds heal. Ancient India used the plant for illnesses and ailments such as headaches, pain, and other disorders. In ancient Egypt it was used to relieve hemorrhoid pain. Medical marijuana is currently being used to treat a wide variety of conditions aside from cancer, including glaucoma, inflammatory bowel disease, migraines, asthma, multiple sclerosis, AIDS and Alzheimer's disease.

THC is one of the few known drugs that has no toxicity. There has never been a single known death due to THC.

Considering its widespread usefulness and complete lack of toxicity, one would think that it would be the most popular medicine worldwide, but anti-drug laws severely limit public access to it. In the US, regulation and restriction of the sale of marijuana as a medicine began as early as 1860. From 1906 onward, cannabis was labeled as a poison, and complete prohibitions began in various states in the 1920s. By the mid-1930s Cannabis was regulated as a drug in every state, including 35 states that adopted the Uniform State Narcotic Drug Act.

Currently, the US federal government has ultimate authority over the nation's drug laws, despite efforts since the 1970s to overturn marijuana prohibition at the state level. Enforcement efforts vary widely from state to state. Despite a campaign of world-wide suppression, the recreational use of cannabis has been a staple of popular culture since the 1960s, and the product remains easily obtainable on the black market in most countries.

The medical use of marijuana is not a new concept, and has been studied in the US for at least 40 years. In the early 1970s, cannabinoids were shown to slow tumor growth and prolong survival of mice innoculated with Lewis lung adenocarcinoma cells.[1]

Some states have legalized the use of marijuana for medical purposes. There are a few medical therapies that have been approved in Canada which incorporate the components of marijuana and other substances to create an oral medicine for certain conditions, including multiple sclerosis and cancer related pain.

In the United States the FDA (Food & Drug Administration) has approved a couple of medical therapies that use components of marijuana to create a medicine that is taken orally for systems related to anorexia and nausea related symptoms with cancer chemotherapy patients.

Synthetic cannabinoids are sold as prescription drugs in some countries. Examples are Marinol in America and Canada, and Cesamet in America, Canada, Mexico, and the UK. These oral medications have a longer half-life than natural marijuana products, and need to be taken only twice daily to maintain their effects. The effects of natural THC wear off within 2 to 3 hours.

Probably the most well known proponent of the use of marijuana oil to cure cancer is Canadian Rick Simpson. He cured cancer in both himself and many of his acqaintances, and unsuccessfully lobbied the Canadian government to legalize the use of marijuana as a cancer treatment. He was finally forced to leave Canada, and currently resides in Holland.

Biochemistry of Cannabinoids

The diverse effects of cannabinoids are mediated through the activation of cellular receptors that are normally activated by a group of endogenous proteins, the endocannabinoids. Two cannabinoid receptors have been isolated and cloned from mammalian tissues. One, the "central" CB_1 receptor, is found mainly in the brain, especially in the basal ganglia, limbic system, including the hippocampus. They are also found in the cerebellum and in the human reproductive system. CB_2 receptors are located almost exclusively in the immune system, with the highest concentration in the spleen.

There are three classes of cannabinoids: compounds such as cannabidiol are found only in the cannabis plant; endogenous cannabinoids (endocannabinoids) such as anandamide and 2-arachidonoylglycerol are produced in animal and human bodies; and synthetic cannabinoids, such as 212-2, WIN-55, JWH-133, and (R)-methanandamide (MET), are lab-created compounds with chemical similarities to either plant-derived or endogenous cannabinoids.[2]

There is some question as to whether cannabinoids have an anti-cancer effect on all cells, or just those with cannabinoid receptors.

Recently, a firm in Israel called Tikkun Olam developed a species of marijuana lacking THC, but still containing all the other medicinal cannabinoid compounds, such as cannabidiol, present in the original variety of the plant. Tzahi Klein, head of development at Tikkun Olam, stated that the plant has no psychoactive effects. If this cultivar becomes widely available, it could open the door for legal cultivation of marijuana, as hemp is grown legally now. It may be slightly less effective due to the lack of THC. However, cannabidiol has a stronger effect than THC against cancer. It would also be more tolerable for patients who have to continue working while undergoing cancer treatment, as it would not interfere with mental functions.

Industrial hemp also has a low level of THC, but these plants are bred for fiber and seed oil, and have varying amounts of cannabinoids.

Studies

There are numerous anecdotal accounts of a wide variety of cancers cured by the use of marijuana.

Many in-vivo and vitro studies exist, but large human studies have not yet been performed.

In animal and in-vitro studies, cannabinoids inhibit proliferation of a multitude of tumor cell lines: gliomas, leukemia, lymphoma, cancers of the breast, prostate, skin, lung, cervix and uterus, colorectal, gastric adenocarcinoma, neuroblastoma, thyroid epithelioma, pancreatic adenocarcinoma, oral cancer, and biliary tract cancer (cholangiocarcinoma). Cannabinoids cause apoptosis of tumor cells, and some studies also show inhibition of angiogenesis.[3-32]

The anti-cancer effect of marijuana is due to multiple chemicals, not just THC. An extract of the whole plant may have more effect than a single compound, or a single, synthesized version of one compound. Many plants have an anti-cancer effect due to a synergistic combination of many chemical compounds, not just one.

Several compounds in marijuana besides THC inhibit cancer cell growth. The effect is seen in numerous human tumor cell lines, including breast, prostate, and colorectoral carcinoma. Researchers assessed the anti-tumor activity of various non-psychoactive cannabinoids, including cannabidiol (CBD), cannabigerol (CBG), and cannabichromine (CBC) *in vivo* and *in vitro*. They found that CBD is a more potent inhibitor of cancer growth than other cannabinoids, including THC. The compound halted the spread of breast cancer cells by triggering apoptosis. Cannabigerol and CBC also showed anti-tumor effects, but lacked the potency of CBD. "These results suggest the use in cancer therapy for cannabidiol," investigators concluded.[33]

Cannabidiol causes apoptosis in glioma cells *in vitro* and tumor regression *in vivo* through activation of caspases and reactive oxygen compounds independent of cannabinoid cell receptors.[34]

Another study found that delta-(9)-tetrahydrocannabinol enhanced breast cancer growth and metastasis specifically in cells which had few cannabinoid receptors by suppressing the antitumor immune response. This suggests that cannabinoids may increase the incidence of cancer in cells that lack cannabinoid receptors.[35]

However, most studies show that cannabinoids inhibit human breast cancer cells in-vitro, so the above study may apply only to a few cell lines which lack cannabinoid receptors.

Human Studies

A small Phase I trial of 9 terminally ill patients with recurrent glioblastoma multiforme not responsive to conventional treatment was performed to test the safety of intracranial administration of THC. Intratumoral administration of THC was associated with decreased tumor cell proliferation in 2/9 patients. The therapy did not prove toxic, but only 2 patients were still alive after 1 year. Mean survival time was 24 weeks. The expected survival time from time of diagnosis for patients with glioblastomas is 6-12 months; however, these patients were already well into this time frame when they were admitted to the study.[36]

Instructions

In curing cancer, oral consumption of marijuana oil (hashish oil) is used. In skin cancer, it is also topically applied. Smoking the plant is ineffective.

There are various methods for extracting marijuana oil, some of which require a fair level of expertise to be performed safely in a kitchen, and involve the use of flammable solvents. "Honey oil" extractors, which are sold on the internet, are probably safer to use.

Do not mistake hash oil, which is effective and probably illegal (depending on your jurisdiction), with hemp seed oil, which is a legal product sold in health food stores as a dietary supplement. Hemp oil is a fatty acid supplement which is not known to have any direct effect against cancer, though it may improve general health.

Rick Simpson's website has more information on this subject.

http://www.cannabisculture.com/articles/5169.html

Caution

Obviously, one should never drive or operate machinery while using psychoactive drugs.

Some studies have linked the long-term heavy use of marijuana to memory loss and increased rates of psychosis. However, these findings have been contested by other studies which do not show these effects.

The possibility of legal prosecution must be weighed as well.

References

(1) Guzman M, "Cannabinoids: potential anticancer agents," Nat Rev Cancer 2003; 3: 745–55

(2) Sami Sarfaraz, et al., "Cannabinoids for Cancer Treatment: Progress and Promise," Cancer Res January 15, 2008 68; 339

(3) Petrocellis et al. "The endogenous cannabinoid anandamide inhibits human breast cancer cell proliferation." Proceedings of the National Academy of Sciences of the United States of America 95: 8375-8380 1998.

(4) Guzman et al. "Delta-9-tetrahydrocannabinol induces apoptosis in C6 glioma cells." FEBS Letters 436: 6-10 1998.

(5) Baek et al.. "Antitumor activity of cannabigerol against human oral epitheloid carcinoma cells." Archives of Pharmacal Research: 21: 353-356 1998

(6) Ruiz et al.. "Delta-9-tetrahydrocannabinol induces apoptosis in human prostate PC-3 cells via a receptor-independent mechanism." FEBS Letters 458: 400-404 1999

(7) Mimeault et al. "Anti-proliferative and apoptotic effects of anandamide in human prostatic cancer cell lines." Prostate 56: 1-12. 2003

(8) Manuel Guzman. "Cannabinoids: potential anticancer agents (PDF)." Nature Reviews Cancer 3: 745-755

(9) Casanova et al. "Inhibition of skin tumor growth and angiogenesis in vivo by activation of cannabinoid receptors." 2003. Journal of Clinical Investigation 111: 43-50.

(10) Sarfaraz et al. "Cannabinoid receptors as a novel target for the treatment of prostate cancer." Cancer Research 65: 1635-1641 2005.

(11) Powles et al. "Cannabis-induced cytotoxicity in leukemic cell lines." Blood 105: 1214-1221 2005

(12) Pastos et al. "The endogenous cannabinoid, anandamide, induces cell death in colorectal carcinoma cells: a possible role for cyclooxygenase-2." Gut 54: 1741-1750 2005.

(13) Pastos et al. "The endogenous cannabinoid, anandamide, induces cell death in colorectal carcinoma cells: a possible role for cyclooxygenase-2." Gut 54: 1741-1750 2005.

(14) Natalya Kogan. "Cannabinoids and cancer." Mini-Reviews in Medicinal Chemistry 5: 941-952 2005.

(15) Cafferal et al. "Delta-9-Tetrahydrocannabinol inhibits cell cycle progression in human breast cancer cells through Cdc2 regulation." Cancer Research 66: 6615-6621 2006.

(16) Di Marzo et al. "Anti-tumor activity of plant cannabinoids with emphasis on the effect of cannabidiol on human breast carcinoma." Journal of Pharmacology and Experimental Therapeutics Fast Forward 318: 1375-1387 2006.

(17) Jia et al. "Delta-9-tetrahydrocannabinol-induced apoptosis in Jurkat leukemic T cells in regulated by translocation of Bad to mitochondria." Molecular Cancer Research 4: 549-562 2006.

(18) Carracedo et al. "Cannabinoids induce apoptosis of pancreatic tumor cells via endoplasmic reticulum stress-related genes." Cancer Research 66: 6748-6755 2006.

(19) Gustafsson et al. "Cannabinoid receptor-mediated apoptosis induced by R(+)-methanandamide and Win55,212 is associated with ceramide accumulation and p38 activation in mantle cell lymphoma." Molecular Pharmacology 70: 1612-1620 2006.

(20) McAllister et al. "Cannabidiol as a novel inhibitor of Id-1 gene expression in aggressive breast cancer cells." Molecular Cancer Therapeutics 6: 2921-2927 2007.

(21) Preet et al. "Delta9-Tetrahydrocannabinol inhibits epithelial growth factor-induced lung cancer cell migration in vitro as well as its growth and metastasis in vivo." Oncogene 10: 339-346 2008.

(22) Liu et al. "Enhancing the in vitro cytotoxic activity of Ä9-tetrahydrocannabinol in leukemic cells through a combinatorial approach." Leukemia and Lymphoma 49: 1800-1809 2008.

(23) Michalski et al. "Cannabinoids in pancreatic cancer: correlation with survival and pain." International Journal of Cancer 122: 742-750 2008 .

(24) Ramer and Hinz. "Inhibition of cancer cell invasion by cannabinoids via increased cell expression of tissue inhibitor of matrix metalloproteinases-1." Journal of the National Cancer Institute 100: 59-69 2008.

(25) Gustafsson et al. "Expression of cannabinoid receptors type 1 and type 2 in non-Hodgkin lymphoma: Growth inhibition by receptor activation." International Journal of Cancer 123: 1025-1033 2008.

(26) Sarafaraz et al. "Cannabinoids for cancer treatment: progress and promise." Cancer Research 68: 339-342 2008.

(27) Cafferal et al. "Cannabinoids reduce ErbB2-driven breast cancer progression through Akt inhibition." Molecular Cancer 9: 196 2010

(28) Marcu et al. "Cannabidiol enhances the inhibitory effects of delta9-tetrahydrocannabinol on human glioblastoma cell proliferation and survival." Molecular Cancer Therapeutics 9: 180-189 2010.

(29) Whyte et al. "Cannabinoids inhibit cellular respiration of human oral cancer cells. Pharmacology 85: 328-335 2010

(30) Leelawat et al. "The dual effects of delta(9)-tetrahydrocannabinol on cholangiocarcinoma cells: anti-invasion activity at low concentration and apoptosis induction at high concentration." Cancer Investigation 28: 357-363 2010.

(31) Foroughi et al. "Spontaneous regression of septum pellucidum/forniceal pilocytic astrocytomas -- possible role of cannabis inhalation." Child's Nervous System 201127: 671-679.

(32) Aviello et al. "Chemopreventive effect of the non-psychotropic phytocannabinoid cannabidiol on experimental colon cancer." Journal of Molecular Medicine 2012 Aug;90(8):925-34. Epub 2012 Jan 10.

(33) Alessia Ligresti, et al., "Antitumor Activity of Plant Cannabinoids with Emphasis on the Effect of Cannabidiol on Human Breast Carcinoma," Journal of Pharmacology and Experimental Therapeutics, September 2006 vol. 318 no. 3 1375-1387

(34) Massi P, Vaccani A, Bianchessi S, et al. "The non-psychoactive cannabidiol triggers caspase activation and oxidative stress in human glioma cells." Cell Mol Life Sci, 2006; 63: 2057–66

(35) McKallip RJ, Nagarkatti M, Nagarkatti PS. "Δ-9-tetrahydrocannabinol enhances breast cancer growth and metastasis by suppression of the antitumor immune response." J Immunol 2005; 174: 3281–9

(36) M Guzmán, et al., "A pilot clinical study of 9-tetrahydracannibinol in patients with recurrent glioblastoma multiforme." British Journal of Cancer (2006) 95, 197–203

Modified Citrus Pectin

Modified citrus pectin (MCP) is a water-soluble carbohydrate found in the pulp and rinds of fruits such as apples, grapefruits, oranges and plums. It has a powerful ability to enhance the cytotoxic ability of T-cells and Natural Killer (NK) cells in their ability to prevent metastasis.

The substance cannot be obtained by directly eating the fruit, as the long chain form must be modified to produce shorter chains of sugar so that it absorbs more easily from the gastrointestinal tract.

Pectins are a viscous, gel-forming dietary fiber found in plant cell walls, especially citrus fruits and apples. They are polysaccharides (complex sugars) which vary in the length of their polysaccharide chains, from 300 to 1,000 monosaccharides (simple sugars). Pectin is depolymerized through a treatment with sodium hydroxide and hydrochloric acid, which breaks the long chains into shorter segments comprised predominantly of D-polygalacturonates, which the body can absorb.

MCP has many anti-tumor functions: it enhances the immune system, making it useful in the treatment of autoimmune disease and cancer; it inhibits cancer cell adhesion, making tumors less likely to form a mass isolated from the rest of the body; and it binds to galectin-3 sites, reducing tumor growth, tissue invasion and metastasis.

It removes toxic material and radioactive waste from the body, thus preventing the initiation of cancer. Its activity as a metal chelator is backed by clinical research.[1]

It also lowers cholesterol.

Studies

According to an in-vivo study on mice implanted with human breast or colon cancer cells, "MCP, given orally, inhibits carbohydrate-mediated tumor growth, angiogenesis, and metastasis in vivo, presumably via its effect on galectin-3 function."[2]

MCP reduces PSA markers in men with prostate cancer.[3]

One in-vivo study was performed on the effects of quercetin and MCP on the size and weight of colon cancer tumors in mice. Both substances showed anti-tumor effects.

Fifty mice were divided into 5 groups. Group 1, the control group, received 1 ml distilled water. The remaining 4 groups were given low-dose quercetin(0.8 mg/ml), high-dose quercetin (1.6 mg/ml), low-dose MCP (0. 8 mg/ml) or high-dose MCP (1.6 mg/ml) on a daily basis, starting on the first day the tumor was palpable by researchers (usually eight days post-implantation). Significant reduction in tumor size was seen by day 20 in all groups compared to controls. The groups fed low-dose quercetin and MCP had a 29% and 38% reduction in tumor size, respectively. The high-dose groups had an even more impressive reduction in size, 65% in the quercetin group and 70% in the MCP group.

Researchers concluded, "This is the first evidence that MCP can reduce the growth of solid primary tumors, and the first research showing QC has antitumor activity."[4]

Instructions

Modified citrus pectin is most often used as an adjuvant to other cancer therapies to prevent metastasis. The usual dose is 15 grams per day in three divided doses of 5 grams each.

MCP is marketed under the brand name Pecta-Sol. It is also referred to as citrus pectin, depolymerized pectin, fractioned pectin, modified pectin, and pH-modified pectin. However, not all brands are equal in activity or percentage of product actually absorbed by the body. Pecta-Sol is a reputable brand.

It has no known side effects.

Suppliers

You can buy Pecta Sol on Ebay for as low as $18.

References

(1) Eliaz I, et al., "The effect of modified citrus pectin on urinary excretion of toxic elements." Phytotherapy Res, 2006 Oct;20(10):859-64.

(2) Nangia-Makker, P., et al., "Inhibition of human cancer cell growth and metastasis in nude mice by oral intake of modified citrus pectin."J. Natl Cancer Inst., 2002 Dec 18;94(24):1854-62.

(3) Guess, B.W., "Modified citrus pectin (MCP) increases the prostate-specific antigen doubling time in men with prostate cancer: a phase II pilot study." Prostate Cancer Prostatic Dis. 2003;6(4):301-4.

(4) Hayashi A., "Effects of daily oral administration of quercetin chalcone and modified citrus pectin on implanted colon-25 tumor growth in Balb-c mice." Altern Med Rev., 2000 Dec;5(6):546-52.

Mustard Vegetables

Some scientists claim that members of the cabbage family of vegetables can not only prevent cancer, but in many cases cure it. The mustard family includes mustard itself as well as broccoli, cauliflower, bok choy, cabbage and Brussels sprouts.

The medicinal properties of cabbage were valued by ancient societies, and poultices of raw ground-up cabbage were used as a treatment for breast cancer by ancient Romans. This was described by Cato the Elder.

The preventative effects of eating cabbage have been shown by numerous studies around the world. The highest preventative effect is seen against cancers of the lung and the gastrointestinal tract.[1]

Members of the mustard family are so effective in fighting cancer because of the presence of the group of sulfur-containing chemicals called glucosinolates. These cancer-fighting chemicals are formed from precursor compounds during crushing of cruciferous vegetables.

Two cancer-fighting compounds are diindolylmethane (chemical name 3,3'-Diindolylmethane, also referred to as DIM) and its precursor, indole-3-carbinol (I3C), a natural part of glycobrassicin which is found in all members of the mustard family of vegetables.

The compound sulphoraphane, particularly abundant in young sprouts of broccoli and cauliflower, stimulates the production of liver enzymes which deactivate carcinogens. An enzyme called myrosinase transforms a precursor compound, glucoraphanin (a glucosinolate), into sulforaphane upon damage to the plant, such as from chewing.

Brussels sprouts also contain a lesser-known compound called sinigrin (the chemical name is allylglucosinolate or 2-propenylglucosinlate) which causes apoptosis in pre-cancerous cells.[2] According to scientists at the Institute of Food Research in Norwich, the effect is so powerful that even the occasional meal of sprouts can eliminate these cells.[3]

I3C

Indole-3-carbinol is an estrogen blocker, which prevents the hormonal stimulation that leads to cancers of the reproductive tissues, such as breast, ovarian, and uterine cancer.[4]

I3C causes apoptosis in breast cancer cells, but not in normal breast cells.[5]

It does so through inactivation of the Akt signalling pathway, which activates NF-kappaB, a well-known endogenous tumor promoter.[6]

I3C prevents bone metastasis of breast cancer cells due to inhibition of NF-kappaB as well as downregulation of genes involved in cancer cell tissue invasion and spread.[7]

I3C leads to apoptosis in multiple cells lines of tumors, including cervical,[8] colon,[9] nasopharyngeal[10] and prostate cancer.[11]

Diindolylmethane (DIM)

In an in-vitro study, human cancer cells MCF-7 (breast cancer), T47-D (human ductal breast epithelial tumor) and Saos-2 (osteosarcoma) all underwent apoptosis when exposed to DIM.[12]

DIM was found to have strong antiproliferative effects on human endometrial cancer cells, partly by activation of 2 estrogen-responsive genes.[13]

An in-vivo study found that DIM caused apoptosis and decreased growth in implanted prostate tumors in a dose-dependent fashion. Doses of 2.5, 5 and 10 mg/kg DIM were used, leading to tumor cell proliferation of 45%, 37% and 33% respectively compared to tumors in a control group.[14]

Arizona Cancer Center researcher Cynthia Thomson has been awarded a $3 million grant from the NIH to study whether DIM can enhance the anti-cancer effects of the breast cancer drug tamoxifen in high-risk women or those previously treated for early-stage breast cancer.

Sulphoraphane

Exposure of breast cancer cells to sulphoraphane blocks cell division by disruption of cellular microtubules, intracellular protein structures used for cell division.[15,16]

Sulphuraphane administered to human breast cancer cells in-vitro reduced the population of stem cells by 65% - 80%, as measured by a stem cell marker. Additional experiments were performed using mice implanted with breast cancer cells. Daily injection of sulforaphane (50 mg/kg) for two weeks reduced the number of stem cells in the mouse tumors by more than 50%. Sulforaphane's ability to eliminate breast cancer stem cells also prevented tumor growth in a second group of mice implanted with tumor cells taken from the group of sulphuraphane-treated mice.[17]

While broccoli contains small amounts of sulphoraphane, broccoli sprouts contain levels 20 times higher than those found in mature heads of broccoli. They are tasty and can be added to salads or used to garnish sandwiches. Eat them raw, as cooking Broccoli sprouts destroys the enzyme *myrosinase* which converts the inactive compound Glucoraphanin to
the active compound, Sulforaphane.

It can be used alongside conventional therapy, and may enhance its effectiveness.

Forms of Supplements

This is one of the many instances when positive in-vitro studies do not necessarily translate into positive results from oral consumption. Test substances can be applied directly to cell cultures, but in humans, chemicals must pass through the digestive system before reaching their cellular targets.

Both I3C and DIM are available as supplements, but one authority on these substances, Dr. Michael Zelig, recommends an enhanced form of DIM (which he has patented and independently tested), for several reasons.[18]

Large amounts of diindolylmethane are found in cruciferous plants following crushing. The precursor molecule, I3C, is only briefly present, primarily during the digestive process. I3C is soluble but extemely reactive, creating more than 20 "condensation products" (including DIM) when mixed with stomach acid and plant enzymes freed by crushing the plant source.

DIM is formed from a chemical reaction which combines 2 I3C molecules. The resulting diindolylmethane is a "di-indole", or double molecule, created from two I3C molecules.

Due to its chemical instability, I3C requires careful storage, avoiding heat, moisture and light to slow its rapid breakdown and maintain shelf-life. It requires gastric acid for conversion to active products. It is more irritating to the stomach than DIM because of its chemical reactivity. It tends to interact with food components, especially vitamin C, limiting its conversion into DIM and other active compounds. Also, the condensation reaction may take more time than food typically spends in the human digestive tract.

One study found that following an oral dose of I3C, only DIM (and no I3C whatsoever) was found in the blood of test subjects. The same study also found that more than 90% of the orally administered I3C was converted into non-DIM condensation products with various chemical structures, absorption rates and biochemical activities.[19]

Some of these byproducts produce undesirable effects, such as indolocarbazole (or ICZ), which has a chemical structure and activity resembling dioxin. It has been linked to oxidative DNA damage[20] and unwanted estrogen metabolites.[21,22]

I3C supplements have been linked to induction of cytochrome enzymes, which affects the metabolism of many medications.[23] DIM has shown no such effects.[24]

Also, DIM but not I3C has been shown to promote healthy levels of estrogen and unbound testosterone, leading some alternative practitioners to use it to treat symptoms of andropause, perimenopause and PMS.

Crystalline DIM is poorly absorbed by the gastrointestinal tract, but a new patented microencapsulated formulation called Bio-Response greatly increases the absorption.[25] It is currently being used in some early clinical trials.[26]

Instructions

If using microencapsulated DIM (recommended), dose is 150 mg 1-2 times daily.
I3C dose is 300-400 mg daily.

Suppliers

Microencapsulated DIM is available from the manufacturer, Bio-Response, $39 for 60 capsules of 150 mg.

http://www.bioresponse.com/

Supplements of I3C can be purchased from the Life Extension Foundation as well as from other sources. Sulphoraphane supplements are also available in various strengths and prices. Vitacost sells both I3C and sulphoraphane.

References

(1) Jane V Higdon, et al, "Cruciferous Vegetables and Human Cancer Risk: Epidemiologic Evidence and Mechanistic Basis." Pharmacol Res. 2007 March; 55(3): 224–236.

(2) Tracy K.Smith, Elizabeth K.Lund and Ian T.Johnson, "Inhibition of dimethylhydrazine-induced aberrant crypt foci and induction of apoptosis in rat colon following oral administration of the glucosinolate sinigrin." Carcinogenesis vol.19 no.2 pp.267–273, 1998

(3) "Why your best friend could be a Brassica." Institute of Food Research

(4) Shyam N Sundar et al., "Indole-3-Carbinol Selectively Uncouples Expression and Activity of Estrogen Receptor Subtypes in Human Breast Cancer Cells." Molecular Endocrinology December 1, 2006 vol. 20 no. 12 3070-3082

(5) Rahman KM, Aranha O, Sarkar FH, "Indole-3-carbinol (I3C) induces apoptosis in tumorigenic but not in nontumorigenic breast epithelial cells." Nutr Cancer. 2003;45(1):101-12.

(6) Elena P. Moiseeva, Louise H. Fox, Lynne M. Howells, Louis A. F. Temple and Margaret M. Manson, "Indole-3-carbinol-induced death in cancer cells involves EGFR downregulation and is exacerbated in a 3D environment." Apoptosis 2006 May;11(5):799-812.

(7) Rahman KM, Sarkar FH, Banerjee S, Wang Z, Liao DJ, Hong X, Sarkar NH, "Therapeutic intervention of experimental breast cancer bone metastasis by indole-3-carbinol in SCID-human mouse model." Mol Cancer Ther. 2006 Nov;5(11):2747-56.

(8) Chen DZ, Qi M, Auborn KJ, Carter TH, "Indole-3-carbinol and diindolylmethane induce apoptosis of human cervical cancer cells and in murine HPV16-transgenic preneoplastic cervical epithelium."J Nutr. 2001 Dec;131(12):3294-302.

(9) Hudson EA, Howells LM, Gallacher-Horley B, Fox LH, Gescher A, Manson MM, "Growth-inhibitory effects of the chemopreventive agent indole-3-carbinol are increased in combination with the polyamine putrescine in the SW480 colon tumour cell line." BMC Cancer. 2003 Jan 14;3:2. Epub 2003 Jan 14.

(10) Xu Y, Zhang J, Dong WG. "Indole-3-carbinol (I3C)-induced apoptosis in nasopharyngeal cancer cells through Fas/FasL and MAPK pathway." Med Oncol. 2011 Dec;28(4):1343-8. Epub 2010 Jul 14.

(11) Nachshon-Kedmi M, Yannai S, Haj A, Fares FA, "Indole-3-carbinol and 3,3'-diindolylmethane induce apoptosis in human prostate cancer cells." Food Chem Toxicol. 2003 Jun;41(6):745-52.

(12) Ge X, Yannai S, Rennert G, Gruener N, Fares FA, "3,30 - Diindolylmethane induces apoptosis in human cancer cells." Biochem Biophys Res Commun 1996;228:153–158.

(13) Leong H, Firestone GL, Bjeldanes LF, "Cytostatic effects of 3,30 - diindolylmethane in human endometrial cancer cells results from an estrogen receptor-mediated increase in transforming growth factor-a expression." Carcinogenesis 2001;22:1809 – 1817.

(14) Maya Nachshon-Kedmi, Fuad A. Fares, and Shmuel Yannai, "Therapeutic Activity of 3,30 –Diindolylmethane on Prostate Cancer in an InVivo Model." The Prostate 61:153-160 (2004)

(15) Steven J.T.Jackson and Keith W.Singletary, "Sulforaphane: a naturally occurring mammary carcinoma mitotic inhibitor,which disrupts tubulin polymerization."Carcinogenesis vol.25 no.2 pp.219-227, 2004

(16) Jackson SJ, Singletary KW. "Sulforaphane inhibits human MCF-7 mammary cancer cell mitotic progression and tubulin polymerization." Journal of Nutrition. 2004;134:2229-2236.

(17) Li Y., et al., "Sulforaphane, a dietary component of broccoli/broccoli sprouts, inhibits breast cancer stem cells." Clin Cancer Res, 2010 May 1;16(9):2580-90

(18) Michael A. Zeligs, M.D. "The Cruciferous Choice: Diindolylmethane or I3C?," Phytonutrient Supplements For Cancer Prevention and Health Promotion

(19) Arneson, DW, Hurwitz, A, McMahon, LM, and Robaugh, D, " Presence of 3,3'-Diindolylmethane in human plasma after oral administration of Indole-3-carbinol." Proceedings of the American Association for Cancer Research, 1999 Mar; (40): #2833.

(20) Park JY, Shigenaga MK, Ames BN, "Induction of cytochrome P4501A1 by 2,3,7,8-tetrachlorodibenzo-p-dioxin or indolo(3,2-b)carbazole is associated with oxidative DNA damage." Proc Natl Acad Sci U S A. 1996 Mar 19;93(6):2322-7.

(21) Liehr JG, Ricci MJ, Jefcoate CR, et al., "4-Hydroxylation of estradiol by human uterine myometrium and myoma microsomes: Implications for the mechanism of uterine tumorigenesis." Proc. Natl. Acad. Sci. USA 1995 Sept 92:9220-9224.

(22) Ritter CL, Prigge WF, Reichert MA, et al., "Oxidations of 17beta-estradiol and estrone and their interconversions catalyzed by liver, mammary gland and mammary tumor after acute and chronic treatment of rats with indole-3-carbinol or beta-naphthoflavone." Can J Physiol Pharmacol 2001; 79(6):519-32.

(23) Stresser, DM, "Report: Examination of potential for absorbable diindolylmethane to induce and inhibit cytochrome P450 isoforms." Gentest Corporation, data on file, BioResponse LLC, 1999.

(24) NIH Chemoprevention Branch, "Safety study of diindolylmethane (BioResponse-DIM) versus Indole-3-carbinol in rats." on File, BioResponse, LLC, 2000.

(25) Jacobs, I.C., and Zeligs, M.A., "Facilitated absorption of a hydrophobic dietary ingredient: Diindolylmethane." Proceedings of the Controlled Release Society 1998.

(26) Heath EI, et al., "A biomarker trial of BR-DIM (BioResponse 3,3'-Diindolylmethane) in patients with prostate cancer who undergo prostatectomy." J Clin Oncol 29: 2011 (suppl; abstr e15185)

Oleander/Anvirzel

Nerium Oleander is a poisonous tree shrub that bears white, pink, red, or purple flowers with leathery leaves. The shrub grows in mild climates and is often kept as an indoor houseplant. Ingredients used for medical treatment and research are extracted from the leaves and used in controlled doses.

The history of oleander shows it has many medicinal uses, and it is recommended for treatment of muscle cramps, menstrual pain, skin & heart conditions, and cancer. Folk medicine uses, which date back thousands of years, use parts of the shrub to create tea, and patients sometimes eat nectar from the plant. Oleander Extract has been used against cancer, AIDS, hepatitis C and other viral illnesses, lupus and malaria.

The plant contains more than 500 biologically active substances, cardioglycosides and polysaccharides, such as oleandrin and neandrin, which act synergistically. Anvirzel, a patented hot water extract of oleander, contains a full spectrum of these substances, as do the folk remedies. It was found to be safe in Phase I clinical trials. However, it has not passed Phase II trials due to lack of funds for such studies, and is therefore approved by the FDA for "compassionate" use only in exceptional cases, for patients who have exhausted conventional therapies or who are considered terminal.

A Russian ethanol extract of oleander, sold under the name Xenavex, contains fewer compounds and is said to be less effective against cancer. Xenavex was promoted mainly to treat congestive heart failure, and not for cancer. It has properties similar to digoxin, another heart medication. It is high in cardioglycosides oleandrin and oleandrigenin, not polysaccharides.

Oleander has also been used in higher doses to make rat and fish poison, and insecticide. It is toxic to the heart in high doses.

Anvirzel crosses the blood-brain barrier.

History

Anvirzel was created by Dr. H. Ziya Ozel, a Turkish surgeon whose attention was drawn to oleander due to its use in Turkish folk medicine. He initially invented Nerium Oleander Extracts (NOE), and used forms of it for the treatment of cancer, AIDS, and immune system diseases for more than 3 decades in Turkey. In 1992 Dr. Ozel obtained an American patent (US# 5,135,745) for his extract of nerium oleander. In 1995 he signed an agreement with a U.S. venture capital firm, Pharmaceutical Ventures Trust, today known as Ozelle Pharmaceuticals, Inc. (OPI), to complete the necessary procedures to obtain FDA approval for NOE, which was sold under the trade name Anvirzel.

Ozel's personal research found that Nerium Oleander Extract was successful in 70% of cancer patients who had not undergone chemotherapy, and 30% successful in cancer patients who had been subjected to chemo. Success rates improve when oleander extract is combined with other medicinal plants such as Cat's Claw, Pau D'Arco, and ABM mushrooms. A Brazilian product called OPC combines oleander extract with these 3 ingredients, but is fairly expensive, at least $300 per bottle. The manufacturer's website also states that tests are currently underway using a combination of oleander extract with an African plant called Sutherlandia Frutescens, which supposedly has better synergistic action than ABM mushrooms .

Studies

In an in-vitro test oleandrin against colon cancer cells, researchers found "significant activity against colorectal cancer cell lines, by mechanisms disparate from currently used anticancer drugs, but at concentrations generally considered not achievable in patient plasma."[1]

Oleander extracts were shown to be cytotoxic to lines of human leukemia cells in-vitro.[2]

Oleandrin caused G2/M cell cycle arrest and autophagy (self-digestion) of human pancreatic tumor cells.[3]

Oleandrin caused a build-up of reactive oxygen compounds (free radicals) within human melanoma cells, resulting in "a loss in cellular viability, proliferation and cellular defense mechanisms such as GSH content." This effect could be blocked by incubation of the cells with acetyl-n-cysteine, an antioxidant and precursor to GSH. GSH, or reduced glutathione, is a natural cellular antioxidant which protects cells from oxidative damage.[4]

Anvirzel and oleandrin displayed anti-tumor effects against 2 lines of human prostate cancer cells.[5]

In general, the levels of oleander extracts used in the in-vitro tests were higher than those that could safely be obtained in blood plasma of human subjects.

Oleander extracts sensitized PC-3 prostate cells to radiation, an effect which is greater with longer exposure times (at least 24 hours prior to and also during radiotherapy). Apoptosis induced by radiation was dependent on activation of caspase-3.[6]

Clinical trials by an independent lab commissioned by Nerium Biotechnology Inc., a manufacturer of oleander-based skin lotions, found the product to be extremely safe for skin lesions as it is not absorbed through the skin, and cardiac glycosides do not appear in blood plasma after topical application. The lotion was tested on actinic keratosis (Nerium-AS), acne (Nerium-ACW & Nerium ACA) and various bacterial and viral skin disorders (NeriumDerm).[7,8,9]

A small phase I clinical trial of oleandrin extract PBI-05204 showed tumor response in 3/15 patients with cases of bladder, colorectal, and fallopian tube cancer. Minimal toxicity was observed.[10]

Caution

Since 1985, there have been 3 deaths reported in association with the use of oleander extracts. However, researchers performing intramuscular injections of oleander extract into animals have found the substance to be safe even at 10 times the usual therapeutic dosage.[11]

Cardiac toxicity can build up over time. Use as a medicine only as long as required, not as a long term health tonic. Patients with any pre-existing heart conditions should use extreme caution with oleander. Some manufacturers advise frail patients with heart conditions to take mineral supplements containing magnesium and potassium before using oleander.

Do not make home-brewed oleander tea from plants for oral consumption, as it is impossible to be sure what dosage it contains.

Instructions & Suppliers

Based in in-vitro tests, oleander extract may be a useful adjunct to radiotherapy. The manufacturer of Anvirzel also claims that their product lessens the side effects of chemotherapy.

The oldest, most thoroughly tested oleander product on the market is Anvirzel. It is a standardized, tested extract of known potency. However, it is fairly expensive, almost $3000 for a 3-month supply. The FDA can legally intercept it in the mail if it is not ordered with their approval.

It may be obtained from Salud Integral in Honduras. Kathy Vega is Director of Patient Services and may be reached at PH: 011 504 220 4575.

http://www.saludintegral.hn/

Oleander pills combined with various mineral supplements claimed to lessen toxicity, called Rose Laurel OPC Plus, are available for $90 from Utopia Silver.

http://cart.utopiasilver.com

The manufacturers of this product advise the use of alpha-lipoic acid and NAC along with their product. However, due to the demonstrated in-vitro blocking action of the antioxidant NAC on one mechanism of oleander, it may be advisable to avoid concurrent use of oleander and antioxidants. This list includes CoQ-10, lipoic acid, vitamins C and E, and NAC.

A new combination of oleander and sutherlandia, Sutherlandia OPC, is available for $60 for 60 capsules each containing 100mg Oleander and 250mg Sutherlandia. Bottles of extract (80% Oleander extract, 20% Sutherlandia extract) are available for $50 for 200ml. http://www.sutherlandiaopc.com/

References

(1) Felth, J; Rickardson, L; Rosén, J; Wickström, M; Fryknäs, M; Lindskog, M; Bohlin, L; Gullbo, J, "Cytotoxic effects of cardiac glycosides in colon cancer cells, alone and in combination with standard chemotherapeutic drugs". Journal of natural products 2009 72 (11): 1969–74.

(2) Turan, N; Akgün-Dar, K; Kuruca, SE; Kiliçaslan-Ayna, T; Seyhan, VG; Atasever, B; Meriçli, F; Carin, M (2006). "Cytotoxic effects of leaf, stem and root extracts of Nerium oleander on leukemia cell lines and role of the p-glycoprotein in this effect." Journal of experimental therapeutics & oncology 6 (1): 31–8

(3) Newman, RA; Kondo, Y; Yokoyama, T; Dixon, S; Cartwright, C; Chan, D; Johansen, M; Yang, P (2007). "Autophagic cell death of human pancreatic tumor cells mediated by oleandrin, a lipid-soluble cardiac glycoside". Integrative cancer therapies 6 (4): 354–64.

(4) Newman, RA; Yang, P; Hittelman, WN; Lu, T; Ho, DH; Ni, D; Chan, D; Vijjeswarapu, M et al (2006). "Oleandrin-mediated oxidative stress in human melanoma cells". Journal of experimental therapeutics & oncology 5 (3): 167–81.

(5) Smith, JA; Madden, T; Vijjeswarapu, M; Newman, RA (2001). "Inhibition of export of fibroblast growth factor-2 (FGF-2) from the prostate cancer cell lines PC3 and DU145 by Anvirzel and its cardiac glycoside component, oleandrin". Biochemical pharmacology 62 (4): 469–72.

(6) Nasu, S; Milas, L; Kawabe, S; Raju, U; Newman, R (2002). "Enhancement of radiotherapy by oleandrin is a caspase-3 dependent process". Cancer Letters 185 (2): 145–51)

(7) ST&T Research Intl. "An open label, non randomized, pilot study to test the safety and efficacy of Nerium-AS, a topical natural Nerium-based solution, (the Test Article) in patients with solar lentigines (Age Spots) and actinic keratosis". 2008c. Report to Nerium Biotechnology, Inc.

(8) ST&T Research Intl. "A double blind product comparison randomized two product study to test the safety and efficacy of a natural topical Nerium based Solutions, Nerium-ACW & Nerium ACA, against a typical Acne OTC product, in volunteers exhibiting mild to moderated Acne Vulgaris". 2008a. Report to Nerium Biotechnology, Inc.

(9) ST&T Research Intl. "An industry-initiated pilot study to test the safety and efficacy of a natural topical Nerium-based antiseptic solution, NeriumDerm, to help promote and speed the healing, reduce symptoms, and/or to mitigate and reduce pain and the spreading of skin irruptions or wounds to outside mouth areas in form of lip lesions, pimples, blemishes, fever blisters, or active cold sore(s) or HSV-1, in otherwise healthy volunteers". 2009. Report to Nerium Biotechnology, Inc.

(10) Henary HA, R Kurzrock, GS Falchook et al., "Final Results of a First-in-Human Phase 1 Trial of PBI-05204, and Inhibitor of AKT, FGF-2, NF-Kb and P70S6K in Advanced Cancer Patients". J Clin Oncol 29; 2011 supplement; abstract 3023

(11) Rhodes JW, "Non-GLP Single Dose Lethality Assessment of Nerium Oleander (NOI) by Intramuscular Administration in the Rat". Southwest Research Institute Project 12-7547-029

Sutherlandia Frutescans

This plant is a member of the legume family, a shrub with bitter, aromatic leaves, and red-orange flowers which appear in spring to mid-summer.

One of the best known multi-purpose medicinal plants in South Africa, Sutherlandia frutescens has a long history of traditional use. South Africa's ancient Zulu warriors named this bush "Insiswa," which means, "the one who dispels darkness," due to its qualities as an anti-depressant. It is also a traditional cancer cure, and Afrikaaners called it "Kankerbos," or "cancer bush." It has numerous other healing properties, and is also useful in treating viral illnesses, diabetes, chronic fatigue, and inflammatory conditions.

Sutherlandia has a direct effect against tumor cells, and also acts as an immune stimulant and anti-oxidant. In addition, it improves quality of life in cancer patients due to its antidepressant and fatigue-fighting effect.

Recently, the plant has been popularized by tradional African healer Credo Mutwa, who is using it to treat AIDS.

Sutherlandia has been shown to be generally safe during a long history of wide traditional use, at least 100 years of use during written history, and a recent clinical trial.

Studies

Anti-inflammatory properties of medicinal plants have been attrributed, at least partly, to their antioxidant activities. A hot water extract of Sutherlandia showed superoxide and hydrogen peroxide scavenging properties at concentrations as low as 10 microg/ml.[1]

The signalling protein NF-kappaB activates genes promoting cell proliferation and preventing apoptosis. It also leads to abnormally elevated expressions of cyclooxygenase-2 (COX-2), a pro-inflammatory molecule implicated in the development and progression of tumors. Methanol extracts of both Sutherlandia and Bambara Groundnut (another medicinal African plant tested) inhibited the DNA binding of NF-kappaB in a dose-dependent manner. Researchers postulated that Sutherlandia inhibited COX-2 expression through suppression of DNA binding of NF-kappaB.[2]

A whole-plant water extract of Sutherlandia frutescens induced apoptosis in two types of tumor cells, cervical carcinoma and CHO (Chinese Hamster Ovary cells) cell lines.[3]

Sutherlandia showed a concentration-dependent growth suppression of several tumor cell lines, with 50% inhibition (IC50) of proliferation of breast cancer, T-cell leukemia, and HL60 (promyelocytic leukemia) cells at 1/250, 1/200, 1/150 and 1/200 dilutions, respectively. However, this study did not show significant antioxidant effects.[4]

A clinical study which examined the safety of Sutherlandia in healthy adults found that consumption of up to 800 mg/day of leaf powder capsules for three months was well tolerated.[5]

Caution

Not recommended to be taken during pregnancy.

Drug interactions have been reported with anti-virals used to treat HIV/AIDS, so do not take concurrently with these medications.

Instructions

Two tablets (600 mg) three times a day after meals. This medication is typically taken long term.

Suppliers

Widely available on Ebay, and from major online vitamin sellers such as iherb.com:

http://www.iherb.com/

A long list of further sources from a website devoted to Sutherlandia:

http://www.sutherlandia.org/sources.html

References

(1) Fernandes AC, Cromarty AD, Albrecht C, van Rensburg CE, "The antioxidant potential of Sutherlandia frutescens," J Ethnopharmacol. 2004 Nov;95(1):1-5.

(2) Na HK, Mossanda KS, Lee JY, Surh YJ, "Inhibition of phorbol ester-induced COX-2 expression by some edible African plants". Biofactors. 2004;21(1-4):149-53.

(3) Chinkwo KA. "Sutherlandia frutescens extracts can induce apoptosis in cultured carcinoma cells". J Ethnopharmacol. 2005 Apr 8;98(1-2):163-70

(4) Tai J, Cheung S, Chan E, Hasman D, "In vitro culture studies of Sutherlandia frutescens on human tumor cell lines". J Ethnopharmacol. 2004 Jul;93(1):9-19

(5) Johnson, Q; Syce, J; Nell, H; Rudeen, K; Folk, WR (2007). "A randomized, double-blind, placebo-controlled trial of Lessertia frutescens in healthy adults". PLoS clinical trials 2 (4): e16

Tea

The herb *Camellia sinensis*, better known as tea, is a beverage used throughout the world. Unfermented green tea is widely consumed in the Orient, where people drink about five cups a day. Westerners tend to consume black tea, which is made by fermenting tea leaves.

Green tea contains epigallocatechin gallate, one of a group of chemicals called "polyphenolic catechins." These catechins are free-radical quenchers that inhibit the growth of cancer and cause lower blood cholesterol levels. It was formerly believed that most of the health benefits reside in green tea, since the fermentation process used to make black tea converts ECGC to theaflavin and thearubigens, but researchers now say the latter compounds are also antioxidants. However, most studies have been done using green tea extract.

Multiple studies have found that regular drinkers of green tea have a reduced risk of breast, esophagus, stomach, colon, and prostate cancer. Green tea extract has been extensively studied for its preventative and curative effect on prostate cancer.

ECGC

Multiple studies show that green tea extract inhibits the growth of various cancer cells in-vitro.

The polyphenol ECGC suppresses the effect of IGF-1 (insulin-like growth factor), a promoter of tumor growth.[1]

ECGC inhibits the release of tumor necrosis factor-alpha, a molecule which promotes tumor formation and progression of malignant cells as well as premalignant cells.[2] It causes apoptosis and cell cycle arrest in cancer cells without affecting normal cells. It also targets biochemical inflammatory pathways NF-κB and COX-2.[3]

A cell study of 250 prostate cancer genes found that ECGC significantly affected 25 genes influencing cancer growth. When rodents with transgenic mouse prostate adenocarcinoma were administered the equivalent of human consumption of 6 cups of green tea per day, no metastasis occurred, tumor growth was inhibited, and survival time was increased. Also, production of vascular endothelial growth factor (VEGF), related to angiogenesis, and enzymes called matrix metalloproteinases (MMP-2 and MMP-9), which are related to the development of metastasis, were inhibited by the green tea extract.

Apoptosis was induced in both androgen-sensitive and androgen insensitive prostate cancer cells.

Pretreatment of prostate cancer cells with green tea extract before exposure to androgen prevented induction of the enzyme ornithine decarboxylase (ODC), an enzyme necessary for the growth of prostate cancer cells. Enzymes called proteasomes allow tumor cell-cycle progression and protect tumor cells against apoptosis. Green tea extract inhibits the activity of these enzymes.

The researchers concluded, "Taken together, our studies and the data from other laboratories suggest that green tea and its constituents induce apoptosis, inhibit cell growth, arrest the progression of the cell cycle, inhibit angiogenesis and metastasis, and importantly, inhibit prostate tumor growth in an animal model in which prostate cancer progresses as in humans."[4]

Other Tea Compounds

A study which examined various polyphenols in green, black and herbal teas found multiple compounds with anti-cancer activity. Researchers evaluated 9 catechins from green tea, three theaflavins from black tea, and aqueous as well as water-ethanol extracts of the tea leaves. All tea extracts reduced the numbers of human cancer cell lines from the breast (MCF-7), colon (HT-29), hepatoma (liver) (HepG2), and prostate (PC-3) as well as normal human liver cells (Chang). The extracts did not inhibit the growth of normal human lung (HEL299) cells.[13]

Human Studies

Breast cancer

A Japanese study comparing 472 women with breast cancer who consumed various amounts of green tea showed that ECGC decreases both the severity of the initial diagnosis and the chance of recurrence. Women with Stage I, II and III breast cancer who drank five or more cups of green tea daily were less likely to have lymph node metastasis. Also, greater tea consumption by patients with Stage I or II breast cancer was associated with a lower rate of recurrence. No effect on recurrence was shown in women with Stage III cancers.[5]

A meta-analysis of five databases from 1998 – 2009 of 5,617 patients also shows that consumption of more than 3 cups of green tea daily lowers rates of recurrence of breast cancer. No effect was seen on breast cancer incidence.[6]

A 5-year prospective population study of approximately 54,000 Japanese women found no correlation between green tea consumption and risk of developing breast cancer. The women were surveyed for their tea consumption habits at the beginning of the study, then followed for 5 years, and re-surveyed.[7]

Some other studies show that green tea does have a preventative effect against breast cancer.[8,9,10]

Generally, it can be said that while there is some conflicting evidence on the preventative powers of green tea in regards to breast cancer, studies show consistently that it mitigates the disease once it has developed.

Leukemia

A Phase II trial by Dr. Tait Shanafelt of the Mayo Clinic found that green tea extract caused regression of chronic lymphocytic leukemia (CLL), a disease characterized by excess production of immature lymphocytes, and swollen lymph nodes. 42 test subjects with untreated, early-stage leukemia (stage 0-II) received 2000 mg of ECGC twice daily for up to 6 months, for an average of 6 treatment cycles. One-third of test subjects showed reduced numbers of lymphocytes, and in two-thirds the size of enlarged lymph nodes was reduced by at least 50%. Patients experienced no major side effects from the treatment.[11]

Ovarian Cancer

A study of 254 patients shows that even a few cups of green tea daily results in a significant increase in the survival for patients with squamous cell ovarian cancer. Three-year survival rates were 77.9% (81/104 subjects) for tea drinkers compared to 47.9% (67/140) of non-tea drinkers.[12]

Adjunct to Chemotherapy

Theanine increases concentrations of chemotherapy drugs inside cancer cells, while shielding normal cells from side effects.[14-19]

Instructions

Green tea catechins, especially EGCG, compose approximately 30% of the dry weight of green tea leaves. Typically, one cup of brewed green tea will contain 20-35 mg ECGC.

Since animal studies indicate that the equivalent of 6 cups of green tea per day has biological effects, aim for an ECGC dosage of at least 120-180 mg (or more) per day.

Suppliers

Standardized Green tea extract is widely available in capsules and powder form. The cheapest form is bulk powder available on ebay. Be sure to buy the concentrated, standardized form with a high percentage of ECGC, not just dried green tea powder.

References

(1) Shimizu M, et al., "EGCG inhibits activation of the insulin-like growth factor (IGF)/IGF-1 receptor axis in human hepatocellular carcinoma cells." Cancer Lett, 2008 Apr 8;262(1):10-8)

(2) Okabe S, Ochiai Y, Aida M, Park K, Kim SJ, Nomura T, Suganuma M, Fujiki H, "Mechanistic Aspects of Green Tea as a Cancer Preventive: Effect of Components on Human Stomach Cancer Cell Lines." Jpn J Cancer Res. 1999 Jul;90(7):733-9

(3) J.J. Johnson, H.H. Bailey, and H. Mukhtar, "Green tea polyphenols for prostate cancer chemoprevention: A translational perspective." Phytomedicine,2010 January 17(1) : 3-13)

(4) Adhami VM, Ahmad N, Mukhtar H. "Molecular targets for green tea in prostate cancer prevention." J Nutr. 2003 Jul;133(7 Suppl):2417S-2424S

(5) Kei Nakachi et al., "Influence of Drinking Green Tea on Breast Cancer Malignancy among Japanese Patients." Cancer Science, March 1998, vol 89, issue 3, pages 254-261

(6) Ogunleye AA, et al., "Green tea consumption and breast cancer risk or recurrence: a meta-analysis." Breast Cancer Res Treat 2010 Jan;119(2):477-84. Epub 2009 May 13

(7) Motoki Iwasaki, et al., "Green tea drinking and subsequent risk of breast cancer in a population to based cohort of Japanese women." Breast Cancer Research, 2010 28 October

(8) Shrubsole MJ, Lu W, Chen Z, Shu XO, Zheng Y, Dai Q, Cai Q, Gu K, Ruan ZX, Gao YT, Zheng W, "Drinking green tea modestly reduces breast cancer risk." J Nutr 2009, 139:310-316

(9) Zhang M, Holman CD, Huang JP, Xie X, "Green tea and the prevention of breast cancer: a case-control study in Southeast China." Carcinogenesis 2007, 28:1074-1078

(10) Wu AH, Yu MC, Tseng CC, Hankin J, Pike MC, "Green tea and risk of breast cancer in Asia." Int J Cancer 2003, 106:574-579

(11) T. D. Shanafelt, T. Call, C. S. Zent, B. LaPlant, J. F. Leis, D. Bowen, M. Roos, D. F. Jelinek, C. Erlichman, N. E. Kay; Mayo Clinic Rochester, Rochester, MN; Mayo Clinic Arizona, Scottsdale, AZ, "Phase II trial of daily, oral green tea extract in patients with asymptomatic, Rai stage 0-II chronic lymphocytic leukemia (CLL)." J Clin Oncol 28:15s, 2010 suppl; abstr 6522

(12) Zhang M, Lee AH, Binns CW, Xie X., "Green tea consumption Enhances survival of epithelial ovarian cancer." Int J Cancer. 2004 in November 1910, 112 (3) :465-9

(13) Friedman M, Mackey BE, Kim HJ, Lee IS, Lee KR, Lee SU, Kozukue E "Structure-activity relationships of tea compounds against human cancer cells." J Agric Food Chem 2007 Jan 24;55(2):243-53.

(14) Sadzuka Y, et al., "The effects of theanine, as a novel biochemical modulator, on the antitumor activity of adriamycin." Cancer Lett 1996 105:203-209

(15) Sadzuka Y, et al., "Improvement of idarubicin induced antitumor activity and bone marrow suppression by theanine, a component of tea." Cancer Lett 2000 158:119-24

(16) Sadzuka Y, et al., "Enhancement of the activity of doxorubicin by inhibition of glutamate transporter." Toxicology Lett 2001 123:159-67.

(17) Sadzuka Y, et al., "Efficacies of tea components on doxorubicin induced antitumor activity and reversal of multidrug resistance." Toxicology Lett 2000 114:155-62.

(18) Sugiyama T, et al., "Enhancing effects of green tea components on the antitumor activity of adriamycin against M5076 ovarian sarcoma." Cancer Lett 1998 133:19-26.

(19) Sugiyama T, et al., "Combination of theanine with doxorubicin inhibits hepatic metastasis of M5076 ovarian sarcoma" Clin Cancer Res 1999 5:413-16.)

Turmeric/Curcumin

Turmeric is a yellow spice commonly used as a spice and coloring in Indian cooking. It has been used in Ayurvedic medicine for millenia. Powdered turmeric is sold in grocery stores, and it is one of the main ingredients of curry powder. Chemically, curcumin or diferuloylmethane is a yellow polyphenol extracted from the rhizome of turmeric (*Curcuma longa*).

It is known as an antioxidant which protects against the development of cancer, and in-vitro and animal studies have also demonstrated curative effects. The active ingredient appears to be curcumin, which inhibits the COX-2 enzyme, which causes inflammation. Inflammation is a strong factor promoting tumor development and growth.

In-vitro demonstrated the activity of curcumin against a wide variety of cancer cell cultures. It has been shown to be particularly effective against tumors of the gastrointestinal tract, skin and breast.

Turmeric can be made into a tea or added to food, and turmeric paste can be applied to the skin.

Although there is no standardized dose for turmeric, some herbalists recommend eating a teaspoon of the spice with each meal. Turmeric powder normally contains from 3% to 5% curcumin, but many supplements are standardized to contain 95% curcumin compounds.

Studies

Literally thousands of papers have been published about the medicinal properties of turmeric. It is probably the most extensively documented medicinal plant in existence.
An in-vitro study on several lines of breast cancer cells (estrogen-sensitive, estrogen insensitive, and drug-resistant) showed that curcumin prevented tumor cell proliferation by halting cell reproduction in the G2/S phase of mitosis. Curcumin-induced cell death was caused neither by apoptosis nor by any significant change in the expression of apoptosis-related genes.[1]

Curcumin inhibits tumor growth through multiple biological actions. It affects cellular survival pathways such as those regulated by NF-kappaB, Akt and growth factors, as well as cytoprotective pathways dependent on Nrf2. It inhibits metastasis and angiogenesis. Curcumin is a free radical scavenger and hydrogen donor, and exhibits both pro- and antioxidant activity. It binds metals, especially iron and copper, and functions as an iron chelator. Curcumin is non-toxic, but has limited bioavailability. Researchers concluded, "Curcumin exhibits great promise as a therapeutic agent, and is currently in human clinical trials for a variety of conditions, including multiple myeloma, pancreatic cancer, myelodysplastic syndromes, colon cancer, psoriasis and Alzheimer's disease."[2]

Curcumin has been studied in the treatment of pancreatic cancer. 25 patients with advanced cancer were enrolled in the study, with 21 available for evaluation. Patients were fed 8 grams of curcumin per day. Two patients showed a response. One had ongoing stable disease for more than 18 months, and a second patient displayed a brief but marked tumor regression, 73%, along with a significant increase in cytokine levels.

In regards to absorption of the curcumin, researchers found little if any unconjugated curcumin present in the blood plasma of the patients. However, levels of curcumin became detectable when the plasma was treated with

glucuronidase and sulfatase enzymes to break up conjugated glucuronide and sulfate compounds. This indicates that curcumin is transported in plasma as part of a protein complex, rather than in its free form.

Researchers expressed some doubts about the bioavailability of the curcumin, as the functional levels of curcumin may not have approached those shown to have anti-cancer effect in-vitro. This may account for the low patient response rate, and the researchers stated, "better formulations of curcumin may provide more consistent blood levels with better pharmacologic effect."

Of course, cell cultures can be dosed with high amounts of curcumin since the compound can be applied directly without having to pass through an intestinal barrier and then carried in the blood. In trying to solve this problem, researchers noted that curcumin is hydrophobic (insoluble in water), and therefore cannot be administered in an intravenous solution. As it is lipophilic (oil soluble), it can be encapsulated in a liposome (a soluble fat compound), and perhaps such a form would be suitable for IV administration. The researchers planned to develop such a compound for further clinical trials.[3]

A phase I trial of 11 patients with pancreatic cancer tested the combination of curcumin and gemcitabine chemotherapy. 1/11 patients (9%) had a partial response (7 months), 4/11 (36%) had stable disease (2, 3, 6 and 12 months) and 6/11 (55%) had tumor progression. Researchers recommended a dosage of <8 gm per day due to gastric upset at
higher doses. The supplement used in the study, Curcumin C3 manufactured by the Sabinsa corporation, is an unenhanced form of curcumin.[4]

Curcumin stops pre-malignant lesions from progressing to cancer. Two human studies show curcumin supplementation (2-4 gm per day) causes regression of premalignant lesions of the bladder, cervix, mouth and stomach.[5,6]

A study of patients with familial adenomatous polyposis found that a combination treatment of curcumin 480 mg and quercetin 20 mg three times daily reduced the number and size of precancerous intestinal polyps by 50.9% and 60.4% respectively. Familial adenomatous polyposis is a genetic disorder characterized by the development of hundreds of colorectal polyps, eventually leading to colorectal cancer.[7]

Bioperene

It should be noted that curcumin absorption is greatly increased by the addition of black pepper, which is coincidentally another ingredient, along with turmeric, in common curry powders. The chemical piperene, derived from black pepper, is often included in curcumin supplements to increase absorption. This compound, also called "bioperine", is manufactured by Sabinsa Corporation in New Jersey, and distributed to various supplement companies for inclusion in their products. According to a study funded by the manufacturer, adding 20 mg of piperene to a dose of curcumin increases the absorption of curcumin by 2000%.[8]

Traditionally, curry spices are cooked in oil (curcumin is oil soluble) before being combined with food. The unenhanced curcumin trial did not add pepper or cooking oil to the oral treatment regime, which would have improved absorption, and perhaps produced better results.

NanoCurc

Other researchers have developed an artificial curcumin compound which has higher absorption than unprocessed curcumin. Their nanoparticle-encapsulated curcumin formula, called NanoCurc, shows much greater bioavailability compared with unprocessed curcumin when administered intravenously. Mice implanted with human pancreatic cancer cells were treated with NanoCurc by itself, NanoCurc along with the chemotherapy drug gemcitabine, or only gemcitabine. A placebo group was treated with an inactive polymer.

Inhibition of tumor growth was shown in all three therapies, but was greatest when the combination was used. Even the NanoCurc alone reduced tumor mass by approximately 50%, quite close to the level of response achieved by the chemo alone (though there was a wider range of response to the NanoCurc). The combination therapy caused the greatest decrease in the mass of the main tumor, and caused complete cellular regression of the tumor in 4 of 5 cases. It also completely eliminated tumor metastasis, extensively present in the lungs, peritoneum and lymph nodes of placebo-treated mice. Approximately 18% of mice in the single-treatment groups still had lymph node metastasis.

Researchers concluded, "NanoCurc is a promising new formulation that is able to overcome a major impediment for the clinical translation of curcumin to cancer patients by improving systemic bioavailability, and by extension, therapeutic efficacy."[9]

Meriva

Meriva is a patented combination of curcumin with soy lecithin. This helps curcumin, which is oil soluble, become suspended in water. This boosts absorption by 20-29 times, according to studies.

A 2007 rat study found that Meriva demonstrated superior bioavailability compared to standardized curcumin extract. Meriva improved blood plasma and liver tissue levels by a factor of 20.[10]

In a human study, curcuminoid absorption was 29 times higher for Meriva compared to a standard curcuminoid mixture.[11]

BCM-95

The patented supplement from Europharma, also referred to as Biocurcumax, combines curcumin with other components of turmeric to increase absorption. In human testing, it produced blood levels of curcumin 6.9 times greater than those obtained with unenhanced curcumin supplements, and 6.3 times greater than with a curcumin-lecithin-piperine formula.[12,13]

On the face of it, this absorption rate does not seem as good as that of Meriva, but Europharma claims their product delivers a higher dose per capsule due to the higher content of active ingredient.

Meriva's curcumin compound is one part curcumin, two parts lecithin (phosphatidylcholine), and two parts cellulose, leaving only 100 mg of actual curcumin in a 500-mg curcumin complex. In contrast, each 500 mg dose of BCM-95 has more than 450 mg of full-spectrum curcuminoids.

In Europharm's study comparing the two enhanced curcumin supplements with plain curcumin, researchers measured the average increase of curcumin in the blood stream following each 1-mg dose of supplement. BCM-95 resulted in a 0.34 ng/g blood level increase, measured as nanograms/gram, Meriva produced a 0.15 ng/g increase, and plain curcumin, only a 0.04 ng/g increase.

In summary, per capsule, BCM-95 delivers a higher dose; but Meriva has a greater percentage of absorption. Since stomach upset is the limiting factor in curcumin dosing, and cancer patients are aiming for the highest blood levels possible, the supplement that is most highly absorbed provides the greatest effect within the tolerable amount. They would probably be better off by taking several capsules of Meriva versus a few BCM-95s.

Longvida

This formula, especially developed to cross the blood-brain barrier, was developed by Alzheimer's Disease researcher Dr. Greg Cole (Ph.D.), Professor of Medicine and Neurology at UCLA. Dr. Cole noted that the biological effects of curcumin are due to free curcumin, not the glucuronidated form often used as a laboratory biomarker for curcumin absorption; the latter is a metabolic product with no biological activity. Longvida was shown to raise blood levels of free curcumin.

During human clinical trials of Longvida in patients with Alzheimer's disease, plasma amyloid-beta and biomarkers for inflammation were improved.[14,15]

Curcumin & Resveratrol

In-vitro and in-vivo tests on colon cancer cells showed that curcumin and resveratrol exerted the greatest control on cancer growth when used together, causing a decrease in tumor cell proliferation and an increase in apoptosis. Curcumin also reduced the activity of the transcription factor NF-kappaB, which has been linked to a number of inflammatory diseases including cancer.[16]

Curcumin & Green Tea Extract

Curcumin causes apoptosis in a wide variety of tumor cells through multiple biochemical actions, and this effect is enhanced by green tea extract (epigallocatechin-3-gallate). In-vitro tests on leukemia cells showed that administration of EGCG followed by curcumin was the most effective treatment regime. Due to overlapping biological effects, simultaneous administration resulted in antagonistic effects.[17]

Caution

Patient studies have shown oral tolerance of up to 10 grams of turmeric per day. Gastric upset is the usual side effect of overconsumption, and is the limiting factor in oral dosing.

Turmeric also has anticoagulant effects, and should be used with caution by patients on blood thinners such as warfarin and Plavix. It should not be used for a two week period prior to major surgery. It is also said to aggravate gallstone problems.

Despite its successful use in combination therapy in animal studies, some recent in-vitro and in-vivo research with breast cancer cells indicates that dietary turmeric may interfere with chemotherapy drugs such as cyclophosphamide, camptothecin, mechlorethamine, and doxorubicin. Breast cancer patients should avoid curcumin supplements while undergoing chemotherapy.

Instructions For Use

Enhanced supplements are recommended, as they are much better absorbed and produce higher blood levels. Gastric tolerance is a dose-limiting factor with curcumin, and enhanced supplements provide greater effect at lower doses, circumventing this side effect. For instance, the recommended dose for Meriva is one capsule per day; however, this is just for health maintenance; researchers fed patients as much curcumin as allowed by gastric tolerance, roughly 10 grams per day.

If you must use a standard curcumin supplement, buy one which contains piperene, and take it with oil. Some alternative health practitioners advise mixing the curcumin with oil such as extra-virgin olive oil or coconut oil, then adding 1-2 egg yolks to emulsify the ingredients. Lecithin may also be helpful. Combine using a high-speed mixer.

Curcumin products for intravenous administration may be available from clinical researchers performing human studies.

Oral doses of 3.6 grams per day were used in a colon cancer study to achieve therapeutic levels in local tissues. At this dose, very little curcumin was detected in peripheral blood.

Suppliers

Curcumin with Meriva from Vitamins.com:

http://www.puritan.com/curcumin-521/

Longvida $44.99 for 60 capsules:

http://www.phytosensia.com/

References

(1) Mehta K, et al. "Antiproliferative effect of curcumin (diferuloylmethane) against human breast tumor cell lines." Anticancer Drugs 1997;8:470-81.

(2) Hatcher, H.; Planalp, R.; Cho, J.; Torti, F. M.; Torti, S. V. "Curcumin: from ancient medicine to current clinical trials". Cellular and Molecular Life Science, 2008, 65 (11): 1631–1652

(3) Navneet Dhillon et al., "Phase II Trial of Curcumin in Patients with Advanced Pancreatic Cancer." Clin Cancer Res, July 15, 2008 14; 4491

(4) R. Epelbaum, B. Vizel, G. Bar-Sela, "Phase II study of curcumin and gemcitabine in patients with advanced pancreatic cancer." J Clin Oncol 26: 2008 (May 20 suppl; abstr 15619)

(5) Cheng AL, Hsu CH, Lin JK, et al. "Phase I clinical trial of curcumin, a chemopreventive agent, in patients with high-risk or pre-malignant lesions." Clin Cancer Res October 15, 2004 10; 6847

(6) Carroll RE, Benya RV, Turgeon DK, Vareed S, Neuman M, Rodriguez L, Kakarala M, Carpenter PM, McLaren C, Meyskens FL Jr., Brenner DE, "Phase IIa clinical trial of curcumin for the prevention of colorectal neoplasia". Cancer Prev Res 2011 Mar;4(3):354-64

(7) Cruz-Correa M et al., "Combination treatment with curcumin and quercetin of adenomas in familial adenomatous polyposis." Clin Gastroenterol Hepatol 2006 Aug;4(8):1035-8. Epub 2006 Jun 6.

(8) Shoba, G.; Joy, D.; Joseph, Thangam; Majeed, M.; Rajendran, R.; Srinivas, P. "Influence of piperine on the pharmacokinetics of curcumin in animals and human volunteers." Planta Medica (May 1998). 64 (4): 353–356

(9) Savita Bishtaff et al., "Systemic Administration of Polymeric Nanoparticle-Encapsulated Curcumin (NanoCurc) Blocks Tumor Growth and Metastases in Preclinical Models of Pancreatic Cancer." Mol Cancer Ther; 2010, 9(8); 2255–64

(10) Marczylo TH, Verschoyle RD, Cooke DN, Morazzoni P, Steward WP, Gescher AJ., "Comparison of systemic availability of curcumin with that of curcumin formulated with phosphatidylcholine." Cancer Chemother Pharmacol. 2007 Jul;60(2):171-7. Epub 2006 Oct 19.

(11) Marczylo TH, Verschoyle RD, Cooke DN, Morazzoni P, Steward WP, Gescher AJ., "Comparison of systemic availability of curcumin with that of curcumin formulated with phosphatidylcholine." Cancer Chemother Pharmacol. 2007 Jul;60(2):171-7. Epub 2006 Oct 19

(12) Antony B et al., "A Pilot Cross-Over Study to Evaluate Human Oral Bioavailability of BCM-95CG (Biocurcumax), A Novel Bioenhanced Preparation of Curcumin." Indian J Pharm Sci 2008 Jul-Aug;70(4):445-9.

(13) Dr. J.K. Mukkadan Ph.D, "BIOAVAILABILITY OF CURCU-GEL™ Softsules® Containing (BCM-95TM SG) A HUMAN STUDY."Study Conducted at: Department of Bio-Chemistry. Little flower Medical Research Center, Angamaly, India. (Recognized Research Center of Mahatma Gandhi University, India)

(14) Baum L, Lam C, Cheung S, et al. "Six-Month Randomized Placebo-Controlled, Double-Blind, Pilot Clinical Trial of Curcumin in Patients with Alzheimer's Disease." Letter in J. Clin. Psychopharm., 2008:28(1), 110-114.

(15) Baum L, Cheung SK, Mok VC, Lam LC, Leung VP, Hui E, Ng CC, Chow M, Ho PC, Lam S, Woo J, Chiu HF, Goggins W, Zee B, Wong A, Mok H, Cheng WK, Fong C, Lee JS, Chan MH, Szeto SS, Lui VW, Tsoh J, Kwok TC, Chan IH, Lam CW, "Curcumin effects on blood lipid profile in a 6-month human study." Pharmacol Res. 2007 Dec;56(6):509-14. Epub 2007 Sep 18

(16) Majumdar A.P., "Curcumin synergizes with resveratrol to inhibit colon cancer." Nutr Cancer 2009;61(4):544-53.

(17) Laura S. Angelo and Razelle Kurzrock, "Turmeric and green tea: a recipe for B-Chronic Lymphocytic Leukemia." Clin Cancer Res., 2009 Feb 15;15(4):1123-5.

Vitamins, Minerals & Antioxidants

Alpha Lipoic Acid

Alpha-lipoic acid was discovered in 1937, when scientists found the compound being produced by certain types of bacteria. Since 1939, it has been used and studied for its antioxidant activity. At one time it was thought to be a vitamin (a substance the body needs, but which it cannot synthesize). However, it was later discovered that the human body does produce small amounts of lipoic acid.

It is currently widely consumed as an antioxidant, and is used by doctors to treat peripheral neuropathy in diabetics. It is one-half of the popular supplement ALCAR, along with the amino acid compound acetyl-L-carnitine, a compound which boosts mitochondrial functioning. Considering that mitochondrial dysfunction and anaerobic respiration are the basis of tumor growth, this is an extremely important function.

Alpha-lipoic acid is a powerful antioxidant which scavenges hydroxyl radicals, reducing the inflammation that fuels the growth of cancer. It also directly causes apoptosis of tumor cells.

Alpha-lipoic acid is an unusual substance in that it is soluble in both water and oil.

The formula for alpha-lipoic acid is *1,2-dithiolane-3-pentanoic acid*. Commercially manufactured alpha-lipoic acid contains two isomers (compounds which are mirror images of each other, and turn either right or left). R- and L-lipoic acid are produced in equal proportions in the synthetic manufacturing process.

The body only produces the R-lipoic form, and this is the form which is biologically active. Currently, some alternative medical practitioners advise the consumption of R-lipoic acid only, since it is the bio-identitical form. There are claims that the L-isomer is not inert, but that it actually interferes with the function of the R-isomer. However, this product is relatively new, and scientific studies have achieved good results using the older mixed-isomer product.

The R-isomer has less stability in terms of storage, so chemically "stabilized" forms are preferable. Unstabilized forms tend to form insoluble polymers, especially if stored in warm conditions.

Poly-MVA (Lipoic Acid Palladium Complex)

One patented product, Poly-MVA, combines alpha lipoic acid with palladium, a rare trace mineral. According to the manufacturer of the supplement, this increases gastrointestinal and cellular absorption. It is officially sold on the manufacturer's website to treat cancer in pets. However, it is being used successfully by some alternative practitioners on human cancer patients. Its use is supported only by anecdotal reports from patients.

Alpha-lipoic Acid Studies

In-vitro tests show it causes apoptosis in tumor cells.[1]

Alpha-lipoic acid caused apoptosis in colon cancer cells while leaving normal colon cells unaffected. Apoptosis was initiated by an increased uptake of oxidizable substances into the mitochondria of tumor cells.[2]

Alpha lipoic acid is usually used as an adjunct to other cancer treatments. It can protect the body against the toxic effects of chemotherapy, such as damage to the peripheral nerves and heart.[3]

Some researchers warn that taking it concurrently with chemotherapy may reduce the effectiveness of the conventional treatment.[4] However, other researchers found no reduction in chemotherapy effectiveness when combined with alpha-lipoic acid, and in fact found the combination extended the life of animal test subjects.[5]

One case study has been documented of a patient with terminal metastatic prostate cancer who used alpha-lipoic acid along with low-dose naltrexone therapy. After being followed up 4 years later, he was still healthy and his cancer had not progressed.[6]

Instructions

If using ordinary alpha-lipoic acid, take 300-500 mg three times daily. If using R-lipoic acid, use half the dose.

Suppliers

If cost is a consideration, buy ordinary, mixed-isomer alpha-lipoic acid. It has been thoroughly studied and has been proven to be effective. R-lipoic acid may be worth the extra expense. There is no proof that the exorbitant price of Poly-MVA is worthwhile in terms of improved results.
Mixed-isomer alpha-lipoic acid is widely available and very inexpensive.

Bulk alpha-lipoic powder costs $20 per 100 grams on Ebay. Stabilized R-lipoic acid costs $90 for 100 gms from Geronova.com.

Specialized formulas such as Poly-MVA cost $165 for an 8-oz bottle. The suggested dose for cancer patients is 8 teaspoons per day, or 1.3 ounces. One bottle will last 6 days.

References

(1) Moungjaroen J, Nimmannit U, Callery PS, et al. "Reactive oxygen species mediate caspase activation and apoptosis induced by lipoic acid in human lung epithelial cancer cells through Bcl-2 down-regulation." Journal of Pharmacology & Experimental Therapeutics. 2006;319:1062-1069

(2) Wenzel U. et al., "Alpha-Lipoic acid induces apoptosis in human colon cancer cells by increasing mitochondrial respiration with a concomitant O2-*-generation." Apoptosis 2005 Mar;10(2):359-68.

(3) Gedlicka C, Scheithauer W, Schüll B, Kornek GV. "Effective treatment of oxaliplatin-induced cumulative polyneuropathy with alpha-lipoic acid." J Clin Oncol. 2002;20:3359-3361; Mythili Y. Sudharsan PT. Sudhahar V. Varalakshmi P. "Protective effect of DL-alpha-lipoic acid on cyclophosphamide induced hyperlipidemic cardiomyopathy". European Journal of Pharmacology. 2006;543:92-96.

(4) Lawenda BD, Kelly KM, Ladas EJ, Sagar SM, Vickers A, Blumberg JB. "Should supplemental antioxidant administration be avoided during chemotherapy and radiation therapy?" J Natl Cancer Inst. 2008;100:773-783.

(5) Berger M. et al., "Effect of thioctic acid (alpha-limpoic acid) on the chemotherapeutic efficacy of cyclophosphamide and vincristine sulfate." Arzneimittelforschung, 1983;33(9):1286-8.

(6) Berkson BM, Rubin DM, Berkson AJ. "The long-term survival of a patient with pancreatic cancer with metastases to the liver after treatment with the intravenous alpha-lipoic acid/low-dose naltrexone protocol." Integrative Cancer Therapies. 2006;5:83-89.

Cesium Chloride

Cesium chloride is one of several therapies listed in this book which target the metabolic differences of cancer cells.

Cesium chloride is a salt based element of cesium, which is a rare mineral.

Because cesium has a structure similar to potassium it is absorbed by the cells within the body. Cancer cells function through anaerobic metabolism, and this affects the acid-base balance, or pH, with cancer cells being more acidic (lower pH) than normal. Cesium has been shown to raise the pH level of tumor cells to levels similar to that of normal cells while leaving normal cells unaffected. Acidotic tissues contain low levels of oxygen, whereas tissues that are alkalotic have high levels of oxygen. Normalizing the pH forces the cells to revert to aerobic metabolism, and subsequently the cell cycle ends in apoptosis.

The pH scale ranges from 0 to 14, with numbers below 7 being acidic and above 7 being alkaline. Cancer cells usually have a pH below 6.5. Cesium raises the pH of cancer cells to 8.0 or above. Cells normally have a pH of 7.35.

DMSO is often used along with cesium chloride to increase its penetration.

During therapy patients can be given cesium either in a pill form or through an IV.

History

Scientists first became interested in cesium after observing that regions of the world with high concentrations of alkali metals in the soil had low rates of cancer. In the 1920s, researchers began studying the potential use of cesium as an anti-cancer agent. Cesium therapy was popularized in the 1980s as "high pH therapy."

Studies

Mice implanted with one of two cell lines of prostate cancer (PC-3 or LNCaP) were given cesium chloride. The PC-3 tumors shrank, but the LNCaP tumors were unaffected. Test animals receiving cesium chloride displayed increased water consumption, and developed crystals in their bladders and fibrin clots in their hearts. Researchers concluded, "CsCl may have a therapeutic effect against prostate cancer, but one cannot overlook the acute toxicities also described."[1]

Human Studies

A physicist named A. Keith Brewer performed a clinical trial involving cesium chloride treatment of 30 patients with various terminal cancers. All 30 patients survived their cancers. He also performed animal tests which showed marked shrinkage of tumor masses within 2 weeks.[2]

Dr. H. E. Sartori used cesium chloride therapy on 50 patients in April 1981 at Life Sciences Universal Medical Clinics in Rockville, Md. The patients were all terminal cases who had already undergone standard treatment for their cancers. Half of them were cured by Dr. Sartori.[3]

In 1992, Dr. Sartori's clinic was raided by the FDA and his records seized. He moved to Thailand to continue his practice, but was charged with murder in 2006 after an Australian patient died. Allegations were also made that he had exaggerated his cure rates, as half of his patients died within a year of treatment.[4]

However, since all his patients were terminally ill and already weakened by conventional therapy, it would be expected that all (rather than only half) would have died within that time frame.

Cesium chloride therapy was also used extensively by Dr. Hans Nieper, who practiced in Hannover, Germany. Many U.S. celebrities and executives suffering from cancer travelled to Germany for treatment by Dr. Nieper.

Caution

Use extreme caution if you plan to use cesium chloride on your own. It is advisable to find a doctor who will administer the therapy. Contact a physician immediately if fatigue, palpitations or blood pressure changes occur. A few patients have required hospital admission to treat electrolyte imbalances due to cesium chloride. Supposedly, it has been linked to some deaths.

Cesium chloride displaces potassium in cells, and this can have serious health consequences such as heart arrythmias. Calcium and magnesium levels will also be affected. Uric acid levels will rise as tumors die, and this can cause kidney problems. An anti-gout drug called Xyloprim can be used to treat this.

Have electrolyte tests every 2-3 weeks, and continue to do them for 3 months after discontinuing therapy as the substance accumulates in cells.

It is important to take potassium, calcium and magnesium supplements regularly.

Instructions

The daily dose of cesium chloride is 3 grams total (3,000 mg), divided into two equal doses of 1.5 g (1,500 mg).

Also, take 1200 mg of liquid ionic potassium chloride each day, divided into two equal doses of 600 mg each. Take the potassium at least one hour after the cesium chloride. If potassium is taken at the same time, it competes with cesium chloride for absorption by cancer cells.

Eat foods high in potassium, such as bananas.

Drink plenty of water. Adults over 125 pounds should consume at least half a gallon per day.

Each dose of cesium chloride may be combined with DMSO, 1 tablespoon of 70% concentration. It can be taken orally or spread on skin.

Suppliers

The following website sells cesium chloride and also provides phone support on its use.

http://www.essense-of-life.com/

References

(1) Low JC, Wasan KM, Fazli L, Eberding A, Adomat H, Guns ES, "Assessing the therapeutic and toxicological effects of cesium chloride following administration to nude mice bearing PC-3 or LNCaP prostate cancer xenografts." Cancer chemotherapy and pharmacology, 2007 60 (6): 821–9.)

(2) Keith Brewer, Ph.D., "The High pH Therapy for Cancer, Tests on Mice and Humans." Pharmacology, biochemistry, and behavior 1984, 21 Suppl 1: 1–5.

(3) Sartori HE, (1984). "Cesium therapy in cancer ." Pharmacology, biochemistry, and behavior 1984 21 (Suppl 1): 11–3

(4) Wood, Leonie. "'Cured' cancer patients died, court told." The Sydney Morning Herald. 20 November 2010

Iodine for Breast Cancer

Breast cancer seems to be one of the most important diseases in the public media these days: How to detect it? Prevent it? Reverse it?

Iodine supplementation is one of the key nutritional strategies for accomplishing this goal. Contrary to the beliefs of most people, medical practitioners included, iodine is not a requirement solely of the thyroid gland. Other organs, especially the breast and prostate, also have receptors for iodine and store it in their tissues. Researchers have studied the link between iodine and breast cancer for at least 40 years.

Due to depleted soils, use of iodine-blockers such as bromide in food and fluoride in drinking water, and inadequate intake of seafood, iodine deficiency is widespread in America. Iodized salt is a major source of iodine in the American diet, but the low-sodium diet encouraged by many mainstream health authorities causes people to avoid the use of salt. Iodine consumption by Americans has dropped 50% since the 1970s. People in the U.S. consume an average 240 micrograms (μg) of iodine a day.

In contrast, people in Japan, where seaweed is regularly eaten, consume an average of 1-3 mg of iodine per day (some researchers have estimated a daily intake of up to 13.5-45 mg, but this is likely too high).[1]

Health comparisons between the two countries are disturbing. The incidence of breast cancer in the U.S. is the highest in the world, and in Japan, until recently, the lowest. However, goitres are common in the areas consuming the highest amount of iodine.

Like many nutrients, both too little and too much can have deleterious health effects. Too little iodine in the diet produces permanent mental defects (cretinism) in children, goitre, autoimmune diseases of the thyroid, metabolic sluggishness, and depression in adults. Too much iodine can produce many of the same problems, goitre and autoimmune thyroid disease.

Studies

A number of studies have linked low iodine intake to cancer, especially breast cancer. Paradoxically, primary hypothyroidism, due to its suppressive effects on metabolism throughout the body, is linked to a lower incidence of breast cancer. However, there is a general consensus that low iodine levels are linked to breast cancer.[2]

Increased thyroid volume, which develops as the undernourished thyroid grows larger in an attempt to absorb more iodine, correlates with a higher incidence of breast cancer.[3]

Another study found that geographic differences in iodine intake were inversely associated with a higher risk of female reproductive organ cancers.[3] In the US Goiter Belt, where soil iodine levels are slower, rates of breast cancer are higher.

Iodine has a protective effect against breast cancer. It desensitizes estrogen receptors in the breast, reduces fibrocystic breast disease (a condition associated with an increased risk of breast cancer) and reduces excessive ovarian estrogen production.

Iodine also affects existing breast cancer, causing apoptosis, slowing of cell division, and reducing angiogenesis.[5]

In-vitro tests show that the iodine-rich mekabu seaweed caused greater cell death in three strains of human breast cancer cells than Fluorouracil.[6]

Animal studies from 1996 to 2001 by H. Funahashi show that iodine prevented rats from developing breast cancer after being fed the known carcinogen DMBA. Adding iodine to chemically induced rat breast tumors halted tumor growth. Adding iodine in combination with medroxyprogesterone produced the greatest response. The researchers suggest that the uptake of iodine was enhanced by medroxyprogesterone.[7,8]

David Brownstein, MD., is a holistic physician and author of "Overcoming Thyroid Disorders." He said, "You cannot give breast cancer to rats that have been fed iodine."

Loading tests show breast cancer patients excrete less iodine than normal test subjects, implying an iodine deficiency.[9]

Breast Cancer Choices, Inc., a nonprofit organization researching breast cancer procedures and treatments, is currently conducting an Iodine Investigation Project to evaluate the use of this nutrient in cancer treatment.

Iodine Supplementation

15% of the U.S. adult female population suffers from moderate to severe iodine deficiency.

According to an editorial published in 1998 in the *Journal of Clinical Endocrinology and Metabolism*, 1/3 of Earth's population lives in areas where the soil is deficient in iodine, making it the most common trace element deficiency in the world.[10]

Studies have shown that 15% of the adult female population in America suffers from iodine deficiency, defined as urinary iodine excretion of less than 50 ug/L).[10] In fact, the actual prevalence of suboptimal levels of iodine is likely far greater than 15%, because the official levels of deficiency only take into account the RDA necessary to maintain function of the thyroid gland. Other organs in the body, such as the breast, also require iodine, and the extra-thyroidal store of iodine is approximately 8 mg, as opposed to 6 mg in the thyroid gland itself, for a total body storage of approximately 14 mg.[12]

Caution

Any patient with known thyroid disorders or taking thyroid medication should consult their physician before starting iodine supplementation.

High iodine intake has been linked to autoimmune thyroiditis in some studies, whereas other studies found an inverse correlation, or no correlation at all. Do not take high doses of iodine for long periods of time, ie, for years. Once iodine stores have been replenished, cut back to a maintenance dose.

Some research suggests that iodine and selenium exist in a balance, and that high iodine intake should be accompanied by 200 mcg/day selenium.

If symptoms of thyroid dsyfunction occur, stop iodine immediately, and consult a physician. Have thyroid function tests regularly.

Instructions

Pioneering physicians Guy Abraham, David Brownstein, and Jorge Flechas, MD, have used supplemental iodine to treat more than 4,000 patients. According to them, the thyroid gland needs approximately 6 mg/day of iodine for sufficiency. The breasts need at least 5 mg of iodine; that leaves 2mg (13 mg-11 mg) of iodine for the rest of the body. This 2 mg is still well above the RDA (14x the RDA) of 150 mcg/day of iodine. The protocol suggested by their research is given below.[13-16]

Note that loading tests for iodine are not always an accurate reflection of iodine sufficiency, as a small minority of patients have problems absorbing iodine and will excrete a large portion of the loading dose even if they are severely deficient. Excretion of large amounts of iodine by patients where iodine deficiency is strongly suspected (ie, those with breast cancer or hypothyroidism) points to defects in the cellular transport mechanism. A company called Optimox now manufactures ATP Cofactors which seem to help some patients who cannot absorb iodine efficiently. They also sell Iodoral.

The supplement should contain both iodine (diatomic iodine) and iodide (potassium iodide). Iodine is stored in breast and other tissues, iodide mainly in the thyroid gland.

One well known iodine supplement is Iodoral tablets, a combined iodine-iodide form available in 12.5 and 50 mg strengths. IodinePlus (5 mg iodine plus 7.5 mg iodide) is another example. Lugols solution comes in 2% and 5% strengths; 1 drop of the 5% equals 6.25 mg iodine.

Start with 50 mg per day for breast cancer, or 12.5 mg per day if this dose is not tolerated.

It may take up to a year for the body to replenish its iodine stores. The recommended maintenance dose is one drop of iodoral daily.

Also take vitamin C 3,000 mg per day, 200 mcg selenium (selenomethionine), 500 mg niacin (B3) not niacinamide, 100 mg vitamin B2 3 times daily combined with a comprehensive vitamin and nutritional program.

Avoid high-dose calcium supplements (2000-3000 mg/day).

Bromide stored in tissues may be flushed out by high doses of iodine, resulting in frontal headache, acne, sedation, brain fog, brassy taste, mouth sores, or other symptoms which occur in a small percentage of patients. If this occurs, decrease the dose of iodine and use pulse dosing (take a 48-hour break between doses).

Salt loading may also lessen symptoms. Take ¼ to ½ teaspoon of unrefined sea salt (ie Celtic sea salt) dissolved in ½ cup warm water. Follow with 12-16 oz pure water. If needed, drink more pure water in 30-45 minutes until copious urination occurs. Follow this procedure twice a day.

Suppliers

Iodoral 189 tabs $40 from Iherb

http://www.iherb.com/Search?kw=iodoral&x=0&y=0

References

(1) Theodore T Zava, David T Zava, "Assessment of Japanese iodine intake based on seaweed consumption in Japan: A literature-based analysis." Thyroid Research 2011, 4:14

(2) Venturi, S. "Is there a role for iodine in breast diseases?" The Breast, 2001 Oct;10(5):379-82

(3) PP Smyth, DF Smith, EW McDermott, MJ Murray, JG Geraghty and NJ O'Higgins, "A direct relationship between thyroid enlargement and breast cancer." Journal of Clinical Endocrinology & Metabolism, 1996; 81: 937-41.

(4) Bruce V. Stadel, "Dietary Iodine and the Risk of Breast, Endometrial and Ovarian Cancer." The Lancet, 1976 April

(5) Vega-Riveroll L.,et al., "The antineoplasic effect of molecular iodine on human mammary cancer involves the activation of apoptotic pathways and the inhibition of angiogenesis." San Antonio Breast Cancer Symposium, 2008)

(6) Funahashi H. et al., "Seaweed Preventing Breast Cancer?", Jpn J Cancer Res 2001.

(7) Hiroomi Funahashi MD et al., "Suppressive effect of iodine on DMBA-induced breast tumor growth in the rat." Journal of Surgical Oncology Volume 61, Issue 3, pages 209–213, March 1996

(8) Funahashi H. et al., "Wakame Seaweed Suppresses the Proliferation of 7,12-Dimethybenz(a)-Anthracene-Induced Mammary Tumors in Rats." Jpn J Cancer Res 1999.

(9) Eskin BA. et al., "Identification of Breast Cancer by Differences in Urinary Iodine.", Abstract Number 2150, Presentation AACR Conference 2005).

(10) "Editorial: What's Happening to Our Iodine?" J Clinical Endocrinology and Metabolism. 1998;33:3398-3400.

(11) Hollowell J, Staehling N, Hannon W, Flanders D, Gunter E, Maberly G. "Iodine Nutrition in the United States. Trends and Public Health Implications: Iodine Excretion Data from National Health and Nutrition Examination Surveys I and III (1971-1974 and 1988-1994)." J Clinical Endocrinology and Metabolism. 1998;83:3401-3408

(12) Abraham GE, Flechas JD, Hakala JC. "Orthoiodosupplementation: Iodine Sufficiency Of The Whole Human Body." The Original Internist. 2002;9:30-41.

(13) Brownstein David, Iodine : Why You Need It, Why You Can't Live Without It, (Third Edition) Medical Alternative Press, West Bloomfield, MI 2006

(14) Abraham, GE, "The Historical Background of the Iodine Project." The Original Internist 12(2):57-66, 2005

(15) Abraham, Guy E. "Iodine supplementation markedly increases urinary excretion of fluoride and bromide." Townsend Letter 238 (2003): 108-109

(16) Abraham, G.E., Brownstein, D., "Evidence that the administration of Vitamin C improves a defective cellular transport mechanism for iodine: A case report." The Original Internist, 12(3):125-130, 2005

Quercetin

Quercetin, also known as rutin, is a flavanoid often combined with other ingredients in anti-oxidant and anti-allergy formulas, and is also used to treat cancer, usually in combination with other therapies. It is widely present in the diet from plant sources, and average daily intake of quercetin has been estimated to be approximately 25 mg.[1]

Studies

Quercetin is being promoted as an anti-aging supplement. Laboratory models of aging using a variety of test subjects, from human cell cultures to worms show that quercetin increases lifespan by 5% (fibroblasts)[2], 11-15% (worms)[3-6], up to 60% (yeast).[7]

Quercetin and resveratrol are the main components of a popular antiaging supplement called Longevinex, and seem to act synergistically.

Higher dietary intakes of quercetin are associated with lower risk of developing various cancers. Comparing subjects with the highest intake of quercetin with those of the lowest intake, lung cancer was reduced 51% overall, and 65% in smokers[8]; colon cancer by 32%[9]; gastric cancer by 43% overall and 80% among smokers.[10]

In-vitro, quercetin has been shown to be cytotoxic to breast,[11,12,13] colon,[14,15,16] esophageal,[17,18] gastric,[19] leukemia,[20] melanoma,[21] prostate,[22] squamous,[23,24] and transitional-cell[25] tumor cells.

Quercetin has several independent mechanisms of anti-tumor action.

It directly induces apoptosis by causing G2/M cell cycle arrest. It acts through mitochondrial and caspase-3-dependent pathways.[17,18,26-29]

Quercetin is a tyrosine kinase inhibitor. Tyrosine kinases are enzymes responsible for activating signalling proteins promoting cell growth, such as Epidermal Growth Factor.[30,31,32]

In-vitro, quercetin inhibits the production of heat-shock protein by colon cancer, breast cancer and leukemia.[33,34,35] Therefore, it may be of help when combined with hyperthermia treatment.

Also, heat shock protein is associated with poorer cancer prognosis, as it improves cancer cell survival under adverse conditions such as low circulation and hypoxia, and is also linked to chemotherapy resistance in breast cancer.[36,37]

The anti-inflammatory and anti-allergy action of quercetin is thought to be due to inhibition of cyclooxygenase and to a lesser extent lipoxygenase,[38] causing reduced production of pro-inflammatory mediators. This is the same mechanism of action as that of NSAIDS, which are currently being studied as anti-cancer agents,[39] especially for colon cancer.[40] Cyclooxygenase is known to be increased in some epithelial cancers,[41] and influences angiogenesis.[42]

In-vitro, quercetin significantly reduces the cytotoxicity of NK cells, even at low doses. However, in-vivo, quercetin rats fed 100 mg/kg, a higher dose than is usually consumed by humans, showed increased NK cell activity compared to a control group. No human studies have been performed to sort out these paradoxical results.[43]

Quercetin may be a useful adjunct to some forms of conventional therapy. It sensitizes tumor cells to the effects of several chemotherapy drugs,[44-49] while protecting renal tubular cells from the nephrotoxic effects of cisplatin,[50] and also protects glomerular kidney cells.[51] It may also be protective against local tissue damage due to radiotherapy.[52]

Neutropenia is frequently a dose-limiting factor in chemotherapy, and researchers tested the ability of quercetin to protect neutrophils from the toxic effects of an alkaloid topoisomerase inhibitor, epotoside. The study found that quercetin was protective only when etoposide was at low concentrations, and actually increased neutrophil apoptosis when used with high doses of etoposide.[53]

Human Studies

One small Phase I trial of terminal cancer patients showed partial response in 2/11 participants, a patient with hepatocellular carcinoma and another with stage IV ovarian cancer. Patients were treated with increasing intravenous doses at 3-week intervals, starting at 60 mg/m2, eventually reaching 1700 mg/m2. Kidney toxicity, but not bone marrow suppression, was the dose-limiting factor.[54]

Caution

Quercetin binds to estrogen receptors, and one rat study shows it increases the development of breast cancers in the presence of estrogen.[55]

Quercetin shows mutagenic properties in-vitro, but this has not translated to carcinogenicity in several animal studies. Test animals (rats and hamsters) fed a diet containing as much as 10% quercetin for up to 850 days showed no tissue damage or increased cancer rates.[56,57]

Intravenous and intraperitoneal injections of quercetin 30-50 mg/kg into guinea pigs and rats, and intravenous injections of 100-200 mg/kg into rabbits, produced no signs of toxicity. Researchers concluded, "rutin is nontoxic both acutely and chronically."[58]

Other animal studies confirm these findings.[59,60]

However, one other study using Norwegian albino rats fed 0.1% dietary quercetin for 406 days found 80% intestinal and 20% bladder tumors in treated animals, compared to no tumors in the control group. Survival rates were similar in both groups.[61]
Another study, in which rats were fed 4% quercetin for 728 days, found decreased rates of mammary fibroadenomas, and increased rates of renal tubular adenomas in males only, in the quercetin group.[62]

Scientists do not know currently why these studies produced such different outcomes, though they speculate the unusual results may have been due to differences in the diets (other than the presence of quercetin), or the different lines of test animals used. However, the preponderance of evidence indicates that the health risks of quercetin are negligable.[1]

Instructions

No clinical studies have been performed to establish the most effective oral dose of quercetin. Some alternative practitioners recommend 1000 mg quercetin, dissolved in water with 1000 mg vitamin C to aid its absorption, 3 times daily.

Suppliers

Widely available at local stores and online. Also a component of other alternative therapies, such as Longevinex and Breast Defend.

References

(1) NTP Technical Report (no.409) on the toxicology and carcinogenesis studies of quercetin in F344/N rats. NIH Publication No.91-3140 (1991). U.S. Department of Health and Human Services, Public Health Service, National Toxicology Program, Research Triangle Park, NC.

(2) Chondrogianni N, Kapeta S, Chinou I, Vassilatou K, Papassideri I, Gonos ES. "Anti-ageing and rejuvenating effects of quercetin." Exp Gerontol. 2010 Oct;45(10):763-71.

(3) Surco-Laos F, Cabello J, Gomez-Orte E, et al. "Effects of O-methylated metabolites of quercetin on oxidative stress, thermotolerance, life span and bioavailability on Caenorhabditis elegans." Food Funct. 2011 Aug;2(8):445-56.

(4) Kampkotter A, Timpel C, Zurawski RF, et al. "Increase of stress resistance and life span of Caenorhabditis elegans by quercetin." Comp Biochem Physiol B Biochem Mol Biol. 2008 Feb;149(2):314-23.

(5) Pietsch K, Saul N, Menzel R, Sturzenbaum SR, Steinberg CE. "Quercetin mediated life span extension in Caenorhabditis elegans is modulated by age-1, daf-2, sek-1 and unc-43." Biogerontology. 2009 Oct;10(5):565-78.

(6) Pietsch K, Saul N, Swain SC, Menzel R, Steinberg CE, Sturzenbaum SR. Meta-analysis of global transcriptomics suggests that conserved genetic pathways are responsible for quercetin and tannic acid mediated longevity in C. elegans. Front Genet. 2012;3:48.

(7) Belinha I, Amorim MA, Rodrigues P, et al. "Quercetin increases oxidative stress resistance and longevity in Saccharomyces cerevisiae." J Agric Food Chem. 2007 Mar 21;55(6):2446-51.

(8) Lam TK, Rotunno M, Lubin JH, et al. "Dietary quercetin, quercetin-gene interaction, metabolic gene expression in lung tissue and lung cancer risk." Carcinogenesis. 2010 Apr;31(4):634-42.

(9) Theodoratou E, Kyle J, Cetnarskyj R, et al. "Dietary flavonoids and the risk of colorectal cancer." Cancer Epidemiol Biomarkers Prev. 2007 Apr;16(4):684-93.

(10) Ekstrom AM, Serafini M, Nyren O, Wolk A, Bosetti C, Bellocco R. "Dietary quercetin intake and risk of gastric cancer: results from a population-based study in Sweden." Ann Oncol. 2011 Feb;22(2):438-43.

(11) Singhal RL, Yeh YA, Prajda N, et al. "Quercetin down-regulates signal transduction in human breast carcinoma cells." Biochem Biophys Res Commun 1995;208:425-431.

(12) So FV, Guthrie N, Chambers AF, et al. "Inhibition of human breast cancer cell proliferation and delay of mammary tumorigenesis by flavonoids and citrus juices." Nutr Cancer 1996;26:167-181.

(13) Chien SY, Wu YC, Chung JG, et al. "Quercetin-induced apoptosis acts through mitochondrial- and caspase-3-dependent pathways in human breast cancer MDA-MB-231 cells." Hum Exp Toxicol. 2009;28:493–503

(14) Agullo G, Gamet L, Besson C, et al. "Quercetin exerts a preferential cytotoxic effect on active dividing colon carcinoma HT29 and Caco-2 cells." Cancer Lett 1994;87:55-63.

(15) Kuo SM. "Antiproliferative potency of structurally distinct dietary flavonoids on human colon cancer cells." Cancer Lett 1996;110:41-48.

(16) Ranelletti FO, Maggiano N, Serra FG, et al. "Quercetin inhibits p21-ras expression in human colon cancer cell lines and in primary colorectal tumors." Int J Cancer 1999;85:438-445.

(17) Zhang Q, Zhao XH, Wang ZJ."Flavones and flavonols exert cytotoxic effcts on a human oesophageal adenocarcinoma cell line OE33 by causing G2/M arrest and inducing apoptosis." Food Chem Toxicol. 2008;46:2042–2053.

(18) Zhang Q, Zhao XH, Wang ZJ. "Cytotoxicity of flavones and flavonols to a human esophageal squamous cell carcinoma cell line KYSE-510 by induction of G2/M arrest and apoptosis." Toxicol In Vitro. 2009;23:797–807.

(19) Yoshida M, Sakai T, Hosokawa N, et al. "The effect of quercetin on cell cycle progression and growth of human gastric cancer cells." FEBS Lett 1990;260:10-13.

(20) Yoshida M, Yamamoto M, Nikaido T. "Quercetin arrests human leukemic T-cells in late G1 phase of the cell cycle." Cancer Res 1992;52:6676-6681.

(21) Piantelli M, Maggiano N, Ricci R, et al. "Tamoxifen and quercetin interact with type II estrogen binding sites and inhibit the growth of human melanoma cells." J Invest Dermatol 1995;105:248-253.

(22) Liu KC, Yen CY, Wu RS, et al. "The roles of endoplasmic reticulum stress and mitochondrial apoptotic signaling pathway in quercetin-mediated cell death of human prostate cancer PC-3 cells." Environ Toxicol. 2012 Mar 20. doi: 10.1002/tox.21769. [Epub ahead of print]

(23) Castillo MH, Perkins E, Campbell JH, et al. "The effects of the bioflavonoid quercetin on squamous cell carcinoma of head and neck origin." Am J Surg 1989;158:351-355.

(24) Kandaswami C, Perkins E, Soloniuk DS, et al. "Antiproliferative effects of citrus flavonoids on a human squamous cell carcinoma in vitro." Cancer Lett 1991;56:147-152.

(25) Larocca LM, Giustacchini M, Maggiano N, et al. "Growth-inhibitory effect of quercetin and presence of type II estrogen binding sites in primary human transitional cell carcinomas." J Urol 1994;152:1029-1033.

(26) Tan J, Wang B, Zhu L. "Regulation of survivin and Bcl-2 in HepG2 cell apoptosis induced by quercetin." Chem Biodivers. 2009;6:1101–1110.

(27) Roos WP, Kaina B. "DNA damage-induced cell death by apoptosis." Trends Mol Med. 2006;12:440–450.

(28) Xiao X, Shi D, Liu L, et al. Quercetin suppresses cyclooxygenase-2 expression and angiogenesis through inactivation of P300 signaling. PLoS One. 2011;6(8):e22934.

(29) Granado-Serrano AB, Martín MÁ, Bravo L, Goya L, Ramos S. "Quercetin attenuates TNF-induced inflammation in hepatic cells by inhibiting the NF-κB pathway" Nutr Cancer. 2012 May;64(4):588-98. Epub 2012 Mar 27.

(30) Levy J, Teuerstein I, Marbach M, et al. "Tyrosine protein kinase activity in the DMBA induced rat mammary tumor: inhibition by quercetin." Biochem Biophys Res Commun 1984;123:1227-1233.

(31) Boutin JA. "Tyrosine protein kinase inhibition and cancer." Int J Biochem 1994;26:1203-1226.

(32) Klohs WD, Fry DW, Kraker AJ. "Inhibitors of tyrosine kinase." Curr Opin Oncol 1997;9:562-568.

(33) Hansen RK, Oesterreich S, Lemieux P, et al. "Quercetin inhibits heat shock protein induction but not heat shock factor DNA-binding in human breast carcinoma cells." Biochem Biophys Res Commun 1997; 239:851-856.

(34) Elia G, Amici C, Rossi A, Santoro MG. "Modulation of prostaglandin A1-induced thermotolerance by quercetin in human leukemic cells: role of heat shock protein." Cancer Res 1996;56:210-217.

(35) Koishi M, Hosokawa N, Sato M, et al. "Quercetin, an inhibitor of heat shock protein synthesis, inhibits the acquisition of thermotolerance in a human colon carcinoma cell line." Jpn J Cancer Res 1992;83:1216-1222

(36) Ciocca DR, Clark GM, Tandon AK, et al. "Heat shock protein hsp70 in patients with axillary lymph node-negative breast cancer: prognostic implications." J Natl Cancer Inst 1993;85:570-574.

(37) Oesterreich S, Weng CN, Qui M, et al. "The small heat shock protein hsp27 is correlated with growth and drug resistance in human breast cancer cell lines." Cancer Res 1993;53:4443-4448.

(38) Welton AF, Hurley J, Will P., "Flavonoids and arachidonic acid metabolism." Prog Clin Biol Res 1988;280:301-312.

(39) Taketo MM. "Cyclooxygenase-2 inhibitors in tumorigenesis (part II)." J Natl Cancer Inst 1998;90:1609-1620.

(40) Exon JH, Magnuson BA, South EH, Hendrix K. "Dietary quercetin, immune functions and colonic carcinogenesis in rats." Immunopharm Immunotox 1998;20:173-190.

(41) Hwang D, Scollard D, Byrne J, Levine E. "Expression of cyclooxygenase-1 and cyclooxygenase-2 in human breast cancer." J Natl Cancer Inst 1998;90:455-460.

(42) Tsujii M, Kawano S, Tsuji S. "Cyclooxygenase regulates angiogenesis induced by colon cancer cells." Cell 1998;93:705-16.

(43) Exon JH, Magnuson BA, South EH, Hendrix K. "Dietary quercetin, immune functions and colonic carcinogenesis in rats." Immunopharm Immunotox 1998;20:173-190.

(44) Hoffman R, Graham L, Newlands ES. "Enhanced anti-proliferative action of busulphan by quercetin on the human leukaemia cell line K562." Br J Cancer 1989;59:347-348.

(45) Scambia G, Ranelletti FO, Panici PB. "Quercetin potentiates the effect of adriamycin in a multidrug-resistant MCF-7 human breastcancer cell line: P-glycoprotein as a possible target." Cancer Chemother Pharmacol 1994;34:459-464.

(46) Hofmann J, Doppler W, Jakob A, et al. "Enhancement of the antiproliferative effect of cis-diamminedichloroplatinum(II) and nitrogen mustard by inhibitors of protein kinase C." Int J Cancer 1988;42:382-388.

(47) Sliutz G, Karlseder J, Tempfer C, et al. "Drug resistance against gemcitabine and topotecan mediated by constitutive hsp70 overexpression in vitro: implication of quercetin as sensitiser in chemotherapy." Br J Cancer 1996;74:172-177.

(48) Hofmann J, Fiebig HH, Winterhalter BR, et al. "Enhancement of the antiproliferative activity of cis-diamminedichloroplatinum(II) by quercetin." Int J Cancer 1990;45:536-539.

(49) Scambia G, Ranelletti FO, Panici PB, et al. "Inhibitory effect of quercetin on primary ovarian and endometrial cancers and synergistic activity with cis-diamminedichloroplatinum (II)." Gyn Oncol 1992;45:13-19.

(50) Kuhlman MK, Horsch E, Burkhardt G, et al. "Reduction of cisplatin toxicity in cultured renal tubular cells by the bioflavonoid quercetin." Arch Toxicol 1998;72:536-540.

(51) Yokoo T, Kitamura M. "Unexpected protection of glomerular mesangial cells from oxidant triggered apoptosis by bioflavonoid quercetin." Am J Physiol 1997;273:F206-F212.

(52) Rozenfel'd LG, Abyzov RA, Bozhko GT, et al. "The possibilities of protection against local radiation injuries in ORL-oncologic patients." Vestn Otorinolaringol 1990;2:56-58. [Article in Russian]

(53) Kapiszewska M, "Lifespan of etoposide-treated human neutrophils is affected by antioxidant ability of quercetin." Toxicol in Vitro 2007 Sep;21(6):1020-30. Epub 2007 Mar 19.

(54) Ferry DR, Smith A, Malkhandi J, et al. "Phase I clinical trial of the flavonoid quercetin: pharmacokinetics and evidence for in vivo tyrosine kinase inhibition." Clin Cancer Res 1996;2:659-668.

(55) Singh B, et al., "Dietary quercetin exacerbates the development of estrogen-induced breast tumors in female ACI rats." Toxico Appl Pharmacol 2010 Sep 1;247(2):83-90. Epub 2010 Jun 22.

(56) Hirono I, Ueno I, Hosaka S, et al. "Carcinogenicity examination of quercetin and rutin in ACI rats." Cancer Lett 1981;13:15-21.

(57) Morino K, Matsukura N, Kawachi T, et al. "Carcinogenicity test of quercetin and rutin in golden hamsters by oral administration." Carcinogenesis 1982;3:93-97.

(58) Wilson RH, Mortarotti TG, Doxtader EK. "Toxicity studies on rutin." Proc Soc Exp Biol Med 1947;64:324-327.

(59) Hirose M, Fukushima S, Sakata T, et al. "Effect of quercetin on two-stage carcinogenesis of the rat urinary bladder." Cancer Lett 1983;21:23-27.

(60) Ito N, Hagiwara A, Tamano S, et al. "Lack of carcinogenicity of quercetin in F344/DuCrj rats." Jpn J Cancer Res 1989;80:317-325.

(61) Pamukcu AM, Yalciner S, Hatcher JF, Bryan GT. "Quercetin, a rat intestinal and bladder carcinogen present in bracken fern (Pteridium aquilinum)." Cancer Res 1980;40:3468-3472.

(62) Hirono I. "Is quercetin carcinogenic?" Jpn J Cancer Res 1992;83:313-314.

Vitamin C (Ascorbic Acid)

Vitamin C has been used for decades at high doses as a cancer cure by alternative practitioners. Its use was pioneered by Linus Pauling.

History & Controversy Surrounding Vitamin C For Cancer

Linus Pauling (February 28, 1901 – August 19, 1994) was a visionary American scientist and peace activist with a diverse range of interests, including chemistry, biochemistry and medicine. He is the only person ever awarded 2 unshared Nobel Prizes, and one of only 2 awarded the prize in different fields (Chemistry and Peace)

In the 1960s, Linus Pauling pioneered the use of high-dose vitamins in the treatment of diseases, a protocol called "Orthomolecular Medicine." He himself was reported to take 3 grams of vitamin C daily to prevent colds.

In 1971 he partnered with a British surgeon named Evan Cameron to test this medical theory in clinical practice, and claimed that high-dose vitamin C prolonged the lives of 100 terminal cancer patients by a factor of 4.2 compared to a control group of 1000 patients with similar disease who were given identical treatment except for the absence of vitamin C. The patients in the vitamin C group survived an average of 210 days, compared to an average of 50 days for patients in the control group.[1,2]

These conclusions were criticized by other scientists, who said the patients treated by Pauling were not as sick as the control group to which they were compared, and that the lifespan extension seen was due to the earlier stage of their cancers.[3]

The Mayo Clinic ran its own study of vitamin C, using 10,000 mg oral doses for a brief treatment period of 2.5 months, found this regime produced no curative results, and declared it worthless.[4,5]

Pauling responded by stating that the vitamin C dose used was too low, that therapeutic levels were unachievable through oral administration, and that the treatment period too short (Pauling stressed lifetime maintenance doses). Accusations of academic fraud were made by each side against the other.

Since then, conventional medicine has abandoned the use of vitamin C, though it continues to be used by alternative practitioners.

Cell Studies

Conventional theory held that its action was indirect, based on its antioxidant function preventing DNA damage by scavenging free radicals.

However, a 2007 Johns Hopkins study by Dr. Chi Dang found that vitamin C's antioxidant action may directly interfere with the cellular mechanism allowing a cancer cell to survive in low-oxygen environments.[6]

Over a decade ago, Johns Hopkins researcher Dr. Gregg Semenza discovered that a protein created in the presence of free radicals called HIF-1 (hypoxia-induced factor) allowed cells to metabolize sugar without oxygen, and also promoted growth of new blood vessels to bring in extra oxygen (angiogenesis).[7]

HIF-1 becomes unstable and ceases to function when free radicals are removed by antioxidants. Antioxidants such as vitamin C inactivate HIF-1 by removing free radicals, thus stopping tumor growth. Scientists tested this theory by creating cancer cells which produced a variation of the HIF-1 protein which was stable without the addition of free radicals. In these cells, addition of antioxidants had no effect and the tumor cells continued to grow.

An in-vitro study in 2005 found that ascorbic acid selectively kills some types of cancer cells, but no normal cells, by generating hydrogen peroxide.[8]

A 2008 study by the same author found that intravenous vitamin C caused significant decrease in the growth of ovarian, pancreatic and glioblastoma tumors implanted in mice. The study concluded, "These data suggest that ascorbate as a prodrug may have benefits in cancers with poor prognosis and limited therapeutic options."[9]

Human Studies

A 1974 study on the use of high-dose vitamin C in 50 patients with advanced cancer concluded that the treatment was both simple and safe, and suggested that it be used both as a standard palliative measure in terminal cases, and as a standard adjunct to reinforce conventional cancer treatments in earlier, less advanced cancer.[10]

A patient with reticulum cell sarcoma was treated only with large doses of ascorbic acid. The treatment resulted in dramatic regression of the disease, but a reduction in vitamin C dosage some months later was associated with reactivation of the cancer. Reinstitution of a higher dose of vitamin C induced a second complete remission.[11]

A protocol for the use of vitamin C to treat cancer was published by the Linus Pauling Institute of Science and Medicine, Palo Alto, California. It recommends that an initial course of intravenous vitamin C followed by an oral maintenance oral dose to be continued indefinitely after treatment. The report stresses the importance of continuous as opposed to intermittent administration of vitamin C.[12] A 2006 study by Sebastian Padayatty discussed 3 clinical cases of cancer cured by intravenous vitamin C therapy without the use of conventional cancer therapy. The cases involved renal cell tumor (kidney cancer), transitional cell bladder cancer, and large B-cell lymphoma.[13]

Despite the long controversy surrounding vitamin C therapy, some researchers are re-evaluating its use, and believe that it could be useful in the treatment of cancer.[14]

Dr. Hugh D. Riordan founded and directed the Center for the Improvement of Human Functioning, in Wichita, Kansas (now called as the Riordan Clinic), and also served as Associate Editor of *the Journal of Orthomolecular Medicine.* He is known worldwide for his research on high-dose vitamin C therapy, which the Riordan Clinic provides, along with other alternative treatments for a variety of illnesses including cancer.

In a 1995 paper, Riordan noted that the highest plasma level of vitamin C that can be achieved with oral supplementation is 4.5 mg/dl, whereas cell studies found the lowest effective anti-tumor level to be at least 0.88 mg/dl (for malignant lymphoma), and that therapeutic effects at this level were rare. Usually, plasma levels of 5-40 mg/dl of vitamin C are required in vitro to kill 100% of tumor cells within 3 days. The levels needed to kill 100% of endometrial carcinoma cells and pancreatic carcinoma cells are 30 mg/dl and 40 mg/dl respectively.[15]

A 2003 report by Dr. Riordan provides a detailed description of a clinical protocol developed over 2 decades using high dose intravenous vitamin C in cancer treatment. Researchers found vitamin C to work synergistically with conventional cancer treatment.[16]

Another report by Dr. Riordan examined seven cases of patients treated with intravenous vitamin C for various malignancies. The cancer cases reviewed included renal cell carcinoma (2 patients), colorectal cancer (1), pancreatic cancer (1), non-Hodgkin's lymphoma (2) and breast cancer (1). These patients had either been declared terminal and offered no further treatment options by their oncologists, had personally refused further conventional treatment, or (1 patient) requested that vitamin C be combined with conventional chemotherapy.

Improvements were seen in all cases, including some complete remissions. Researchers found that intravenous vitamin C in a dose of more than 100 grams per day administered by a slow infusion to be non-toxic. Vitamin C did not interfer with the effect of conventional therapy, and may in fact decrease its toxicity.[17]

A Korean study found that quality of life in terminal cancer patients was significantly enhanced by vitamin C therapy. Patients reported significantly less for fatigue, nausea/vomiting, pain, and loss of appetite.[18]

A recent survey on the clinical use of vitamin C therapy finds the practice to be surprisingly widespread, judging by sales of vials of vitamin C for IV use. Researchers surveyed 550 attendees at the 2006 and 2008 conferences of Complementary and Alternate Medicine (CAM) practitioners. Of the 199 practitioners who responded to the survey, 172 practitioners used intravenous vitamin C to treat 11,233 patients in 2006, and 8876 patients in 2008. The average dosage was 28 grams every 4 days, for a total of 22 treatments per patient. Estimated doses used per year (as 25 g/50 ml vials) were 318,539 in 2006 and 354,647 in 2008. Manufacturers report sales of 750,000 vials in 2006 and 855,000 vials in 2008. Common reasons for vitamin C treatment included not only cancer, but also infection and fatigue.

Data was available for 9,328 patients treated. 101 experienced adverse effects, usually minor, such as fatigue/lethargy (59), change in mental status (21) and vein irritation/phlebitis (6). In addition, 2 deaths were documented in patients known to be at risk for side effects from IV vitamin C, but due to confounding factors, the FDA Adverse Events Database was not informative.[19]

Caution

Use with caution in patients with kidney disease or a metabolic disorder called glucose 6-phosphate-dehydrogenase deficiency.

Instructions

The maximum oral dose of vitamin C tolerated by patients is approximately 18 grams per day. This often produces peak plasma concentrations of only 220 μmol/L. Intravenous administration of this same dose produces plasma concentrations about 25 times higher. Larger doses of 50–100 grams given intravenously result in plasma concentrations of about 14 000 μmol/L. In-vitro studies have shown that at concentrations of 1000-5000 μmol/L, vitamin C is toxic to some cancer cells while leaving normal cells unharmed.

If you are planning to use vitamin C against cancer, be sure to get **intravenous treatments**, as oral doses cannot produce the required blood levels.

Suppliers

The Riordan Clinic in Kansas is known to offer intravenous vitamin C therapy.

http://riordanclinic.org/

The Envita cancer clinics also feature this treatment.

http://www.envita.com/cancer/

References

(1) Cameron E, Pauling L, "Supplemental ascorbate in the supportive treatment of cancer: Prolongation of survival times in terminal human cancer." Proceedings of the National Academy of Sciences (October 1976). 73 (10): 3685–9

(2) Cameron E, Pauling L, "Supplemental ascorbate in the supportive treatment of cancer: Reevaluation of prolongation of survival times in terminal human cancer." Proceedings of the National Academy of Sciences (September 1978). 75 (9): 4538–42.

(3) DeWys WD, "How to evaluate a new treatment for cancer." Your Patient and Cancer (1982) 2 (5): 31–36.

(4) Creagan ET, Moertel CG, O'Fallon JR, et al, "Failure of high-dose vitamin C (ascorbic acid) therapy to benefit patients with advanced cancer. A controlled trial." The New England Journal of Medicine (September 1979). 301 (13): 687–90.

(5) Moertel CG, Fleming TR, Creagan ET, Rubin J, O'Connell MJ, Ames MM, "High-dose vitamin C versus placebo in the treatment of patients with advanced cancer who have had no prior chemotherapy. A randomized double-blind comparison." The New England Journal of Medicine (January 1985). 312 (3): 137–41.

(6) Ping Gao, Huafeng Zhang, Ramani Dinavahi, Feng Li, Yan Xiang, Venu Raman, Zaver M. Bhujwalla, Dean W. Felsher, Linzhao Cheng, Jonathan Pevsner, Linda A. Lee, Gregg L. Semenza, Chi V. Dang, "HIF-Dependent Antitumorigenic Effect of Antioxidants In Vivo." Cancer Cell, Volume 12, Issue 3, 230-238, 11 September, 2007

(7) Gregg Semenza, "Targeting HIF-1 For Cancer Therapy." Nature Reviews Cancer 3, 721-732 (October 2003)

(8) Qi Chen, et al., "Pharmacologic ascorbic acid concentrations selectively kill cancer cells: Action as a pro-drug to deliver hydrogen peroxide to tissues." Proc Natl Acad Sci U S A. 2005 September 20; 102(38): 13604–13609

(9) Chen Q, Espey MG, Sun AY, Pooput C, Kirk KL, Krishna MC, Khosh DB, Drisko J, Levine M, "Pharmacologic Doses of Ascorbate Act as a Pro-oxidant and Decrease Growth of Aggressive Tumor Xenografts in Mice." Proc Natl Acad Sci U S A. 2008 Aug 12;105(32):11105-9. Epub 2008 Aug 4

(10) Ewan Cameron and Allan Campbell, "The Orthomolecular Treatment of Cancer. Clinical Trial of High-Dose Ascorbic Acid Supplements in Advanced Human Cancer." Chemico-Biological Interactions, October 1974; Volume 9, Issue 4, Pages 285-315

(11) Ewan Cameron, Allan Campbell and Thomas Jack, "The Orthomolecular Treatment of Cancer: III. Reticulum Cell Sarcoma: Double Complete

Regression Induced by High-Dose Ascorbic Acid Therapy." Chemico-Biological Interactions, November 1975; Volume 11, Issue 5, , p. 387-393

(12) Cameron E, "Protocol for the Use of Vitamin C in the Treatment of Cancer." Med Hypotheses 1991 Nov;36(3):190-4

(13) Sebastian J. Padayatty, "Intravenously administered vitamin C as cancer therapy: three cases." CMAJ March 28, 2006 vol. 174 no. 7 937-942

(14) Ohno S et al., "High-dose vitamin C (ascorbic acid) therapy in the treatment of patients with advanced cancer." Anticancer Res, 2009 Mar;29(3):809-15.

(15) N. H. Riordan, H. D. Riordan, X. Meng, Y. Li and J. A. Jackson, "Intravenous Ascorbate as a Tumor Cytotoxic Chemotherapeutic Agent." Medical Hypotheses (1995), 44, 207-213

(16) Hugh D. Riordan, Ronald E. Hunninghake, Neil H. Riordan, James A. Jackson, Xiao LongMeng, Paul Taylor, et al. "Intravenous Ascorbic Acid: Protocol for Its Application and Use." Puerto Rico Health Sciences Journal (2003) 22:3, 287-290

(17) Riordan HD et al., "Intravenous vitamin C as a chemotherapy agent: a report on clinical cases." P R Health Sci J, 2004 Jun;23(2):115-8.

(18) Yeom CH et al., "Changes of terminal cancer patients' health-related quality of life after high dose vitamin C administration." 2007 Feb;22(1):7-11.

(19) Padayatty SJ, "Vitamin C: intravenous use by complementary and alternative medicine practitioners and adverse effects." PloS One 2010 Jul 7;5(7):e11414

Vitamin E, Tocotrienol

Vitamin E is not a single molecule. It is actually a group of related compounds, four tocopherols and four tocotrienols each designated as alpha, beta, gamma and delta depending on their attached molecules. Alpha-tocopherol is the best-known, and most commercial vitamin E supplements contain this compound alone. However, newer research shows that the other forms each have unique antioxidant, cholesterol-lowering, and anti-cancer effects.

Tocotrienols, especially delta-tocotrienol, are powerful antioxidants with strong anticancer effects.

While alpha-tocopherol (ordinary vitamin E) is the most well-known fat-soluble antioxidant, alpha-tocotrienol has been shown to be 40-60 times more powerful in the prevention of lipid peroxidation (rancidity of fat due to oxidation). Delta-tocotrienol is even more potent; in fact, this little-known compound is the most powerful antioxidant of the entire vitamin E group. Tocotrienols may be more effective in protecting the interior cell membranes, such as those that surround the cell nucleus and mitochondria, because they are more easily incorporated into cell membranes.

Several researchers attribute the anti-cancer effects to diverse biochemical pathways, such as antioxidant activity and suppression of inflammation, the downregulation or degradation of HMG-CoA reductase, the apoptotic pathways of caspase-3 and inhibition of vascular endothelial growth factor (VEGF).[1,2,3,4]

Studies

In an in-vitro study, tocotrienols, alpha-tocopheryl succinate (vitamin E succinate) and delta-tocopherol, caused apoptosis in human breast cancer cells, with estrogen-responsive tumor cells showing greater sensitivity than estrogen-nonresponsive cells. In both cell lines, delta-tocotrienol was the most powerful inducer of apoptosis. Other natural tocopherols showed no effect.

Estrogen-responsive cells showed a half-maximum response for tocotrienols (alpha, gamma, and delta) and delta-tocopherol at 14, 15, 7, and 97 micrograms/ml, respectively. The tocotrienols (alpha, gamma, and delta) and delta-tocopherol caused non-estrogen-responsive cells to undergo apoptosis at concentrations of 176, 28, 13, and 145 micrograms/ml, respectively. The lower the concentration required to produce a response, the more powerful the substance is in fighting cancer.[5]

Another in-vitro study found that tocotrienols inhibit the growth of human breast cancer cells regardless of estrogen receptor status, with gamma-and delta-tocotrienol having the greatest effect. Gamma-tocotrienol showed an inhibitory action three times greater than that of the chemotherapy drug tamoxifen.[6]

Gamma-tocotrienols inhibit cultured mouse melanoma cells in-vitro, and delay tumor progression in mice with melanoma. Treatment increased the survival time of the animal test subjects.[7]

Gamma-tocotrienol suppresses the growth of mouse melanoma, human breast adenocarcinoma and human leukemia cells by causing apoptosis and arrest of cell reproduction at the G1 phase of the cell division cycle.[4]

Tocotrienols can inhibit the growth of prostate tumours and sensitize them to the effects of chemotherapy.

Researcher Dr. Patrick Ling states that existing chemotherapy and hormonal therapy treatment of prostate cancer is insufficient because it fails to kill prostate cancer stem cells, which are responsible for the regrowth of tumours and subsequent chemotherapy resistance. However, his research team discovered a particular form of T3, gamma-tocotrienol (γ-T3), successfully kills cancer stem cells.

"Currently there is no effective treatment for metastatic prostate cancer, because it grows back after conventional therapies in more than 70% of cases," said Dr. Ling.

Dr Ling said in animal trials, γ-T3 completely inhibited tumour formation in more than 70% of the mice implanted with prostate cancer cells and fed the vitamin E constituent in water. In the remaining cases, tumour regrowth was considerably reduced, while tumours regrew in 100% of the control group.

Dr Ling plans human clinical trials in the future.[8]

In addition to antioxidant and anticancer activities, Vitamin E has also been investigated for its ability to lower cholesterol.

Tocopherols have almost no cholesterol-lowering function, but many clinical studies have shown that tocotrienols, especially gamma- and delta-tocotrienol, inhibit the synthesis of cholesterol by the liver. These tocotrienols inhibit the hepatic enzyme HMG-CoA reductase, which is also affected by statins and red yeast rice.[9,10,11]

Instructions

No human studies exist to confirm the dose needed for anti-cancer effects. For cholesterol-lowering action 100 mg per day is suggested by the Life Extension Foundation. Take with food to enhance absorption, and at least one hour away from any other vitamin E supplement.

Half-life in blood plasma for tocotrienols ranged from 2-4 hours[12] (meaning they are completely cleared from the body in 4-8 hours), so 2-3 divided doses may be more effective than one dose daily.

Suppliers

Not all tocotrienol products contain all forms of tocotrienols. Palm oil is rich in gamma-T3, but commercially available tocotrienol is also sourced from other plants, some of which lack gamma-T3 entirely.

Tocotrienols are available from many suppliers. If buying a full-spectrum supplement, be sure to check the source, and buy only the variety made from palm oil, unless the gamma- and delta-T3 content is listed.

Fractionated products such as Delta Gold contain a higher proportion of delta-tocotrienol.

References

(1) Palozza P. et al., "Comparative antioxidant activity of tocotrienols and the novel molecule chromanyl-polyisoprenyl FeAox-6 in isolated membranes and intact cells." Mol. Cell. Biochem., 2006, 287 (1-2): 21-32.

(2) Theriault A, Chao JT, Wang Q, Gapor A, Adeli K. "Tocotrienol: a review of its therapeutic potential." Clin Biochem 1999;32:309-19.

(3) Theriault A, Chao JT, Gapor A, et al. "Tocotrienol is the most effective vitamin E for reducing endothelial expression of adhesion molecules and adhesion to monocytes." Atherosclerosis 2002:160:21-30.

(4) Mo H. et al., "Apoptosis and cell-cycle arrest in human and murine tumor cells Initiated by isoprenoids." J. Nutr., 1999, 129: 804-13

(5) Simmons-Menchaca M, Gapor A, et al. "Induction of apoptosis in human breast cancer cells by tocopherols and tocotrienols." Nutr Cancer 1999;33:26-32.

(6) Guthrie N, Gapor A, Chambers AF, Carroll KK. "Inhibition of proliferation of estrogen receptor-negative MDA-MB-435 and -positive MCF-7 human breast cancer cells by palm oil tocotrienols and tamoxifen, alone and in combination." J Nutr 1997;127:544S-548S

(7) He L. et al., "Isoprenoids suppress the growth of murine B16 melanomas in vitro and in vivo." J. Nutr., 1997, 127:668-74.

(8) Luk SU, Yap WN, Chiu YT, Lee DTW, Ma S, Lee TKW, Wong YC, Ching YP, Yap YL, Ling MT. "Gamma-Tocotrienol as an effective agent in targeting prostate cancer stem cell-like population." International Journal of Cancer. 2011; 128:2182-91.

(9) Pearce BC, Parker RA, Deason ME, Qureshi AA, Wright JJ. "Hypocholesterolemic activity of synthetic and natural tocotrienols." J Med Chem 1992;35: 526-541 and 3595-606.

(10) Qureshi AA, Pearce BC, Nor RM, et al. "Dietary alpha-tocopherol attenuates the impact of gamma-tocotrienol on hepatic 3-hydroxy-3-methylglutaryl coenzyme A reductase activity in chickens." J Nutr 1996;126:389-94.

(11) Qureshi AA, Sami SA, Salser WA, Khan FA. "Dose-dependent suppression of serum cholesterol by tocotrienol-rich fraction (TRF25) of rice bran in hypercholesterolemic humans." Atherosclerosis 2002;161:199-207.

(12) Yap SP, Yuen KH, Wong JW. "Pharmacokinetics and bioavailability of alpha-, gamma- and delta-tocotrienols under different food status." J Pharm Pharmacol 2001;53:67-71.

Combination Formulas – Herbal

Breast Defend

This formula by Dr. Isaac Eliaz is especially formulated for breast cancer. It contains a proprietary blend of plant extract and antioxidants known to exhibit anti-cancer activity, including Scutellaria barbata, curcumin, quercetin, Astragalus root, and a mushroom blend of Coriolus versicolor (Coriolus), Ganorderma lucidum (Reishi), Phellinus linteus, and DIM.

Studies

This formula performs well against breast cancer in animal studies, and human trials are being planned.

In-vitro, Breast Defend combined with Pecta-Sol MCP suppressed invasiveness of breast cancer cells, and a related formula, ProstaCaid, suppressed prostate cancer cells.[1]

In mice implanted with triple-negative human breast cancer, Breast Defend (100 mg/kg for 4 weeks) decreased the development of breast-to-lung metastasis from 67% (control group) to 20% (treatment group). Size of metastatic tumors was also reduced in the treatment group. Anti-metastatic activity was confirmed by down-regulation of several genes in the tumor cells. No toxicity was noted.[2,3,4]

Instructions

Up to 8 capsules daily for acute treatment, then 2 daily for maintenance.

Suppliers

$100 for 120 capsules:

http://www.rockwellnutrition.com

References

(1) Jiang, J., Eliaz, I and Silva, D. "Suppression of Invasive Behavior of Human Breast and Prostate Cancer Cells Synergistic and Additive Effects of Modified Citrus Pectin With Two Poly-botanical Compounds, in the Suppression of Invasive Behavior of Human Breast and Prostate Cancer Cells." Integrative Cancer Therapies. 2012 April 24

(2) Jiang J, Thyagarajan-Sahu A, Loganathan J, Eliaz I, Terry C, Sandusky GE, Sliva D. BreastDefend prevents breast-to-lung cancer metastases in an orthotopic animal model of triple-negative human breast cancer. Oncol Rep. (2012 Jul 26). doi: 10.3892/or.2012.1936.

(3) Dr. Eliaz Interview. (2012, Aug.). Breast Health Project. Retrieved on August 8, 2012 from: http://breasthe.ipower.com/DrEliazInterviewBreastDefend.html

(4) First of its Kind Botanical Formula Shows Promise for Incurable Breast Cancer (2012, Aug. 1). PR Newswire. Retrieved on August 8, 2012 from: http://www.prnewswire.com/news-releases/first-of-its-kind-botanical-formula-shows-promise-for-incurable-breast-cancer-164558366.html

Cancema

Cansema is a black salve or ointment used as an alternative treatment for skin cancer. It is basically an escharotic, a solution that burns the skin away and leaves black dead tissues that eventually fall off.

The skin removal is the signal that the treatment for skin cancer or skin disorder is successful. Cansema is not FDA-approved.

Origin of Cansema

Escharotics were used in the treatment of skin lesions as early as the 1800s. A herb called bloodroot is the key ingredient to an escharotic and even today, it is popularly used in the treatment of sores, eczema, warts, and other skin problems.

The main ingredients of Cansema are zinc chloride, blood root, and chapparal. The bloodroot extract that is used in Cansema is the main ingredient that burns off the tissues of the skin cancer and lesions, thus leaving a black burned out tissue.

Correct proportions of these ingredients must be mixed in preparing the black salve. If the combination is wrong, more tissues will be damaged and this might cause more problems than solutions. The original Cansema was made by Alpha-Omega Labs, but many variations are sold, often using the same name.

When Cansema is applied to the skin, it burns off the skin lesions. After a few days of application, the dead skin cells fall off in the form of black soot and this signals that the skin disorder is cured.

Caution

As with other medications, this product also has some side effects and it is necessary that the correct strength of formula is used; otherwise, severe skin damage might occur. Different strengths or dosage of Cansema are available for several types of skin diseases. Full strength is used in the treatment of skin cancers in humans, but a dosage of mild strength is used for treating pets with skin disorders.

It is believed that Cansema removes only cancerous cells and does not remove the healthy cells. However, if not properly applied and if the incorrect dosage is used, it may leave holes in the skin.

If severe irritation develops, discontinue use. BEC-5 may be a safer alternative.

Suppliers

Cansema is available at the following website, along with a lengthy history of the product and the controversey surrounding it.

Cansema® Black Topical Salve (Original) $24.95 per 0.77 Oz. (22 g.)

http://www.altcancer.com/Products/qblack-salveq.html

Essiac

Essiac tea was popularized in the 1920s by Rene Caisse, a modest Canadian nurse who adapted a herbal cancer cure originated by Ojibway traditional healers. The name "Essiac" is Caisse spelled backwards. After developing the formula, she distributed it to cancer patients, and accepted no payment except donations to keep her clinic running. Rene Caisse died in relative obscurity.

History of Essiac

While working on a hospital ward in 1922, nurse Caisse met a woman with a strangely scarred breast. The woman told Caisse she had suffered from breast cancer 20 years earlier, and had been told she needed a mastectomy. She declined the surgery, and instead accepted an herbal remedy from an Ojibway friend, who taught her how to prepare the mixture. Her tumor disappeared, leaving only a scar.

Caisse asked the patient for the recipe, thinking it would be useful if she ever developed cancer. Shortly afterward, Caisse's aunt was diagnosed with terminal stomach cancer and given six months to live. Caisse asked the physician treating her aunt, Dr. R. O. Fisher, for permission to give her aunt the Ojibway remedy. Her aunt drank the tea daily for two months, was cured of her cancer, and lived for two more decades.

In 1934, Dr. Fisher and nurse Caisse established a cancer clinic in Bracebridge, Ontario, to treat patients with the herbal formula, which she modified somewhat and named Essiac. Thousands of patients, many who had been diagnosed as terminal by their doctors, improved dramatically.

One case involved a woman with inoperable bowel cancer and insulin-dependent diabetes, who was cured of both her diabetes and her tumor. Dr. Frederick Banting, the discoverer of insulin, heard about Essiac and wanted to test it as a possible treatment for diabetes. However, he wanted Caisse and Fisher to shut down their cancer clinic while the tests were underway, and since they refused to do this, the diabetes drug trial was never performed.

In 1942 the clinic shut down due to pressure from the medical community, who claimed Caisse was practicing medicine without a licence. However, Caisse continued to give away her formula to cancer patients until her death in 1978.

Essiac Formula

Essiac consists of four main herbs that grow wild in Ontario, Canada. They are burdock root (Arctium lappa), Turkey rhubarb (Rheum palmatum), sheep sorrel (Rumex acetosella), and slippery elm (Ulmus fulva). Native Canadians used this formula as a treatment for various illnesses and health conditions. As with many folk remedies, slightly different versions of it exist, though usually with the same four basic herbs in different proportions, plus some additional ingredients. However, only one company produces the authorized version used by Caisse.

Essiac is said to have the ability to detoxify the body, relieve pain, strengthen the immune system, and cure cancer. It has been a controversial treatment, and does not have FDA approval, though it has been widely used by cancer patients. Proponents of Essiac claim that the extracts of the herb reduce the size of tumors and help cancer patients live longer.

As a non-standardized plant-based remedy, potency can vary from batch to batch, depending upon the quality and proportion of the ingredients and the method of preparation and handling. It is best to buy the official version, as it uses Caisse's original formula, manufactured under high laboratory standards.

Scientific research identified some components of Essiac effective to an extent, but understanding the synergistic effect of all the ingredients has been difficult. Though it has been stated that Essiac tea can be used alongside different forms of treatment, radiation and chemotherapy may reduce the effectiveness.

Essiac Studies

In 1959 Rene Caisse presented her Essiac formula to Dr. Charles Brusch, M.D., President John F. Kennedy's physician. Caisse began a series of supervised clinical trials on terminal cancer patients and laboratory mice at the Brusch Medical Center in Cambridge, Massachusetts, supervised by Dr. Charles McClure and Dr. Brusch. According to an article in Homemaker's Magazine by Sheila Fraser and Caroll Allen, the researchers concluded after three months that, "On mice [Essiac] has been shown to cause a decided recession of the mass, and a definite change in cell formation.

"Clinically, on patients suffering from pathologically proven cancer, it reduces pain and causes a recession in the growth; patients have gained weight and shown an improvement in their general health. This, after only three months' tests and the proof Miss Caisse has to show of the many patients she has benefited in the past 25 years, has convinced the doctors at the Brusch Medical Center that Essiac has merit in the treatment of cancer. The doctors do not say that Essiac is a cure, but they do say it is of benefit. It is non-toxic, and is administered both orally and by intra muscular injection."

Rene Caisse refused to reveal her formula to the medical establishment because they would give her no assurance that they would use it to treat cancer patients. She stated, "if they did not know what I was using, they could not be in a position to condemn it. I have therefore kept my own counsel." She felt that this led to laboratories associated with the Brusch Center to stop processing their studies. The American Medical Association had forbidden its members to supply unknown medications to patients, and physicians refused to refer their patients to the Brusch clinic. Therefore, the Essiac trials at the clinic ended.

In 1990, Dr Charles Brusch wrote, "Many years have gone by since I first experienced the use of Essiac with my patients. . .suffering from many varied forms of cancer. . . . Rene [Caisse] worked with me and together we refined and perfected her formula. . . . Remarkably beneficial results were obtained even on those cases at the 'end of the road' where it proved to prolong life and the 'quality' of that life.

"In some cases, if the tumor didn't disappear, it could be surgically removed after Essiac with less risk of metastasis resulting in new outbreaks. Hemorrhage has been rapidly brought under control in many difficult cases, open lesions of lip and breast responded to treatment, and patients with cancer of the stomach have returned to normal activity among many other remembered cases. Also, intestinal burns from radiation were healed and damage replaced, and it was found to greatly improve whatever the condition. . . .I endorse this therapy even today, for I have in fact cured my own cancer, the original site of which was the lower bowel, through Essiac alone." (From a notarized letter, April 6, 1990.)

In 1991, Dr. Jim Chan, N.D., obtained Essiac from the Resperin Corp. of Toronto for cancer patients through Canada' emergency drug release program, a government program which supplies officially unapproved medications to terminally ill patients. He maintains it is more effective than conventional cancer therapy, but is not 100% effective. The general health and lifestyle of the patient, and the type and extent of their cancer all contribute to the outcome of treatment. Chan found the highest success rate in patients who began taking Essiac in the early stages of their illness, and had the least chemo or radiotherapy.

Memorial Sloan-Kettering Cancer Center performed animal tests of Essiac in 1959 and the mid-1970s, but could not verifiy any antitumor effects. In 1983, Canadian health authorities arranged tests of Essiac by the U.S. National Cancer Institute (NCI), which found no anti-cancer activity in animal studies. After reviewing 86 case studies, Canadian health officials concluded that there was no evidence that Essiac slowed cancer progression. However, they noted that there were few serious side effects, and that patients reported an increased sense of well-being.

Supplier

In 1977, Rene Caisse signed over all her rights to the original Essiac formula to the Resperin Corporation Limited. Dr. Charles Brusch of Cambridge, MA, witnessed the signing of the legal agreement and swears her original herbal formula was never revealed to anyone other than representatives of Resperin. In return, Resperin gave Rene Caisse assurance that Essiac would continue to be produced and distributed. On May 29th, 1995 Resperin transferred the rights to Essiac® to Essiac Products Inc., and the Resperin corporation was voluntarily dissolved. Today, Essiac® Canada International owns the rights to the Essiac® formula and exports it worldwide.

http://www.essiac-resperin.com/en/index.html

Instructions

Full Program:
Amount: 4 capsules twice daily
Duration: 12 weeks
ESSIAC® required: 12 bottles
Notes:
No food 1 hour before and after consuming ESSIAC®
No juices 30 minutes before and after consuming ESSIAC®
Not to be taken during pregnancy, by nursing mothers or infants

Further Reading

Cynthia Olsen, Jim Khan. Essiac: A Native Herbal Cancer Remedy Kali Press 1998.

Sheila Snow and Mali Klein, Essiac Essentials, Gill & McMillan, 1999

Hoxsey Herbs

Like Essiac, the Hoxsey formula is a version of a Native American cancer treatment.
It is actually composed of 2 distinct formulas, one for external use, the other taken internally.

The external formula, intended for application to skin cancers, consists of a paste compounded out of bloodroot, mixed with zinc chloride and antimony sulfide.

The internal formula is a herbal tonic of licorice root, red clover blossom, buckthorn bark, burdock root, stillingia root, poke root, barberry root, oregon grape root, cascara sagrada bark, prickly ash bark, wild indigo root, with a recent addition of sea kelp. Patients are also given a supplement of potassium iodide. The formula has been modified somewhat over time.

History

Harry Hoxsey (1901-1974) was the son of a rural Illinois veterinarian who used the herbal medicine to treat animals with cancer, and who also surreptitiously treated human cancer patients. The formula had been passed down in Hoxsey's family.

On his deathbed, Hoxsey's father told his son to use the family name for the formula to insure its consistency, to heal as many cancer patients as possible, and not to concentrate on monetary gain. Harry Hoxsey took his father's wishes to heart, and in 1922, opened a clinic in Taylorville, Illinois, where he was continuously persecuted by authorities for practicing medicine without a license.

In an effort to gain official approval for the formula, in 1924 Harry Hoxsey went to Chicago to meet with Dr. Morris Fishbein, head of the AMA and editor of the AMA Medical Journal. The Hoxsey formula was tested on a terminal cancer patient, a Chicago police sergeant Thomas Manix, who was subsequently cured of his cancer. This case was officially documented, and Thomas Manix lived for another decade.

After this demonstrated success, Dr. Fishbein and his associates pressured Harry Hoxsey to sell them his rights to the formula, but he refused out of concern that he would lose control over the formula, and there was no guarantee that it would even be made available to the public. After his refusal to hand over the formula, Hoxsey was subjected to an increasing campaign of harassment by the medical authorities.

In 1936, Hoxsey founded a clinic in Dallas, Texas, which was at the time the largest independent cancer clinic in America. He was immediately confronted by Assistant District Attorney Al Templeton, who caused Hoxsey to be arrested almost 100 times in 2 years. However, Templeton could never make any charges stick, since Hoxsey's patients were happy with the treatment and refused to testify against him. Templeton ceased his campaign against the clinic when his own brother was healed of cancer by Hoxsey's formula. After this, Templeton became an outspoken supporter of the Hoxsey clinic, and worked as Hoxsey's lawyer. When Templeton was elected district judge, it appeared as though Hoxsey finally had official support for his practice, at least on a local level.

Hoxsey promoted his treatment with a book called "You Don't Have To Die," which detailed the attempted suppression of his treatment and his encounters with medical authorities.

Fishbein continued his efforts to drive Hoxsey out of business, and published articles attacking him in the *Journal of the American Medical Assocation (JAMA)*. In 1949, Fishbein published a further article of baseless character assassination called "Blood Money," which was distributed in Hearst Papers' *Sunday Magazine*. Hoxsey sued Fishbein and Hearst for slander and libel, and 50 cancer patients cured by Hoxsey testified in court on his behalf. Hoxsey won the court case, though he was given only a symbolic award of $2 for damages, since the judge found no evidence that Hoxsey had been financially impacted by the *JAMA* articles. The Supreme Court upheld the verdict, ruling that the AMA had used restrictive trade techniques.

Congress upheld this viewpoint with the 1953 Fitzgerald Report, which determined that organized medicine had actively conspired to suppress the Hoxsey formula and 12 other alternative cancer treatments. The resulting public outcry forced Fishbein to resign from his position as head of the AMA.

Hoxsey lobbied for congressional hearings on the effectiveness of his treatments, and a committee of doctors with nutritional and herbal backgrounds asserted that Hoxsey's formula was effective. However, an AMA panel of surgeons and radiologists dismissed this verdict, and refused to do any further investigation on the grounds that they did not want to raise false hopes in cancer patients.

Due to continuing pressure from the medical establishment, the FDA finally closed all 17 of Hoxsey's clinics on the same day in 1960, and after this, Hoxsey retired from active practice. His legacy was carried on by his chief nurse from his Dallas clinic, Mildred Nelson, who opened a practice in Tijuana in 1963, called the Bio-Medical Center.

Ironically, Harry Hoxsey developed prostatic melanoma, and his formula was unable to cure the cancer. He underwent cancer surgery, and died 7 years later.

The Bio-Medical clinic still exists today. In keeping with the wishes of Hoxsey's father, treatments are still affordably priced, approximately $3500-$5000 for an entire course of treatment.

Studies

The herbs in Hosxey's formula have antioxidant, antimicrobial and anti-tumor activity in-vitro.[1,2,3]

Caution

No conclusive independent studies exist to confirm cure rates by Hoxsey therapy. In 1994, an attempt was made to evaluate 39 patients treated at the Tijuana clinic. Medical records were unavailable and tumor staging was based upon patient interviews. Only 16/39 patients were available at the 4-year followup; 10/16 had died, with an average survival of 15.4 months; 6/16 were still alive, with an average survival of 58 months.[4]

Like Essiac, Hoxsey herbs are a traditional herbal remedy which remains popular due to anecdotal reports.

References

(1) Diamond WJ, et al. An alternative medicine definitive guide to cancer. Tiburon: Future Medicine Publishing, Inc., 1997:829.

(2) Tyler VE, Foster S. Tyler's honest herbal. New York: Haworth Herbal Press, 1999:316,72.

(3) Duke, James. "The Herbal Shotgun Shell," American Botanical Council's HerbalGram, No. 18/19, Fall 1988/Winter 1989, pp. 12-13

(4) Austin, Dale, DeKadt. "Long term follow-up of cancer patients using Contreras, Hoxsey and Gerson therapies." Journal of Naturopathic Medicine. 1994;5:74-76

Triphala

Triphala is an Indian herbal mixture used in traditional medicine to treat various illnesses. Triphala is considered a "tridoshic rasayan" with balancing and rejuvenating effects on the three constitutional elements that govern human health: Vata which maintains the nervous system, Pitta which regulates metabolism, and Kapha which supports the body's structural integrity. Triphala is made of Amalaki (Emblica officinalis), Haritaki (Chebulic myrobalan), and Bhibitaki (Beleric myrobalan). The name is translated as "Three Fruits."

Triphala is a traditional part of Ayurveda medicine used for stimulating the activity of the immune system, improving digestion, providing relief for constipation and gas as well as cleaning the gastrointestinal tract. Triphala has also been used in treatment of diabetes and eye disease. It also shows action against cancer.

Studies

An in-vitro study tested the effect of aqueous extract of Triphala on human breast cancer cell line (MCF-7) and a transplantable mouse thymic lymphoma (barcl-95). The triphala caused apoptosis of the tumor cells in a dose-dependant manner, due to an increase in intracellular reactive oxygen species (ROS), or free radicals. Treatment of normal breast epithelial cells, MCF-10 F, human peripheral blood mononuclear cells, and mouse liver and spleen cells, with similar concentrations of Triphala did not produce cytotoxicity or increased ROS.

Further in-vivo tests of oral feeding of Triphala (40mg/kg body weight) to mice transplanted with barcl-95 lymphoma cells showed significant reduction in tumor volume, and apoptosis in tumors subsequently excised from the mice.[1]

An ethanol extract of Triphala was tested on various cancer cell lines, including breast and prostate cancer. Cytotoxicity was shown against all the cell lines. The effective component of the extract was identified as gallic acid, a major polyphenol in Triphala.[2]

Triphala also protected mice from the lethal effects of radiation.[3]

Triphala has been shown to be safe up to very high doses. In mice, Triphala was non-toxic up to an intraperitoneal (within the abdominal cavity) dose of 240 mg/kg, where no drug-induced deaths were observed. The dose required to kill 50% of test animals (LD50) was found to be 280 mg/kg body weight. The optimum radioprotective dose of triphala was 1/28 of its LD50 dose, or 10 mg/kg.[4]

Caution

Do not take during pregnancy

Instructions

Take 2-3 grams triphala powder in warm water daily. Consume the entire amount each evening or divide into 3 doses throughout the day, between meals.

Suppliers

Widely available online as bulk powder or capsules.

http://www.iherb.com

References

(1) Sandhya T, et al., "Potential of traditional ayurvedic formulation, Triphala, as a novel anticancer drug". Cancer Letters, Volume 231, Issue 2 , Pages 206-214, 18 January 2006)

(2) Kaur S et al., "The in vitro cytotoxic and apoptotic activity of Triphala--an Indian herbal drug". J Ethnopharmacol. 2005 Feb 10;97(1):15-20. Epub 2004 Dec 25).

(3) Jagetia GC et al., "Triphala, an ayurvedic rasayana drug, protects mice against radiation-induced lethality by free-radical scavenging". J Altern Complement Med. 2004. Dec;10(6):971-8)

(4) Jagetia GC et al., "The evaluation of the radioprotective effect of Triphala (an ayurvedic rejuvenating drug) in the mice exposed to gamma-radiation". Phytomedicine, 2002 Mar;9(2):99-108)

Combination Formulas - Synthetic

Cancell (Entelev/Cantron/Procel/Taxol)

According to information on the American Cancer Society web site, Cancell is composed of common chemicals, including nitric acid, potassium hydroxide, sodium sulfite, sulfuric acid, and catechol.

Although the formula of Cancell has been modified slightly over the years, according to the label it contains inositol, potassium, sodium, copper, and a bioflavonoid complex.

A main active ingredient is catechol. Cancell works by inhibiting cancer cell metabolism, thus causing tumor cells to starve to death.

History

Entelev was developed by a biochemist named James V. Sheridan.

Working in a chemistry lab with students, he accidentally precipitated chemicals in a beaker into banded layers with the colors of the rainbow, a phenomenon called rhythmic banding, in which the width of each band is 2.7 times the width of the band above it. A month after this event, Sheridan began research on the Debye Theory, published in 1927, which dealt with cellular respiration enzymes.
On the afternoon of September 6, 1936, Sheridan had a vivid dream while napping. In the dream, the mathematically precise layers of the rhythmic banding represented discrete metabolic levels of cells. Each color stood for an enzyme at a specific oxidation level. The

electrons in the Debye theory represented the energy in the cellular respiration cycle moving from glucose to oxygen. The dream suggested to Sheridan the possibility of manipulating cellular energy flow to influence cell health and growth.

Sheridan postulated that cancer cells function at a lower energy level than normal cells, and that it was possible to shut down their energy production altogether. Rather than trying to re-differentiate the tumor cells towards a more normal metabolism, Sheridan tried to push them further towards de-differentiation, to the point where they could no longer produce enough energy to survive. At that point, they could be removed by the body's natural mechanisms for cellular renewal.

By 1936 Sheridan developed a formula he called Entelev. Sheridan, a devout man, believed his dream had been a gift from God, and therefore he gave away Entelev freely to cancer patients who asked for it, without any financial compensation. The rainbow on the Cantron bottle is the color of the rainbow, symbolizing Sheridan's dream.

Over time, Entelev was also promoted under other names, including Cancell, Cantron, Procel and Taxol.

In the 1940s, James Sheridan successfully tested his formula on animals.

During the 1960's, while working at Battelle Laboratories, the testing centers for the National Cancer Institute, Sheridan performed an in-vitro test of Entelev. According to NCI records, the two-day test produced a large decrease in the size of tumor cells, but only a small number of dead cells. Many medical professionals who evaluated the test are of the opinion that if the Entelev had been administered for a longer period of time, the shrunken cells would also have died.

However, a longer trial was not allowed. The NCI evaluates new anti-tumor products by comparing them to standard chemotherapy drugs, which have direct and immediate cytotoxic action. If a compound takes longer to work, and does not perform in exactly the same time frame as conventional chemotherapy, it is said to have failed. Therefore, the NCI gave the Entelev trial a response of negative results. The NCI refused to consider that a longer period of time might have shown Entelev to be superior to chemotherapy in the long run.

Entelev acts by reducing the amount of energy produced by the adenosine triphosphate by mitochondria in each cell. In normal cells the reduction is not sufficient to disrupt their functioning, but cancer cells are already operating in a low-energy mode, and a further decrease causes them to die.

This is a slower process than standard chemotherapy, but it avoids systemic poisoning and harm to the entire body.
Subsequent to the NCI testing, Sheridan attempted to have his product tested at private labs, but these facilities wanted nothing to do with the controversial product, and refused to perform the tests.

In May of 1983, Sheridan, who was advancing in age, had worked with his formula for 47 years and was no nearer to obtaining official recognition. Therefore, he gave his formula to Don Wilson, an author and lecturer on health-related topics. A few weeks after handing over the formula, Sheridan's free distribution of Entelev was stopped by a cease and desist order from the FDA.

Wilson initially thought of publishing Sheridan's entire manufacturing process for the public to read, but decided against it due to the complicated and hazardous manufacturing process. In 1984, Wilson enlisted the help of Professor Orz Feather and chemist Ed Sopcak, and began producing Sheridan's formula under the name Cantron. Jerome Godin, a marketing specialist with a long history in alternative health care, also joined the team at this time.

In addition to working for the Cantron project, Feather and Sopcak began making small batches of the formula to distribute themselves, outside of Cantron. In June or July of 1985, approximately 2 years after the Cantron project was initiated in the summer of 1983, Ed Sopcak decided to give his version of Sheridan's formula its own brand name, *Cancell. The product was given away free of charge until 1992, at which time a federal judge cited Sopcak for contempt of a 1989 permanent injunction ordering him to cease and desist from making or distributing *Cancell.

The Cantron company was raided by the FDA in 1994. After this, the Dietary Supplement Health and Education Act of 1994 was passed in America, spelling out more clearly what alternative health care suppliers were allowed to do, and the company was allowed to continue business as long as they carefully avoided making health claims for their products.

Sheridan's formula has been modified slightly over the years, but thousands of patients have claimed success with all versions.

Since 1989, it has been illegal in the United States to produce, sell, or give away Sheridan's product as a treatment for any disease. While the formula cannot be sold as a medication to fight cancer, it is still available from Medical Research Products under the name of Cantron. The Federal Drug Administration has not prosecuted the company, since the product is being marketed simply as a dietary supplement. Currently the company is being run by Gerome Godin.

The makers of Cancell claim that more than 15,000 patients have used their product successfully, and that it is safe and effective in treating 50% to 80% of all cancers. If this is true, then James Sheridan is right and Entelev truly is a gift from God.

Instructions For Use

Avoid sugar, Vitamin C, Vitamin E, Selenium, C0Q10, and any other cellular energy boosters when taking Cancell.

Other alternative therapies said to be compatible with Cancell are laetrile, germanium 132, grape seed extract and noni. However, the company website cautions against taking Cancell with ANY other product.

Willard's Water (water treated with charged colloidal particles which aids the absorption of Cancell), as well as bromelain and pancreatin (pineapple and pancreatic enzymes that dissolve necrotic tissue and the protective capsule surrounding tumors), all improve the effectiveness of Cancell.

Like paw-paw and graviola, Cancell works by starving cancer cells. It must be taken on a regular basis, every 4 hours, preferably down to the minute, with no breaks or drug holidays. Even a brief break will allow tumors to recover from periods of starvation. Take it for at least 2-3 months. As James Sheridan said, "It takes time to work... 7 to 9 weeks is typical and some cases take up to 3 months or more to see a response."

Supplier

$190 - $125 for a 32 oz bottle (discounts for bulk purchases)

http://cantron.com/

DMSO

DMSO (Dimethyl sulfoxide) is an industrial solvent that is a by-product of manufacturing paper. It was first discovered in the mid- to late nineteenth century and has been used as an industrial solvent for more than a century. In the 1950s, it was discovered that DMSO protected cells from the damage due to freezing. In the 1960s, researcher Dr. Stanley Jacob investigated other medicinal uses of the substance. Clinical trials of DMSO were begun in 1965 but were stopped due to safety concerns. However, in the 1970s, DMSO was approved for use as a veterinary anti-inflammatory treatment in dogs and horses, and as a prescription drug for a type of bladder inflammation called interstitial cystitis in humans.

According to many alternative practitioners, DMSO can help normalize cellular respiration and cause cancer cells to revert to normal. It can also protect tissues from side effects due to conventional cancer treatments.

In-vitro, DMSO can cause cancer cells to redifferentiate and mature, but this occurs only at a dosage level that would be toxic in a human body. It can cause eye damage and even death in high doses. Some alternative practitioners recommend combining it with hematoxylon to reduce toxicity.

DMSO is a solvent that can help other treatments, both alternative and conventional, enter tissues and cells.

Studies

DMSO has a strong affinity for cancer cells, and can carry substances into them. None-cancerous tissues are not affected. In one study, a marker dye and chemotherapeutic agent combined with DMSO accumulated preferentially in cancer cells. A 1966 clinical trial by Dr. E.J. Tucker of Houston, Texas, of 37 pre-terminal cancer patients found that the combination of DMSO and hematoxylon along with standard cancer therapy caused improvement in 70.5% of cases. DMSO-hematoxylon alone resulted in improvement in 38.1 percent of patients, compared to only 5.4% of patients treated with conventional therapy.[1]

For half a century, Dr. Tucker was a Fellow of the American College of Surgeons, a member of the Orthopedic Board of the International College of Surgeons, an honorary life member of the American Medical Association, and one of the rare recipients of the "Award of Merit" by the AMA for his developments in bone grafting. He was a highly respected member of the traditional medical establishment. However, he managed to publish only one paper on the use of DMSO to treat cancer, due to criticism by colleagues and expulsion from the boards of two hospitals for administering the treatment.[2]

DMSO can be used to potentiate chemotherapy, allowing the drugs to kill more cancer cells with less collateral damage to healthy tissue. According to research by the Oregon Health Sciences University DMSO can be used as a carrier molecule for adriamycin, vinblastine, 5-fluorouracil, and cisplatin. It has also been combined with methotrexate.

DMSO does not bind to every form of chemotherapy, and current research is scarce. Unfortunately, studies about this potentially useful compound have been strongly discouraged by the government.

Some alternative clinics that have employed the combination therapy have been able to reduce chemotherapy dosage by 90%. However, in America such clinics have been prosecuted and shut down by the FDA.

DMSO has also been combined with cesium chloride.

Caution

Do not use during pregancy or while nursing.
Do not use in combination with any electromedicine device, as some of these devices affect cell membranes and make them more porous, allowing DMSO and any molecules it has carried to escape into surrounding tissues.

The most common side effects are headaches, and burning and itching on contact with the skin. Severe allergic reactions have been reported. It can also cause a strong garlic-like taste and odor on the breath and skin. In high concentrations it can cause eye damage, and can even be fatal. Industrial-grade DMSO can be contaminated with other substances. DMSO is a solvent that can increase the absorption of contaminants, toxins, and medicines, with unpredictable results.

DMSO increases the effects of anti-coagulants, steroids, heart medicines, sedatives, and other drugs. Use caution using DMSO if taking other medications.

Do not allow DMSO to come into contact with eyes.

DMSO is a highly effective solvent and is known to be safe only on contact with inert containers such as rigid plastic, glass, ceramic, metal or wood container.

DO NOT USE ORDINARY RUBBER OR LATEX GLOVES WITH THIS PRODUCT.

DMSO will dissolve them and carry toxic substances through the skin. It is highly advisable to use gloves of some kind when handling DMSO to prevent severe wrinkling of the skin of the hands.

It is important to test any brand of gloves to be sure it is safe with DMSO. Soak the tip of the glove in DMSO, and also fill the tip of a glove finger with DMSO, and leave it for 24 hours. Then, check the glove inside and out. If the glove is entirely intact after that time period, it is safe to use.

Dosage

For home use, DMSO is usually applied to the skin. If taken orally, be sure to combine it with plenty of water to avoid dehydration. It is likely to cause gastric upset if taken orally.

The usual oral dosage of DMSO is 1-2 teaspoons (5 - 10 ml) per day. It is rapidly absorbed and reaches a blood level peak in 4 hours, becoming undetectable after 120 hours. Mix with juice to disguise the unpleasant taste.

DMSO is readily absorbed when applied on skin, though with slightly less bioavailability than oral doses. Peak blood levels occur after 4-8 hours. DMSO should not be rubbed into skin, just patted or painted on in a thin coating. If skin irritation occurs, use a more dilute solution of DMSO.

The optimal concentration of DMSO for topical treatments varies from 50-80% DMSO. Skin of the face and neck is more sensitive to topical DMSO than other parts of the body, so the maximum concentration of DMSO for application here should not exceed 50%. Topical applications of DMSO should not exceed 70% in areas of the skin with poor circulation.

It is best to begin topical DMSO treatments at low concentrations until skin tolerance builds up. The skin should be dry, clean, and unbroken.

Aloe Vera gel can relieve the skin irritation that sometimes occurs as a result of DMSO application.

If using DMSO as part of a cesium cloride protocol, it is advisable to get expert advice. A company called Essence of Life provides a variety of products tailored to various cancers, and also provides counselling on how to use them. It is best to phone the company before buying in order to get an individualized regime. The contact number is listed on the website.

http://www.essense-of-life.com/

DMSO-Hematoxylon Protocol

This formula, for intravenous or other administration, is recommended by Dr. Morton Walker, who wrote a book on Dr. Tucker's research and other uses of DMSO. This medication should be administered only under medical supervision.

From a chemical supply store, obtain 25 grams of Hematoxylon HX-0025. Place in 80cc bottle. Fill bottle ¾ full of DMSO, place stopper in bottle and shake until all dye is dissolved. Then, fill bottle to fill line with DMSO.

Start treatment by adding .5 cc of the prepared DMSO solution to a 250 ml bottle of 5% dextrose. For diabetics, normal saline may be substituted for dextrose. Administer intravenously at 47 drops/minute

Increase the concentration dosage by 10% daily until tolerance is reached. Too high a dose will cause the patient to develop a high fever 35 minutes after treatment. Use Demerol or 50 mg Benadryl 30-40 minutes before treatment to counteract this side effect.

The intravenous solution may also be taken orally. Do not eat or drink immediately before or after consuming the solution. DO NOT use this route of administration for stomach cancer, as the rapid death of a stomach tumor will leave a hole in the stomach lining similar to that of a perforated ulcer; use intravenous treatments for gastrointestinal tumors instead.

For lung cancer, it may be administered in a nebulizer. The source mentions a Bennet Respirator Machine, 2cc of saline solution and 4 drops of DMSO solution. Inhale for 10 minutes twice a day, with at least 2 hour intervals between treatments.

For bone cancer, consume at least 2 gm of bone meal tablets daily along with the treatment.

For skin or facial tumors, start with a solution diluted by ½ and apply directly to tumor. Paint the skin twice daily. Increase strength of solution as tolerated by patient.

While undergoing treatment, tests of kidney function should be done biweekly. Patient should not consume alcohol or other liver toxins.

References

(1) E. J. Tucker, M.D., F.A.C.S., and A. Carrizo, M.D, "Haematoxylon Dissolved in Dimethylsulfoxide [DMSO] Used in Recurrent Neoplasms." International Surgery, June 1968, Vol 49, No. 6, p. 516-527)

(2) Dr. Morton Walker, "DMSO-Nature's Healer". 1993, ISBN 0-89529-548-2)

Off-Label Drugs

Aspirin/Acetylsalicylic Acid

Aspirin, an anti-inflammatory analgesic used for decades as an anti-coagulant to prevent heart attacks, also inhibits the development of cancer.

Studies

According to Oxford researcher Peter Rothwell, aspirin can reduce cancer metastasis by 40-50%, with adenocarcinomas showing the greatest inhibition. The effect occurred independent of age and sex of the patients, but smokers received the greatest benefit. Aspirin reduced death due to cancer in patients who developed adenocarcinoma, especially those without metastasis at diagnosis.[1]

Other studies, including research by Rothwell in 2007, 2010 and 2011, found that even a low dose of 75mg per day reduced the long-term risk of developing some cancers, especially those of the esophagus and proximal (but not the distal) colon.

However, the effect only appeared after several years of aspirin treatment. Professor Rothwell claimed that the long gap between aspirin consumption and cancer prevention was due to the fact that aspirin prevented cancer at a very early stage, and that patients show clinical disease many years later.[2]

At least 5 years of treatment were needed to lower the risk of esophageal, brain, pancreatic, and lung cancer, and the effect was even more delayed for stomach, colorectal, and prostate cancer. The greatest preventative action occurred against adenocarcinomas. Benefit was unrelated to aspirin dose, sex of patients, or smoking, but increased with increasing age.[3]

Caution

ASA causes gastrointestinal upset and bleeding.

Instructions

Take 75 mg per day.

Suppliers

Widely available in both brand name and generic form online and in pharmacies.

References

(1) Peter M. Rothwell, et al., "Effect of daily aspirin on risk of cancer metastasis: a study of incident cancers during randomised controlled trials." The Lancet, Early Online Publication, 21 March 2012)

(2) Peter M. Rothwell, et al., "Long-term effect of aspirin on colorectal cancer incidence and mortality: 20-year follow-up of five randomised trials., The Lancet, Vol 376, Issue 9754, Pages 1741 - 1750, 20 November 2010)

(3) Peter M. Rothwell, et al., "Effect of daily aspirin on long-term risk of death due to cancer: analysis of individual patient data from randomised trials." The Lancet Vol 377 Issue 9759, Pages 31 - 41, 1 January 2011)

Cimetidine

Cimetidine (sold under the brand name Tagamet) is a drug used since the 1970s to reduce the production of stomach acid in the case of gastric ulcers. It was initially a prescription product but is now sold over the counter.

Stomach acid is secreted when histamine binds to the H2 receptors on the surface of parietal cells, or oxyntic cells, located in the epithelium of the stomach. Cimetidine binds to the H2 receptors, blocking the binding of histamine, thus preventing the subsequent production of acid.

The use of cimetidine as an anti-cancer agent was first proposed in 1979 after the remission of metastatic cancer in two patients who were coincidentally using the drug. Since then, many studies assessing the use of cimetidine to treat a variety of malignancies have produced varied and inconclusive results.

The initial theory explaining the anti-cancer action of cimetidine was that it caused stimulation of the immune system. Histamine inhibits the function of the immune system, so to suppress its production would prevent immunosuppression. Cimetidine also blocks the action of T-suppressor cells.

This may be part of the explanation, but researchers also believe that cimetidine directly affects tumor cells by preventing their adhesion to the walls of blood vessels. Metastasis starts when a tumor cell circulating in the blood attaches itself to the wall of a blood vessel and begins to multiply. Cancer cells attach to a molecule called E-selectin, which lines the blood vessels, by means of their own cell surface binding molecules (ligands), called Lewis X and Lewis A. Cimetidine blocks the production of E-selectin (ELAM-1), thus preventing cancer cells from adhering. Instead, they are eventually eliminated by the body.

As long as a tumor has Lewis X and Lewis A ligands, cimetidine will block its spread. However, not all tumors have them. According to various studies, approximately 70% of colorectal tumors have Lewis X and Lewis A ligands. Other studies have also found them in breast and pancreatic cancers, which may indicate that cimetidine will block metastasis of these forms of cancer.

Given the amount of clinical evidence proving increased survival rates when cimetidine is administered, it is surprising that it is not more widely used as a cancer treatment.

Studies

In one cimetidine trial, the ten-year survival rate of patients who had undergone the surgical removal of a colorectal cancer was increased from 49.8% to 84.6% when they were treated for a year after surgery with cimetidine as an adjuvant to the chemotherapy agent 5-fluorouracil. Tumors not possessing Lewis antigens did not show response to cimetidine.[1]

However, a double-blind study of 192 colon cancer patients by the British Stomach Cancer Group found increases in survival time only for Dukes Stage C (Stage III) colon cancer.[2]

In 1988, researchers reported that post-operative treatment with cimetidine improved survival in patients with all stages of stomach cancer, increasing median survival from 316 to 459 days.[3] However, in a large study of 442 stomach cancer patients, cimetidine (400 mg to 800 mg twice daily) was not found to have a statistically significant effect on survival time. 5-year survival rates were 21% for patients treated with cimetidine versus 18% for patients treated with a placebo.[4]

Other studies have demonstrated significantly enhanced survival rates in patients with various types of cancer who received cimetidine. Treatment with cimetidine was reported to be beneficial for patients with gastric cancer, melanoma and renal cell cancer. However, other researchers have failed to confirm these findings.

In summary, cimetidine has been conclusively proven to be useful in treating Dukes Stage C (Stage III) colon cancer, and tumors with Lewis X and Lewis A ligands. It is of questionable use for other cancers.

Genzyme Genetics is an American company which can test for the presence of Lewis X and Lewis A ligands on tumours.

Caution

May cause dizziness and drowsiness, especially when combined with alcohol.

Instructions

Test for Lewis X and Lewis A ligands to determine whether cimetidine will be useful.

Dosage: 400-800 mg twice daily.

Suppliers

Widely available in both brand name and generic form online and at pharmacies.

References

(1) Matsumoto et al. "Cimetidine increases survival of colorectal cancer patients with high levels of sialyl Lewis-X and sialyl Lewis-A epitope expression on tumour cells," Br J Cancer. 2002 January 21; 86(2): 161–167.

(2) Svendsen LB, "Cimetidine as an adjuvant treatment in colorectal cancer. A double-blind, randomized pilot study". Dis Colon Rectum, 1995 May; 38(5):514-8.

(3) Tonnesen H, Knigge U, Bulow S, Damm P, Fischermann K, Hesselfeldt P, Hjortrup A, Pedersen IK, Pedersen VM, Siemssen OJ, Svendsen LB, Christiannen PM (1988) "Effect of cimetidine on survival after gastric cancer." Lancet 2: 990–992

(4) Langman MJ, Dunn JA, Whiting JL, Burton A, Hallissey MT, Fielding JW, Kerr DJ (1999) "Prospective, double-blind, placebo-controlled randomized trial of cimetidine in gastric cancer." British Stomach Cancer Group. Br J Cancer 81: 1356–1362

DCA (Dichloroacetate)

Dichloroacetic acid or DCA, is an analogue of acetic acid in which two of the three hydrogen atoms of the methyl group are replaced by chlorine atoms. This substance is not patentable because it was synthesized as long ago as 1864, so it is now in the public domain. However, a patent has been filed for its use as a cancer treatment.

Since there is no incentive for any pharmaceutical company to study the use of this compound as a cancer treatment, research is being funded by Canadian public agencies, the Canada Foundation for Innovation, the Canadian Institutes for Health Research (CIHR), the Canada Research Chairs program, and the Alberta Heritage Foundation for Medical Research.

DCA was initially used to treat metabolic disorders such as congenital lactic acidosis. DCA increases the activity of the enzyme pyruvate dehydrogenase through its inhibition of the enzyme pyruvate dehydrogenase kinase, and therefore decreases lactate production by shifting metabolism of pyruvate from glycolysis towards oxidation by the mitochondria.

This is important because cancer cells create energy through anaerobic metabolism, and their mitochondria are inactive. Once the mitochondria are reactivated and their normal function is restored, the cancer cell dies (undergoes apoptosis) instead of continuing its uncontrolled growth. DCA has no effects on normal, non-cancerous cells. The often-reversible nature of cancer is in direct conflict with the established dogma that cancer cells are permanently damaged due to genetic mutation.

The connection between anaerobic metabolism and cancer was first exposed in 1931 by Dr. Warburg, who won his first Nobel Prize for proving cancer is caused by anaerobic cellular respiration. He stated in an article entitled *The Prime Cause and Prevention of Cancer* that, "the cause of cancer is no longer a mystery, we know it occurs whenever any cell is denied 60% of its oxygen requirements.

"Cancer, above all other diseases, has countless secondary causes. But even for cancer, there is only one prime cause. Summarized in a few words, the prime cause of cancer is the replacement of the respiration of oxygen in normal body cells by a fermentation of sugar.

"All normal body cells meet their energy needs by respiration of oxygen, whereas cancer cells meet their energy needs in great part by fermentation. All normal body cells are thus obligate aerobes, whereas all cancer cells are partial anaerobes."

Dr. Evangelos Michelakis, a professor at the University of Alberta Department of Medicine, found that dichloroacetate (DCA) causes regression in several types of tumors, including breast, lung, and brain cancer. DCA caused significant decrease in tumor growth both in-vitro and in animal studies.

DCA has been used for years to treat cancer in animals. It is not officially approved for human use, but it is sold online, ostensibly for veterinary use.

In Toronto, Canada, Akbar and Humaira Khan have been using DCA off-label to treat cancer patients since March 2007 at their private clinic, Medicor Cancer Centres. In treating various types of tumors they have found "varied positive responses to DCA including tumor shrinkage, reduction in tumor markers, symptom control, and improvement in lab tests." They report 2 cases of patients who added DCA to conventional chemotherapy and experienced complete remission of metastatic cancer. The clinic posts progress updates on their website:

http://www.medicorcancer.com/dca-data.html

Animal studies at the University of Alberta, Canada, found that DCA "induces apoptosis, decreases proliferation, and inhibits tumor growth, without apparent toxicity."[1]

In a 2010 study, DCA was used to treat glioblastomas in 5 cancer patients and 49 excised tumor tissue samples. The lives of glioblastoma patients were extended in 4 of the 5 cases, and in-vitro studies showed that DCA normalized cell metabolism, caused apoptosis of cancer cells and decreased angiogenesis.[2]

"This preliminary research is encouraging and offers hope to thousands of Canadians and all those around the world who are afflicted by cancer, as it accelerates our understanding of and action around targeted cancer treatments," said Dr. Philip Branton, Scientic Director of the CIHR Institute of Cancer.

There are online forums to support patients who want to use dca:

http://www.thedcasite.com/

There are 2 clinics known to incorporate DCA into their cancer protocols, the Medicor clinic in Toronto, Canada, and the CHIPSA clinic in Mexico.

Caution

DCA can cause hepatoxicity (liver damage) at high doses, though none was seen by the Alberta researchers at the doses they used. Patients using DCA without clinical monitoring may not know their livers are failing in time to prevent permanent liver damage.

DCA can also cause peripheral neuropathy (painful or tingling sensation in the extremities), which is reversible upon stopping the DCA. Thiamine supplements can prevent this to a limited extent. Also, continual longterm use may not be needed in cancer treatment.

DCA can sometimes stimulate tumor growth. In a 2010 study, it was found that for human colorectal tumours grown under hypoxic conditions in mice, DCA produced a decrease rather than an increase in apoptosis, enhancing cancer growth. However, under conditions of normal oxygen, DCA suppressed tumor growth.[3]

Tests on mice show that long-term use (more than a year) of high doses of DCA (more than 77 mg/kg/day) increases the risk of liver cancer.

Beware of Scammers

In 2010, a professional con artist named Hazim Gaber was sentenced to 3 years in prison, fines and restitution after pleading guilty to charges of selling fake DCA through his website, DCAadvice.com. The website was cleverly set up, purporting to be connected with the University of Alberta, and even contained a photo and biography of Dr. Michelakis.

According to court documents, Gaber charged customers $23.68 for 10 grams of the purported DCA, $45.52 for 20 grams and $110.27 for 100 grams, plus shipping.

In fact, he sent victims a white powder that was found by laboratory testing to contain dextrose, lactose or starch, and no DCA whatsoever. Additionally, each package contained a fraudulent certificate of analysis from a non-existent laboratory, along with instructions on how to dilute and ingest the bogus DCA.

http://cnews.canoe.ca/CNEWS/Crime/2010/05/11/13915966.html

Instructions

The DCA dose given to patients by the Alberta researchers was 12.5 mg/kg twice daily for a month. At this point, the dose was increased to 25mg/kg twice daily, then decreased by 50% in a stepped fashion as side effects (peripheral neuropathy) developed. At 6.25 mg/kg twice per day, no patient had significant neuropathy.

Suppliers

It is safest to obtain pharmaceutical grade DCA by asking your doctor to prescribe it off-label (it is already approved to treat metabolic disorders). The doctor can then monitor the cancer patient for any liver damage.

If you intend to proceed independently, be sure to purchase sodium dichloroacetate, **not** dichloroacetic acid, which is highly acidic.

Also, do not buy Industrial Grade sodium dichloroacetate, as it may be contaminated, especially by the industrial solvent toluene.

As this drug may be dangerous when used unsupervised, and scammers have been proven to exist, we cannot vouch for any non-physician suppliers. Buyer beware.

References

(2) Bonnet S, Archer SL, Allalunis-Turner J, Haromy, et al. "A mitochondria-K+ channel axis is suppressed in cancer and its normalization promotes apoptosis and inhibits cancer growth." Cancer Cell 2007 Jan;11(1):37-5

(3) Michelakis ED et al., "Metabolic Modulation of Glioblastoma with Dichloroacetate." Sci Transl Med 12 May 2010: Vol. 2, Issue 31, p. 31-34

(4) Siranoush Shahrzad et al., "Sodium dichloroacetate (DCA) reduces apoptosis in colorectal tumor hypoxia." Cancer Letters (2010) Volume: 297, Issue: 1, 75-83

Noscapine

Noscapine is a non-opiate alkaloid (a poppy derivative) which comprises 1-10% of opium's alkaloid content. It lacks significant pain-killing properties, but has been marketed as a cough medicine for 40 years. As a cough medicine, it has been widely consumed by the public without ill effect. Alternative practioners have been using it as an anti-cancer medication at approximately 100 times the dose used as an anti-tussive.

It is a tubulin stabilizer, which inhibits cancer growth by interfering with microtubules, major cytoskeletal structures that maintain genetic stability during cell division. Substances that prevent microtubule functioning often lead to apotosis during mitosis.[1]

Though it has the same biochemical effect as vinca alkaloids and taxane drugs such as paclitaxel and docetaxel, which are also tubulin stabilizers, it is effective even against tumors which have developed resistance to taxanes. Also, unlike these drugs, it is non-toxic to normal cells.

Noscapine binds to tubulin and changes its configuration, preventing microtubule assembly and increasing the time that microtubules spend idle in a paused state, unlike other tubulin inhibitors such as the taxanes and vinca alkaloids which change the polymerization of microtubules.[2]

Overexpression of hypoxia-inducible factor-1 (HIF-1) is frequently found in solid malignancies due to low levels of oxygen, and it correlates with more advanced disease stages, increased tumor angiogenesis and worse prognosis. Noscapine has been shown to inhibit the production of this factor in cell studies.[3]

Studies

In mouse studies, noscapine inhibited both growth and metastasis of implanted human prostate cancers by approximately 60% at an oral dose of 300 mg/kg.
In-vivo and in-vitro studies have found noscapine effective against a wide range of human and murine cancers including breast cancer, lymphoma, melanoma and thymoma. Unlike chemotherapy, it has no negative effects on normal tissue with high rates of cell proliferation such as bone marrow, gastro-intestinal tract or spleen.[4,5]

Noscapine also crosses the blood-brain barrier, and inhibits the growth of gliomas.[6]

Noscapine causes apoptosis in drug-resistant ovarian cancer cells, and causes these cells to become sensitive to cisplatin. It is effective on its own, and it is also a useful adjunct to chemotherapy.[7,8]

Researchers have developed noscapine analogue, such as 9-aminonoscapine, 9-bromonoscapine, and 9-nitro-noscapine, with higher tubulin inhibition than noscapine itself.[9,10,11] Also, such an analogue can be patented and sold at a higher profit than noscapine itself.

Clinical Trials

In 2003, a phase I/II clinical trial was begun at the USC/Norris Cancer Center of noscapine for patients with refractory non-Hodgkin's lymphoma and chronic lymphocytic leukemia. It was ended early due to lack of funding, but preliminary results in 2005 from 12 patients found 2 cases of stabilized disease and 1 partial response.

There is an ongoing phase I trial of noscapine for multiple myeloma at the Center for Lymphoma and Myeloma/Weill Cornell Medical College and Columbia University Medical Center.

http://inclinicaltrials.com/refractory-multiple-myeloma/

Clinical trials of noscapine for prostate cancer are planned by Dr. Barken of the Prostate Cancer Research and Educational Foundation (PC-REF) in San Diego, California.

Website with further information about noscapine:

http://www.noscapine.org/

Caution

Do not combine with MAO inhibitors, alcohol or sedatives. May increase the anticoagulant effect of warfarin.

Instructions

400 mg daily, or as directed by a physician.

Suppliers

Available by prescription.

References

(1) Ye K, Ke Y, Keshava N, Shanks J, Kapp JA, Tekmal RR, Petros J, and Joshi HC (1998) Opium alkaloid noscapine is an antitumor agent that arrests metaphase and induces apoptosis in dividing cells. Proc Natl Acad Sci USA 95: 1601-1606.

(2) Shiwang Li, et al., "Noscapine Induced Apoptosis via Downregulation of Survivin in Human Neuroblastoma Cells Having Wild Type or Null p53." Proc Natl Acad Sci, 1998, 17;95(4):1601-6

(3) Newcomb EW, "Noscapine inhibits hypoxia-mediated HIF-1alpha expression and angiogenesis in vitro: a novel function for an old drug." Int J Oncol, 2006 May;28(5):1121-30.

(4) Yong Ke, et al., "Noscapine inhibits tumor growth with little toxicity to normal tissues or inhibition of immune responses." Cancer Immunology, Immunotherapy Volume 49, Numbers 4-5 (2000

(5) Landen JW, Lang R, McMahon SJ, Rusan NM, Yvon AM, Adams AW, Sorcinelli MD, Campbell R, Bonaccorsi P, Ansel JC, Archer DR, Wadsworth P, Armstrong CA, Joshi HC. "Noscapine alters microtubule dynamics in living cells and inhibits the progression of melanoma." Cancer Res. 2002 Jul 15;62(14):4109-14.

(6) Landen JW, Hau V, Wang M, Davis T, Ciliax B, Wainer BH, Van Meir EG, Glass JD, Joshi HC, Archer DR. "Noscapine crosses the blood-brain barrier and inhibits glioblastoma growth." Clin Cancer Res. 2004 Aug 1;10(15):5187-201.

(7) Zhou J, Gupta K, Yao J, Ye K, Panda D, Giannakakou P, Joshi HC, "Paclitaxel-resistant human ovary carcinoma cells undergo C-Jun NH2-terminal kinase-mediated apoptosis in response to noscapine." J Biol Chem. 2002 Oct 18;277(42):39777-85. Epub 2002 Aug 14.

(8) Su W, "Noscapine sensitizes chemoresistant ovarian cancer cells to cisplatin through inhibition of HIF-1α." Cancer Lett 2011 Jun 1;305(1):94-9. Epub 2011 Mar 21.

(9) Harish Joshi, et al., "Novel Noscapine Analogs as a Potential Cancer Therapeutic." Emory University, posted on 08/23/2012

(10) Harish Joshi, et al., "Development of a Novel Nitro-Derivative of Noscapine for the Potential Treatment of Drug-Resistant Ovarian Cancer and T-Cell Lymphoma." Molecular Pharmacology June 2006 vol. 69 no. 6 1801-1809

(11) Karna P, et al., "A novel microtubule-modulating noscapinoid triggers apoptosis by inducing spindle multipolarity via centrosome amplification and declustering." Mol Cancer Ther. 2006 Sep;5(9):2366-77

Tetracycline

Tetracycline, an old and commonly-used antibiotic, has the surprising side effect of inhibiting tumors, and is especially good at preventing bone metastasis.

Studies

Tetracycline and its derivatives doxycycline and minocycline prevent bone metastasis, a common sequelae of many types of cancer, especially of the breast and prostate. It inhibits matrix metalloproteinases, enzymes such as collagenase which allow tumors to spread by degrading the extracellular collagen matrix that connects intact normal tissue.[1]

Doxycycline causes mitochondrial inhibition and apoptosis of tumor cells in-vitro and enhances their sensitivity to chemotherapy drugs.[2]

Tetracyclines are naturally osteotropic, that is, they are selectively absorbed by bone, making them especially useful in preventing bone metastasis. Doxycycline reduced bone metastasis from breast cancer in mouse test subjects.[3]

Dr. Gurmit Singh, a longterm researcher into the effect of tetracyclines on cancer, is planning a clinical trial on breast cancer patients at the Hamilton Regional Cancer Centre in Ontario, Canada, funded by the Canadian Breast Cancer Research Initiative. The study will probably begin sometime in 2012.

COL-3 (Metastat)

A number of chemically modified tetracyclines have been created to treat cancer. One of them, COL-3, has been the subject of recent clinical trials. The reasons for creating these modified tetracylines are to avoid the gastrointestinal toxicity common to these drugs, to extend the half-life in human plasma, and to enhance metalloproteinase inhibition at lower concentrations.[4] The fact that ordinary tetracyclines are not patentable, and therefore not profitable, may be another factor driving the development of derivatives.

Col-3 was used in 2001 as a Phase I trial in 35 patients with metastatic cancer. Photosensitivity (a common side effect with tetracycline and its derivatives) was the major dose-limiting side effect, as well as drug-induced lupus, and anemia. Disease stabilization occurred in 3 patients for periods of greater than 26 months in hemangioendothelioma, 8 months in Sertoli-Leydig cell tumor, and 6 months in fibrosarcoma.[5]

In a 2006 phase II trial, COL-3 was used to treat 75 patients with AIDS-related Kaposi's Sarcoma. Thirty-three patients, or 44%, had more than 50 malignant lesions. Patients given COL-3 in a dose of 100 mg/day showed a 29% remission rate, compared to 41% in the group receiving 50 mg/day.[5] Researchers concluded, "COL-3, when administered as 50 mg/d, is both active and well tolerated in the treatment of AIDS-related KS. COL-3 is a promising agent for the treatment of this opportunistic neoplasm of AIDS."[6]

Caution

Tetracyclines can be taken safely at low doses for long periods of time (they are often taken for years at a time to treat acne). However, they can cause gastric upset. Take with food to prevent this.

Do not take expired tetracycline. It can cause Fanconi syndrome, a kidney disorder.

Longterm antibiotic use will deplete beneficial intestinal bacteria. Use probiotic supplements.

Instructions

Clinical trials of tetracyclines to determine the appropriate dose to treat cancer have not yet been done. COL-3 has not yet been approved by the FDA, but may be available in clinical trials.

However, standard doses of ordinary tetracycline antibiotics for infectious diseases are given below.

Doxycycline : 100-200 mg twice daily , or 2-5 mg/kg/day in 2 divided doses.

Minocycline : 100 mg twice daily, or 2 m/kg/day in 2 divided doses. Do not exceed 400 mg in a 24 hour period.

Tetracycline : 250-500 mg every 6 hours, or 25-50 mg/kg/day in divided doses every 6 hours.

Suppliers

Available by prescription or from online pharmaceutical companies.

References

(1) Duivenvoorden WC, Hirte HW, Singh G, "Use of tetracycline as an inhibitor of matrix metalloproteinase activity secreted by human bone-metastasizing cancer cells." Invasion and Metastasis 1997, 17(6):312-322

(2) Sagar J, Sales K, Taanman JW, Dijk S, Winslet M. "Lowering the apoptotic threshold in colorectal cancer cells by targeting mitochondria." Cancer Cell Int. 2010 Sep 6; 10:31. Epub 2010 Sep 6

(3) Saikali Z Singh G, "Doxycycline and other tetracyclines in the treatment of bone metastasis." AntiCancer Drugs, 2003 Nov;14(10):773-8.

(4) Manuel Hidalgo, S. Gail Eckhardt, "Development of Matrix Metalloproteinase Inhibitors in Cancer Therapy." Journal of the National Cancer Institute, Vol. 93, No. 3, February 7, 2001

(5) Michelle A Rudek, et al., "Phase I Clinical Trial of Oral COL-3, a Matrix Metalloproteinase Inhibitor, in Patients With Refractory Metastatic Cancer." Journal of Clinical Oncology, January 15, 2001 vol. 19 no. 2 584-592

(6) Bruce J Dezubeaff, "Randomized Phase II Trial of Matrix Metalloproteinase Inhibitor COL-3 in AIDS-Related Kaposi's Sarcoma: An AIDS Malignancy Consortium Study." Journal of Clinical Oncology March 20, 2006 vol. 24 no. 9 1389-1394

12. Diets For Cancer Prevention and Treatment

Many medical experts in the field of traditional cancer treatment as well as many alternative practitioners believe that adhering to a certain diet and lifestyle will help in the battle against cancer.

Beans, lentils and peas contain saponis, which in many cases will stop the reproduction of cancer cells; protease inhibitors, which often have been proven to stop the division of cancer cells; and phytic acid, which many medical professionals feel tests have shown has often been known to slow down the production of tumors.

Fruits and berries are known to be an excellent source of vitamin C and phytonutrients, which many medical professionals believe are major combatants against cancer.

Carrots, orange squash, yams and leafy green vegetables contain carotenoids, which act as antioxidants and aid in detoxification. Studies show that carotenoids are especially effective in preventing and fighting cancer of the breast, lung, skin and stomach (however, current smokers should avoid beta-carotene supplements).

Other vegetables which have proven to be effective against cancer are broccoli, cauliflower, cabbage, Brussels sprouts, bok choy and kale. These are believed to be especially effective against cancers of the mouth, pharynx, larynx, esophagus and stomach.
Garlic is believed by many medical professionals to be effective in slowing and sometimes even stopping cancers of the prostate, bladder, colon and stomach.

Grapes, green tea, and fermented soy foods are also considered to be cancer preventatives.

Carbohydrate Restricted Diet

Since elevated insulin levels fuel tumor growth, it might be expected that low-carbohydrate diets which reduce insulin would also reduce tumor growth. Also, tumor cells have a very primitive metabolism, and can generate energy only by fermenting sugar. Normal cells can switch to producing energy from ketones derived from fat, but tumor cells lack this ability. If they have no sugar, they starve.

One must differentiate between a low carbohydrate diet, which still allows cells to function by metabolizing sugar; and a no-carbohydrate, or ketogenic diet, which forces cells to generate energy through metabolism of fat.

Animal Studies

Scientists have tested a variety of diets for their effect on cancer, from low-carbohydrate to low-fat. The majority of animal studies indicate a positive result from carbohydrate restriction, though one group of researchers found no effect at all from any diet variation they tested. Many of the studies have been done using mice injected with human prostate cancer cells.

Mice innoculated with human prostate cells were divided into 3 test groups. One group was fed a very high-fat/no-carbohydrate ketogenic diet (NCKD: 84% fat, 0% carbohydrate, 16% protein). Another group was fed a low-fat/high-carbohydrate diet (LFD: 12% fat, 72% carbohydrate, 16% protein). A third group was fed a version of the standard Western diet, high-fat/moderate-carbohydrate diet (MCD: 40% fat, 44% carbohydrate, 16% protein). NCKD and LFD mice had tumors 33% smaller than those in the MCD group. Mice in the NCKD group had the longest survival times, followed by the LFD group.

"Low-fat mice had shorter survival and large tumors, while mice on the Western diet had the worst survival and biggest tumors. In addition, though both the low-carb and low-fat mice had lower levels of insulin, only the low-carb mice had lower levels of the form of IGF capable of stimulating tumor growth," said lead researcher Dr. Stephen Freedland, a urologist at Duke University Medical Center.[1]

The same experiment was repeated by another group of researchers. In this case, mice on the LFD diet had the longest survival times, followed closely by the NCKD group. The MCD group survival time was again the worst.[2]

A diet high in refined carbohydrates caused increased tumor size, and activation of insulin-related biochemical pathways leading to increased tumor growth in mice inoculated with human prostate cancer cells.[3]

This study found no difference in survival between groups of tumor-innoculated mice on carbohydrate restricted diets (10-20% of calorie intake) compared completely carbohydrate-free ketogenic diets.[4] Carbohydrate restriction resulted in less tumor growth and longer lifespans in mice inoculated with a variety of tumors. The effect was enhanced by addition of a chemotherapy drug (CCI-779) or an anti-inflammatory (Celebrex).[5]

Human Studies

A few small human studies seem to confirm the animal research.

The first human research on the ketogenic diet was conducted in 1995 by oncologist Linda Nebeling.[6] Three children with brain cancer were placed on a high-fat, ketogenic diet. Ten years later, one of the subjects was still alive, and still on the ketogenic diet.

Since 2007, Dr. Melanie Schmidt and biologist Ulrike Kämmerer, at the Würzburg hospital in Germany, have been enrolling cancer patients in a Phase I clinical study of the ketogenic diet. Patients are placed on a diet which bans all carbohydrates, and provides energy only from high-quality plant oils, such as flax and hempseed, and protein from soy and animal sources. Only terminally ill patients who have exhausted all conventional therapy have been permitted to enter the study. Patients with multiple types of cancer have been studied, including those with pancreatic tumors and glioblastomas. Participants are screened to select those whose tumors show high glucose metabolism in PET scans.

A few of the participants were so sick they died almost immediately after entering the study. Several left the study because they missed high-carbohydrate foods such as chocolates and soda. However, five patients who adhered to the diet for 3 months all survived, their physical condition stabilized or improved, and their tumors grew less quickly, stopped growing, or shrank.

In a case report of one patient, a woman with glioblastoma multiforme was placed on a ketogenic diet. After 2 months, no brain tumor tissue could be seen using PET scanning or MRI imaging. However, after suspension of the diet for 10 weeks, an MRI scan showed evidence of tumor recurrence.[7]

References

(1) Freedland SJ, Mavropoulos J, Wang A, et al., "Carbohydrate restriction, prostate cancer growth, and the insulin-like growth factor axis." The Prostate 2008;68(1): 11-9.

(2) Mavropoulos JC, Buschemeyer WC, 3rd, Tewari AK, et al., "The effects of varying dietary carbohydrate and fat content on survival in a murine LNCaP prostate cancer xenograft model." Cancer Prevention Research 2009;2(6): 557-65.

(3) Venkateswaran V, Haddad AQ, Fleshner NE, et al., "Association of Diet-Induced Hyperinsulinemia With Accelerated Growth of Prostate Cancer (LNCaP) Xenografts." Journal of the National Cancer Institute 2007;99(23): 1793-800.

(4) Masko EM, Thomas JA, 2nd, Antonelli JA, et al., "Low-carbohydrate diets and prostate cancer: how low is "low enough"?" Cancer prevention research 2010;3(9): 1124-31.

(5) Ho VW, Leung K, Hsu A, et al., "A Low Carbohydrate, High Protein Diet Slows Tumor Growth and Prevents Cancer Initiation," Cancer research 2011;71(13): 4484-93.

(6) Linda Nebeling, "Effects of dietary-induced ketosis on tumor metabolism, nutritional status, and quality of life in pediatric oncology patients." Nutrition, 1992

(7) Giulio Zuccoli, Norina Marcello, Anna Pisanello, Franco Servadei, Salvatore Vaccaro, Purna Mukherjee and Thomas N Seyfried, "Metabolic management of glioblastoma multiforme using standard therapy together with a restricted ketogenic diet: Case Report." Nutrition & Metabolism 2010, 7:33

Gerson Diet

This cancer detoxification diet was created by German physician Max Gerson, who practiced in Germany before emigrating to New York and starting a medical practice there in 1938. The diet was part of what is called the Gerson Therapy, and it is an alternative choice for treatment of chronic diseases as well as a possible cure for cancer. Gerson believed that cancer develops when changes occur in cell metabolism due to the buildup of toxic substances in the body. The purpose of the organic-based therapy was to reverse the results of exposure to environmental elements, which Gerson believed affected those who had chronic diseases including diabetes, cancer, and arthritis.

Gerson was born in 1881 and suffered from migraine headaches. He altered his diet to one based on raw and organic plants and fruits, and was relieved of his headaches. After going into private practice in Germany, he started prescribing a natural form of therapy to migraine patients, similar to what he had used to cure himself.

The treatment was successful among many of his patients. Those who had other pre-existing conditions reported a positive outcome not only with their migraines but with other symptoms as well. He started treating cancer patients in the late 1920s after seeing positive results from clinical studies done previously.

Gerson received criticism for his treatment practices by his peers, even though he reported good results with patients including those who suffered from tuberculosis.

After 30 years of clinical practice, Gerson stated that he had developed a successful cure for advanced cancer. He believed that cancer patients showed ineffective immune responses and tissue damage, especially of the liver; and that destruction of cancerous tissues could lead to toxicity and death due to liver failure. His therapy consisted of a low sodium, high potassium diet, with no fats or oils and minimal animal products. Raw vegetable and fruit juices and raw liver provided oxidizing enzymes to help normalize liver functions. Iodine and niacin supplements were also added. Caffeine enemas were used to dilate the bile ducts, helping the liver to excrete toxins, and also to remove toxins across the colonic wall. He concluded, "The therapy must be used as an integrated whole. Parts of the therapy used in isolation will not be successful. This therapy has cured many cases of advanced cancer."[1]

Modern Gerson Therapy includes drinking raw plant based juices with dietary supplements including flaxseed oil, iodine, potassium, vitamins A, B3 and C, pancreatic enzymes and the stomach enzyme pepsin. Gerson's original raw liver extract has been replaced by supplements of vitamin B12 and Coenzyme Q10. Patients are given coffee or chamomile enemas.

The results of Gerson's therapy attracted interest from other medical researchers and patients, and in the 1970's the Gerson Institute was established to help promote the therapy.

Gerson published several papers about his success in treating hundreds of cancer patients. These claims were criticized on the grounds of inconsistent and incomplete record keeping in Gerson's clinic.

Some medical practitioners say that his therapy is not effective, while others suggest it may help lengthen the life expectancy and quality of life of cancer patients.

Studies

Gerson himself published a number of papers about cases in his own practice. In a preliminary report he concluded, "In all of these patients, while no actual cure has occurred, nevertheless improvement was manifested not only in general bodily health but also in many cases the tumors themselves diminished in size."[2] Some cases showed complete remission of their cancer.[3] Gerson published a book detailing 50 cases.[4]

Independent studies also exist.

In one small randomized study of the Gerson diet, two groups of patients who had undergone surgery (18 with metastatic colon cancer, and 38 with breast cancer) were divided into diet and non-diet groups. All patients also continued with conventional therapy. In the colon cancer patients, survival time was 28.6 months in the diet group, compared to 16.2 months in the nondiet group. In the breast cancer group, side effects of chemotherapy, pain and pleural effusion were lessened in the diet group.[5]

A retrospective study compared the 5-year survival rates of 153 patients with various stages of melanoma, who were treated with the Gerson diet, to the average survival time for melanoma patients treated with conventional therapy. Patients treated with the Gerson diet showed markedly increased survival.[6]

Case studies of 6 patients treated with a combination of the Gerson diet and conventional therapy found evidence that the diet was associated with improved patient outcomes, and longer than expected survival times.[7]

References

(1) Gerson M. "The cure of advanced cancer by diet therapy: a summary of 30 years of clinical experimentation." Physiol Chem Phys 10 (5): 449-64, 1978

(2) Gerson M. "Dietary considerations in malignant neoplastic disease: preliminary." Rev Gastroenterol 12: 419-25, 1945

(3) Gerson M. "Effects of a combined dietary regime on patients with malignant tumors." Exp Med Surg 7 (4): 299-317, illust, 1949

(4) Gerson M. "A Cancer Therapy: Results of Fifty Cases and The Cure of Advanced Cancer by Diet Therapy." San Diego, Calif: The Gerson Institute, 2002.

(5) Lechner P, Kroneberger L Jr., "Experiences with the use of diet therapy in surgical oncology." Aktuel Ernahrungsmed 2 (15): 72-8, 1990

(6) Hildenbrand GL, Hildenbrand LC, Bradford K, Cavin SW, "Five-year survival rates of melanoma patients treated by diet therapy after the manner of Gerson: a retrospective review." Altern Ther Health Med. 1995;1(4):29-37

(7) A. Molassiotis, RN, PhD, and P. Peat, RGN, DiplPallCare, "Surviving Against All Odds: Analysis of 6 Case Studies of Patients With Cancer Who Followed the Gerson Therapy." Integrative Cancer Therapies 9(1); 2007 pp.80-88.

Macrobiotic Diet

Michio Kushi, a well-known promoter of macrobiotics, stated that it is "the universal way of life with which humanity has developed biologically, psychologically, and spiritually and with which we will maintain our health, happiness, and peace." Macrobiotics is not only a diet, but also a philosophy and a lifestyle.

Macrobiotic diets are vegetarian-based with the incorporation of whole grain ingredients such as brown rice along with cooked vegetables. Early versions of the diet were strictly vegetarian and quite limited in food selection.

The modern macrobiotic diet consists of 50-60% organically grown whole grains, 20-25% locally grown organic fruits and vegetables, and 5-10% soups containing seaweed, vegetables and soy products such as miso. Occasional elements may include white fish, nuts and seeds, pickles, Asian condiments and mild herbal teas. Red meat, dairy, eggs, coffee, sugar, aromatic herbs, processed foods, vegetables of the nightshade group (potatoes, tomatoes, peppers), spinach, beets, zucchini, and avocadoes are discouraged. Produce not locally available (such as pineapples in the continental United States) are also forbidden.

The macrobiotic diet also recommends specific cooking methods. Cooking utensils should be made of non-reactive material such as glass, wood, stainless steel, enamel or ceramic. Teflon pans are not allowed. Cooking should be done over direct heat, without the use of microwaves or electricity. The diet does not contain artificial dietary supplements. Food should be chewed until it is fluid in order to aid digestion. Since food is thought to be sacred, it is prepared and consumed in a peaceful setting.

Those familiar with the macrobiotic diet see it as a way of living rather than just a diet program. Like many diets, it requires a good balance of foods in order to produce good results. The macrobiotic diet carries the risk of nutrition deficiencies, especially in children. Common deficiencies include iron and vitamin B-12.

The diet combines Buddhist elements with dietary components based on avoiding toxins from everyday foods such as meats, dairy products, and foods high in oil. It is based on simplicity and food restriction.

The diet varies depending on the needs of the individual along with their age and level of daily activity.

The diet is popular in certain areas of the world, with additional variations depending on the gender of the person and the climate in which they live. The word macrobiotic has Greek roots with the word meaning "long life." The term reflects on the concept of looking forward to long term health with a spiritual significance. Many people see the macrobiotic diet as a way of common sense living and not a form of therapy.

Some cancer patients claim their cancer went into remission because of the macrobiotic diet. Components of the diet have shown effects in cancer treatment and prevention, such as vegetarianism against cancers of the reproductive tract. Vegetarian women have lower levels of estrogen, which is protective against breast cancer. Another anticancer effect of the macrobiotic diet may be due to its inclusion of seaweed containing fucoidan, a sulfated polysaccharide present almost exclusively in brown seaweed; and fucoxanthin, the carotenoid which gives brown seaweed its color.

Diets rich in whole grains, fruits, and vegetables have been proven beneficial to health, and though the claim that such a diet can cure cancer is controversial, it certainly will help lower the risk of numerous degenerative diseases.

Studies

An anecdotal report of cancer cured by a macrobiotic diet can be found in the 1982 book, *Recalled by Life: The Story of My Recovery from Cancer*, an autobiography by Dr Anthony Sattilaro. The author, who was diagnosed with metastatic prostate cancer at age 49, adhered to a macrobiotic diet for one year and was completely cured of his cancer. He continued the diet, and was still cancer-free at a follow up 3 years later.

Other stories can be found in such books as *Healing Miracles from Macrobiotics* by Dr J. Kohler; *The Cancer Prevention Diet* by M. Kushi; *Macrobiotic Miracle: How a Vermont Family Overcame Cancer* by V Brown and S Stayman; *Recovery from Cancer* by E. Nussbaum; *Physician, Heal Thyself* by H. Faulkner; and *Cancer-Free: 30 Who Triumphed Over Cancer Naturally* by The East West Foundation with A. Fawcett and C. Smith. [1-6]

The stories of both Sattilaro and Kohler describe an initial period in which all animal products and fruit were avoided, with their reintroduction at a later period.

A retrospective study found that cancer patients who followed a macrobiotic diet had longer survival times and better quality of life than would be expected statistically.

Study subjects were 101 patients with pancreatic cancer who had sought advice about macrobiotics from a certified counselor during a 4 year time period. Of the 101 subjects, researchers successfully contacted 28 of them, or their next of kin. In 23/28 cases, a macrobiotic diet had been followed for at least 3 months. Median survival time of these 23 was 13 months after initial diagnosis, compared to 3 months for pancreatic cancer patients enrolled in the NCI Surveillance, Epidemiology, and End Results (SEER) program.

Also, 9 patients with prostate cancer who followed a macrobiotic diet had a median survival time of 228 months, compared to 72 months in matched control subjects.[7]

References

(1) Kohler JC, Kohler MA. Healing miracles from macrobiotics: a diet for all diseases. West Nyack (NY): Parker Publishing; 1979.

(2) Kushi M, Jack A. The cancer prevention diet: Michio Kushi's nutritional blue print for the prevention and relief of disease. New York: St Martin's Press; 1993.

(3) Brown V. Macrobiotic miracle: how a Vermont family overcame cancer. Tokyo: Japan Publications; 1984.

(4) Faulkner H. Physician, heal thyself. Becket. (MA): One Peaceful World Press; 1993.

(5) Nussbaum E. Recovery from cancer. Garden City Park (NY):Avery Publishing Group; 1992.

(6) East West Foundation, Fawcett A, Smith C, Kushi M. Cancer-free: 30 who triumphed over cancer naturally. New York: Japan Publications; 1992.)

(7) Carter JP, Saxe GP, Newbold V, Peres CE, Campeau RJ, Bernal-Green L., Hypothesis: dietary management may improve survival from nutritionally linked cancers based on analysis of representative cases." J Am Coll Nutr 1993 Jun;12(3):209-26).

Mediterranean Diet

This diet follows the traditional eating habits of the mediterranean region, such as Spain. The diet is plant-based, with legumes, nuts, grains and fish, little red meat, and the sparing use of olive oil. It is relatively low in fat, especially saturated fat. Most of the fat in this diet is olive oil, or omega-3 fat from plants or fish.

It is associated with a lower risk of developing cancer, especially breast cancer. However, there are no studies claiming it cures existing cancer.

Nutritional Typing

The following dietary recommendations come from William Kelley, a dentist who was one of the inventors of nutritional typing, and Nick Gonzalez, an alternative physician who studied Kelley's research. Kelley discovered that different cancers responded best to different diets.

Solid tumors, such as those of the breast, colon, liver, lungs, pancreas, prostate, stomach, uterus and ovaries, responded best to a largely vegetarian diet. Immune system cancers such as leukemia, lymphoma, myeloma, or sarcoma (a connective tissue cancer related to immune cancer) tended to do better on a diet high in fat and meat.

Within these two broad groups, there were many variations; the recommended vegetarian diets ranged from 80% raw to 80% cooked ingredients. In his non-vegetarian diets, some had minimal animal protein, others contained fish, some also featured red meat.

Paleolithic Diet

The African explorer, Dr. David Livingstone, suggested that cancer is a "disease of civilization." Similarly, the "Rule of 20 years" was formulated by Thomas L. Cleave, a surgeon captain who observed a consistent pattern of negative health effects caused by consumption of refined carbohydrates such as white sugar and flour. Cleave studied primitive cultures and observed that they were free of diseases such as heart disease, high blood pressure and diabetes until about 20 years after their societies were introduced to refined starches.

Keeping this in mind, the paleolithic diet attempts to thwart cancer by turning back to the "natural" human diet.

The Paleolithic diet was developed in the mid-1970s by Dr. Walter L. Voegtlin, a gastroenterologist who wrote "The Stone Age Diet."

The concept is based on the idea that humans would be healthier if they followed the eating habits of their stone-age ancestors in the Paleolithic era, approximately 2.5 million years ago, before the existence of modern agriculture.

The diet features free-range meats and eggs, wild fish, nuts, and organic fruits and vegetables, cooked as minimally as possible. Grains and legumes, being products of agriculture, are excluded from the diet, as are sugar, dairy and refined flour.

While it is true that primitive peoples do not display the chronic health problems of modern civilized man, there are many factors behind this besides diet. First of all, they exercised daily in order to survive. Females reached menarche later, and had several offspring starting at a young age due to the lack of birth control, leading to lower estrogen levels. They lived in an unpolluted environment.

The animals eaten by stone-age humans were wild and free-range, not corn-fed, with a lower percentage and different chemical composition of body fat. Available fruits were not the swollen, high-sugar hybrids found in the modern supermarket, but rather small, fibrous, tart in flavor and full of phytochemicals. Vegetables and fruits were plucked from the natural environment, not cultivated in mineral-depleted soils. Refined flour, sugar and oils did not exist. Cigarettes and alcohol were unknown.

All these lifesyle and dietary factors contributed to a lower risk for cancer.

It is extremely difficult to recreate all these conditions and find matching products in the local supermarket. However, it may be said that any diet that leaves out refined flour and sugar is a large step in the right direction, as these 2 components of the modern diet are most closely linked to the development of degenerative diseases. Dairy consumption has also been linked to cancer.

So far, there are no clinical studies using the paleolithic diet as a cancer cure, though if history is any indication, it will at least have preventative value.

13. Frequency-Based Technology

This category of cancer treatment covers a range of devices such as those by Royal Rife, Hulda Clark, Bob Beck, and the Resonant Light Generator.

There is increasing evidence that cancer is caused by parasites or viruses.
Early researchers such as Royal Rife, Virginia Livingstone, and Hulda Clark pioneered the idea that cancer is caused by microorganisms, and some even claimed to have seen and identified them. The most likely suspect seems to be a pleomorphic nano-bacterium, but others have been identified as well.

Theoretically, eliminating the causative microbe will cure the resultant cancer. Limited success has been achieved using antibiotics against cancer-causing microbes, perhaps due to antibiotic resistance, and the fact that many are viruses which are not susceptible to any antibiotics.

The earliest frequency technology predates all modern antibiotics. One way to cure cancer is to destroy these infectious agents responsible for causing it, which these machines claim to do through targeting their cellular frequency.

Every living organism has a certain frequency, and interrupting this frequency can kill the organism, just as an opera singer can shatter glass with the voice through resonance. Royal Rife referred to this frequency as the "Mortal Oscillatory Rate" of an organism.

According to the manufacturers of these devices, the frequencies produced devitalize microorganisms linked to the development of cancer, while leaving normal tissue unaffected.

Of course, this technology also targets bacteria and viruses associated with ordinary infectious diseases. The Beck machine was initially developed as an electomagnetic treatment for HIV/AIDS, before it was found to be useful for cancer as well.

The theory that frequencies could destroy microbes was originated by Royal Rife in the 1930s. He used frequencies specifically targeted to each species of microbe.

A modern example of the bacteriocidal properties of electricity was provided in 1990 by Dr. Stephen Kaali and Dr. Willain Lyman. They discovered that a small electric current prevented viruses from being able to enter cells and multiply, thus rendering them harmless. A current flow in the range of 50-100 microamperes (uA) produced the best results against the HIV virus. Their in-vitro studies culminated in a patent for an implantable blood electrification device intended for the treatment of HIV/AIDS (patent #5,139,684 issued on August 18, 1992).

Other studies have shown the effectiveness of small amounts of electricity against bacteria and fungus.

Most practitioners who promote these machines recommend that they be used regularly for 2-3 months for effects to be seen. The main problem would seem to be how far the frequency or current would penetrate living tissue. However, with constant use against an arterial location, such as the radial artery at the wrist, all the blood in the body could be exposed to the frequency and at the very least the blood would be cleared of pathogens, considerably lightening the load on the body's immune system.

While Royal Rife had documented successful clinical trials of his device, his original machine and the exact plans for it were destroyed. Many versions of frequency-based machines based on Rife's general research have been built by others, but one cannot be sure they have the precise same frequency output or effectiveness. The machines mentioned here all have testimonials supporting them.

This is not secretive, proprietary multi-million-dollar technology. The scientific theory behind it is easy to understand. Anyone with training in electronics can build these machines for relatively little money, since the specifications and plans are easy to find on the Internet. However, most patients will probably find it easier (and safer, considering the risk of electric shock from poorly assembled electronic devices) to buy them ready-made from reputable suppliers.

Caution

Use of machines generating electric currents should be strictly avoided by patients with pacemakers.

Dr Royal Rife

Dr. Royal Raymond Rife invented the original "Rife Machine," a frequency generator used to cure terminally ill cancer patients through selective electronic frequency treatment programs.

Royal Raymond Rife (1888-1971) was born in Elkhorn, Nebraska. After studying bacteriology at Johns Hopkins University, Rife invented technology still currently used in the fields of electronics, optics, radiochemistry, ballistics, biochemistry, and aviation. Rife was the pioneer of bioelectric medicine.

Rife received an honorary Doctorate by the University of Heidelberg for his work, and was given 14 major awards and honors for his research. For a time, he worked in Germany with Carl Zeiss, of Zeiss Optics.

Rife's inventions include a heterodyning ultraviolet microscope, a Rife frequency machine, a micromanipulator and micro-dissector. He was a versatile and gifted scientist, and when he needed an instrument for his research that was unavailable, he would invent it.

By 1920, Rife had finished building the world's first microscope using monochromatic light with resolution so fine it was capable of viewing living viruses. By 1933, his work on this technology culminated in the Rife Universal Microscope, an instrument with nearly 6,000 different components and a magnification factor of 60,000. Using his incredible invention, Rife became the first person to see a living virus.

Rife's microscope functioned by focusing 2 different waves of the same ultraviolet light frequency, producing interference where the waves merged. This interference created in effect a third, longer wave falling within the visible electromagnetic spectrum. This technique, called "heterodyning", was widely used in early radio broadcasting.

The correct frequency of light was determined by viewing the microbe to be examined with a slit spectroscope attachment. Block quartz prisms were rotated until the wavelength created matched the frequency of the organism being studied, at which point it would come into view. Each type of microorganism had a unique frequency specific to its species.

This allowed Rife to visualize microbes without killing them, a feat which modern electron microscopes could not duplicate, as these machines only view dead microbes. Rife observed microbes actively invading live tissues, and also changing form as they went through their life cycle.

Until very recently, the Universal Microscope was the only microscope capable of viewing live viruses. The University of

Manchester announced in 2011 the invention of a "nanoscope" using ordinary white light focused by tiny 'microspheres' (small spherical particles). It can visualize items as small as 50 nanometers in size, resolution 20 times as good as standard light microscopes. Finally, today's scientists are catching up to Rife's work, done 80 years ago.

In 1920, Royal Rife identified a virus he felt was linked to cancer. To prove his theory that viral infection could initiate cancer, Rife made thousands of unsuccessful attempts to transform normal cells into cancer cells. He finally succeeded in isolating a strain of virus, which he named *Cryptocides primordiale*, that consistently produced tumors in animal test subjects.

Rife not only used specific frequencies to visualize microorganisms, but also to kill them. By increasing the intensity of the frequency which resonated with each species of microbes, Rife exaggerated their natural oscillations until their structural integrity was destroyed and they died. Rife called this frequency, which was harmless to other tissues, the "mortal oscillatory rate," or "MOR" of microbes.

Rife spent years testing which frequencies could be used to destroy common species of pathogenic organisms including polio, herpes, spinal meningitis, influenza and tetanus. These experiments were using the Rife Microscope in conjunction with the Rife Frequency Machine.

In 1934, the University of Southern California created a Special Medical Research Committee to bring end-stage cancer patients from Pasadena County Hospital to Rife's San Diego Laboratory and clinic for experimental treatment with Rife's frequency generator. The researchers included pathologists and doctors who were to examine these terminal patients 90 days after treatment with Rife's equipment.

After the 90 days of treatment, the Committee found that 86.5% of the patients had been completely cured. The remaining 13.5% of the patients were cured within the next month. Rife's technology produced a cure rate of 100%.

In 1934 at the Scripps Institute in La Jolla, California, Rife performed clinical trials on 16 terminally ill cancer patients, curing all of them.

Rife's work was funded by some private trusts, and he had little experience with the medical establishment and its tactics. He was slandered and harassed by the AMA, and scientists who supported his work were either bribed to abandon him, or else died in mysterious circumstances.

In 1932, Dr. Arthur Kendall, director of Medical Research at Northwestern University, made a speech to the Association of American Physicians at Johns Hopkins University about Rife's success in treating cancer. Dr. Thomas Rivers, a microbiologist who was director of the Rockefeller Institute (a primary source of funding for medical research) and Dr. Hans Zinsser, denounced Kendall to the audience as a fraud.

In 1939 a frivolous lawsuit was filed by Philip Hoyland, an agent of pharmaceutical companies, against the Beam Ray Corporation, the only company manufacturing Rife's frequency instruments. Hoyland lost the lawsuit, but legal bills bankrupted the company, and production of Rife's equipment ceased. Hoyland admitted to accepting a $10,000 bribe from Hahn Realty Group, agents of the AMA, to sue Beam Ray.

The multi-million dollar Burnett Lab in New Jersey was destroyed by arson, just before its scientists could announce public confirmation of Rife's theories. Unknown vandals destroyed Rife's precious virus microscopes and stole some of the parts. Finally, police conducted an illegal raid of Rife's lab and confiscated 50 years of research.

In 1971, Royal Rife died in povery, his amazing discoveries largely suppressed by the medical establishment and forgotten by the public. Fortunately, a handful of humanitarian doctors and engineers reconstructed the frequency instruments invented by this genius.

Today's newer 'Rife' technology uses a variety of frequency

generators to target cancer-causing organisms through the use of hand-held, footplate, or applied electrodes. Proper frequency exposure for sufficient time is essential to success.

Suppliers

You can buy a Rife Generator for $1725 by typing in your browser:

"Rife generator notarized testimonials"

http://www.frequencyrising.com/rifemachine_testimonials.htm

Hulda Clark – The Zapper

Dr. Hulda Regehr Clark was born on October 18th, 1928 in Rosthern, Saskatchewan, Canada.

She initially studied at the University of Saskatchewan, Canada, where she received a Bachelor of Arts degree in 1950, Magna Cum Laude. Dr. Clark also earned a Master of Arts degree, with High Honors from the University of Saskatchewan.

After two years of study at McGill University, she attended the University of Minnesota where she was awarded a Doctorate degree in 1958, with a major in zoology and a minor in botany. Dr. Clark operated a nutritional consulting practice in the late 1960's in additon to her work as a university researcher at the University of Indiana. In 1974, after Federal research funds were eliminated, she worked as a nutritional consultant on a full time basis. She received a degree in naturopathy from the Clayton College of Natural Health. She specialized in private research of all human illness, especially cancer.

Her search for the basic cause of cancer led her to focus on a combination of factors, from microorganisms and parasites, to heavy metals, solvents and radioactivity. She came up with many solutions to cleanse the human body of these invaders, including the use of herbs, essential oils, orthomolecular therapy and frequency therapy. She stressed the importance of dental health, as well as awareness of environmental pollution.

Her most important discovery was a frequency generator called the "zapper", a hand-held, battery operated, multi-frequency generator built by her son in 1994. Initially, the device was intended to kill intestinal flukes, but it was found to kill all pathogens.

Like many alternative practitioners, Hulda Clark was prosecuted by the FDA, and she was forced to move her practice from America to Mexico.
Her clinic was the subject of continual controversy, due to issues of cleanliness of her premises, cost of her treatments, and her embrace of unorthodox practices (even by the standards of alternative medicine) such as treatment for "oral cavitation".

Some patients gave satisfied testimonials of cancer cures, others complained bitterly of high expenses coupled with lack of results.

Hulda Clark died at the age of 80 due to complications of multiple myeloma, a type of bone marrow cancer, according to a copy of her death certificate posted online. Ironically, the longtime cancer researcher could not cure herself.

Caution

There have been no clinical trials of the zapper. However, zappers do not interfere with chemo, radiation and surgery. There is some compelling evidence on the web pertaining to the efficiency of the zapper, and many positive testimonials. Do your own research.

Our suggestion is to buy the Zapper, since it is very economical and has no side effects, but use it only as an adjunct to other treatment.

Instructions

Use the zapper once a day.

Suppliers

Ebay or other websites.

Bob Beck Protocol

The late Dr. Robert Beck, who died in 2002, had a PhD in physics and taught at the University of Southern California. He was inspired by the research of Lyman and Kaali to produce his own blood electrification machine. He initially designed the machine to treat HIV/AIDS, but many cancer patients use the machine as well, as it targets a wide range of microorganisms.

Beck found that the direct application of electricity to the skin produced cell damage, so he modified his device to use a low-voltage AC current that avoided this problem.

The Beck machine, also called the "Beck Zapper," generates a bi-phasic square wave, meaning that the waveform voltage has a positive half and a negative half, with the current reversing direction each half cycle. Square waves produce a large number of harmonics, which are multiples of the original frequency. Odd harmonics are multiples of the original frequency by odd numbers such as 3, 5, 7, while even harmonics are multiples of 2. For example, the odd harmonics of a 4 Hertz (Hz) square wave would be 12 Hz, 20 Hz, 28 Hz, and upward into the radio frequency range.
Beck reccommended the application of his electrodes to the arteries in the wrist. He invented the "Beck Protocol," which also involves use of a magnetic field pulser, colloidial silver, and the consumption

of ozonated water and an alkaline diet to augment the results of blood electrification.

The magnetic field pulser was added to the regime because Dr. Beck found that AIDS viruses embedded in deep tissues such as bone marrow were unaffected by blood electrification. The magnetic pulser contains a large induction coil that emits a strong magnetic field automatically once every 3 seconds. The shape and polarity of this magnetic spike has the same effect on microorganisms as the electric current.

Use of Equipment

Do not use the blood electrification machine and the magnetic pulser at the same time, as the blood electrifier will be damaged. Use the magnetic pulser first, to break up colonies of microbes living in deep tissues, then use the electrifier 15 to 30 minutes later to deactivate them in the blood. Take the colloidial silver 15 minutes after completing these 2 treatments. Drink copious amounts of water, preferably ozonated water, throughout the treatment period.

Caution

This device is not recommended for use during radiation or chemotherapy, or concurrent with the use of any potentially toxic drugs. One reason for this is that the body has to eliminate the remains of killed microorganisms, and adding the burden of toxic drugs may overload the liver and kidneys. Also, the machine may increase the cellular absorption and effects of drugs.

While using the Beck machine, strictly avoid strong prescription drugs, strong over-the counter medication such as aspirin or Tylenol, vitamins (especially vitamin A), enzymes, garlic, seasoning herbs (many have medicinal effects), smoking, recreational drugs, and alcohol. *Not for use by patients with pacemakers or pregnant women.*

Beck zappers can be purchased for approximately $70-$300, magnetic field pulsers for approximately $300-$350.

Two reputable vendors are Sota Instruments and BioElectric. Their machines have different instructions for use. According to some alternative practitioners, the Sota is closer to the original specifications than the BioElectric. Bioelectric describes their unit as having improvements over the original.

http://educate-yourself.org/be/beckdevicesdesc.shtml

Resonant Light Generator

According to the Canadian manufacturer of this machine, "Sound is actually slow-moving light. Light, inversely, is fast-moving sound. The resultant configuration of integrating the two is known as "resonant light", and when the meld of these two is done correctly, a signal is created that can target and destroy pathogenic microorganisms. This integration along with RF (radio frequency) gave birth to a piece of equipment known as a photon emission resonant light device: the Phorle™."

The manufacturer's website credits Royal Rife as being the inspiration for their design. This machine changes targeted audio frequencies into a modulated radiofrequency (RF) signal. This RF signal is then processed, via a tuning circuit, through an Argon-gas-filled glass tube, creating a plasma wave. This plasma wave emits a specific output of sound, light, and RF energy. Energy frequencies produced a range from 1HZ to 999,999Hz, accurate within .001Hz.

The Canadian Resonant light generator website has glowing reviews from users. Fourteen of these devices were bought by a British anti-cancer organization because they were so effective in the treatment of childhood cancer. Kids Integrated Cancer Treatment is a UK nonprofit organisation dedicated to providing support to families with children who are fighting cancer and other serious diseases.

Supplier

Not cheap, at $5600 each

http://www.resonantlight.com

14. Clinic Treatments

Acupuncture

Acupuncture is a medical procedure in which needles are stuck into the body in various places, and sometimes connected to electricity, sound waves or some other technique in order to cure health problems.

Practitioners of acupuncture say that its goal is to keep the "chi" or life force in the body flowing properly.

The overall opinion of most traditional medical health organizations is that acupuncture does not do anything to fight cancer, although it may help to reduce the pain and nausea involved with cancer and the traditional treatments used against cancer.

There are, however, non-traditional medical health organizations which claim that acupuncture can not only be effective in minimizing symptoms, but that it can cure cancer in cases in which traditional methods have been ineffective. There are anecdotal reports of cancer patients who claim to have been completely cured by acupuncture.

If you decide to make use of acupuncture, make a careful study of the clinics and practitioners offering this service. You will want to make sure that the treatment is being offered by someone who is considered a professional in the field. Do your own research and don't be afraid to ask questions.

Acupuncture does not interfere with conventional cancer therapy. You might want to make use of traditional chemotherapy and/or radiation therapies to fight the cancer, and use acupuncture to fight the nausea and pain involved.

Prices for acupuncture treatments vary.

Hyperthermia

Hyperthermia is an ancient healing technique for a variety of diseases. Ancient Greeks, Romans, and Egyptians used heat to treat breast masses, and traditional healers in ancient India employed regional and whole-body hyperthermia.[1] Native Americans had sweat lodges which were used for both medicinal and ceremonial purposes.

Hyperthermia, either full-body or localized, is one of the oldest therapies against cancer. It has long been noticed that "spontaneous" remissions of cancer occurred after high fevers. The Issels clinic in Germany has used this mode of treatment for decades in conjunction with other therapies.

During the first half of the 20th century, numerous theories regarding the underlying causes of cancer were postulated. Many such theories originated from incidental laboratory findings or from interesting single-patient case presentations. However, many of these early cancer hypotheses seemed to contradict each other, even though many theories had an underlying factual basis.

Early on, proponents of many different cancer therapies abounded. While Virginia Livingston was developing her theory on *cancer-causing bacteria*, William Coley was developing an interest for the potential existence of *cancer-treating bacteria*.

Initially trained as an orthopedic surgeon, Dr. Coley later developed an interest in cancer therapy, specifically targeting bone cancers, such as deadly osteosarcoma. His role in pioneering the field of cancer immunotherapy has had a marked impact on current understanding of cancer immunology; however, some of his findings also established a link between hyperthermia and improved cancer survival.

Dr. Coley had come across a case report of a patient with osteosarcoma achieving full remission after an episode of erysipelas, which is a type of bacterial skin infection caused by a *streptococcus* species.

Subsequent attempts to expose cancer patients to the infectious agent, and therefore erysipelas, appeared to produce a cure or prolonged remission in some patients, which, at the time, was considered quite successful. Dr. Coley initially theorized that the bacterium itself was the agent causing the cancer to regress.

However, further research revealed that the actual mediators of cancer regression were several inflammatory cytokines produced in response to the pathogen, many of which induce a febrile response.

The role of fever in humans is still poorly understood, and its necessity questioned. However, it is known that, in many animals, such as laboratory rats, exposure to pathogenic bacteria will result in an immediate febrile response. Furthermore, if the rats are prevented from producing such febrile response, their survival rate and ability to fight the infection is significantly decreased.

Because the ability to increase core body temperature in response to an infection seems evolutionarily conserved throughout the Animal Kingdom, febrile reactions appear to play an important role in survival. Specifically, it is thought that the elevated temperature characteristic of a fever can enhance immune system function to combat both bacterial and oncological threats.

Interest in elevated cellular temperature as a possible cancer therapy gained momentum in the 1970's as laboratory evidence showed cancer cells to be more vulnerable to heat-mediated cellular injury and death than their normal counterparts.

However, early attempts to introduce hyperthermia therapies *in vivo* faced significant challenges, such as how to deliver a consistent target temperature to a well-defined target tissue. In spite of many roadblocks, early uses of thermal energy applied to superficial cancers produced encouraging evidence.

Today, current technology allows for more predictable heating patterns as well as improved safety and monitoring in this specific form of cancer treatment.

How exactly does heat target cancer cells? The exact mechanism is not fully understood. However, we do know that all human cells are potentially vulnerable when exposed to increased cellular temperatures.

Some researchers say that cancerous cells are not inherently more sensitive to the effects of heat, and that *in vitro,* normal cells and cancer cells show the same responses to heat. However, the vascular disorganization of solid tumors creates an unfavorable microenvironment of low oxygen, higher concentration of acid (low pH), and insufficient nutrients, giving normal cells greater tolerance to heat stress.[2,3]

Temperature elevations can induce changes in the shape of cellular proteins, potentially causing irreversible loss of function as well as the initiation of cellular suicide pathways.

Furthermore, elevated cellular temperatures also place the cellular DNA at risk of injury, which can lead to activation of cellular death. In response to even mildly elevated temperatures (>39.5°C), healthy cells produce Heat Shock Proteins (HSPs), which act to shield the cell from potential thermal energy-induced injury.

HSPs allow normal cells to function at higher temperatures by maintaining protein shape & function.

Fortunately, cancer cells usually cannot adapt well to elevated temperatures. The cancer cells within a large tumor that are the toughest to kill with conventional therapies also happen to be the most susceptible to hyperthermia. These cells are usually located at the center of large tumors, where blood, oxygen, and nutrient supplies are limited. These cells are thus less able to utilize resources towards the production of HSPs, and therefore less capable of protecting themselves against applied heat.

Hyperthermia can thus preferentially target cancer cells to a greater extent than normal healthy cells. Increased temperatures can also increase the blood supply to some portions of the tumor, which will help target cancer cells through standard therapy. Oxygenated areas of tumors are much more susceptible to chemotherapy and radiation and therefore are more easily eradicated.

Other potential mechanisms of hyperthermia-mediated cancer destruction seem to result from enhancement of the immune system due to elevated body temperatures.

Tumors rely on stealth to evade the host's immune system. Hyperthermia-induced cellular damage appears to also induce the expression of specific cellular proteins unique to cancer cells, making them more easily detectable by the immune system. Hyperthermia also enhances the ability of immune cells to travel to cancer sites as well as their overall killing potential.

Hyperthermia has been tested in Phase III cancer clinical trials and has shown significant success against many forms of cancer. Often, hyperthermia is provided along with some form of radiation and/or chemotherapy. It is usually used as an adjunct to other therapies, not as a cure in and of itself.

Hyperthermia can be combined with gene therapy such as heat shock protein 70 promoter.

When combined with radiation, hyperthermia is particularly effective at increasing the damage to acidic, hypoxic areas of a tumor.

Hyperthermia induces biochemical pathways causing increased sensitivity of cancer cells to radiotherapy.[4]

It is selectively toxic to dividing cells, and is most effective when applied at the same time, or within an hour, of radiotherapy.[5]

Research is being conducted to improve delivery methods for hyperthermia. Challenges related to hyperthermia relate to preferentially heating cancerous tissue while maintaining the surrounding tissue at temperatures below 42 degrees celsius, and avoiding "hot spots" of overheated tissues. Over the past 2 decades, technologies for hyperthermia have included direct application of heat, radiofrequency, microwave and ultrasound energy. Ultrasound is the most frequently used technology, with both direct, single-beam as well as multiple focused beams being employed.[6]

The use of delivery systems, such as vests, allows for a more customized approach in this new type of cancer therapy. Furthermore, MRI-based thermal maps can now be obtained, which accurately depict both the tumor areas and the relative tissue temperatures. Ultimately, these features ensure that a consistent temperature can be delivered for more consistent results.

Studies

Dozens of successful clinical trials have been performed using hyperthermia as an adjunct treatment.

Five randomized clinical trials of hyperthermia were performed between 1988 and 1991. Patients had advanced primary or recurrent breast cancer, treated with local radiotherapy in preference to surgery. The overall response rate for radiotherapy alone was 41%, compared to 59% for the combined treatment.[7] Multiple studies exist showing successful use of hyperthermia to treat breast cancer.[8,9,10]

A meta-analysis of 4 randomized phase III clinical trials using radiotherapy alone or combined with hyperthermia to treat patients with chest-wall recurrence of breast cancer found a response rate of 41% and 61% respectively. Overall complete response rate for hyperthermia and radiation was 61% compared to 41% for radiation alone. Thermal dose correlated with tumor response, and subsequently with time to local recurrence and overall survival time.[11]

Radiotherapy plus hyperthermia was compared to radiotherapy alone in the Dutch Deep Hyperthermia Trial, a randomized, prospective study involving patients with advanced bladder, cervical, and rectal cancer. The 3-year survival rates were 27% for patients receiving radiotherapy alone, compared to 51% for those receiving radiotherapy and hyperthermia, according to a report published in April 2000 in *The Lancet*. [12]

Hyperthermia was found to be especially effective in treating cervical cancer. The Dutch Deep Hyperthermia Trial documented a 51% vs. 31% 3-year survival rate of 114 patients from 1990 – 1996 with locally advanced cervical cancer treated with hyperthermia plus radiation compared to those treated with radiation alone. The researchers concluded, "Hyperthermia in addition to standard radiotherapy of locally advanced cervical tumours results in therapeutic gain and is cost-effective." [13]

According to a follow up study, the 12-year survival rate of the two groups of patients was 20% vs. 37%. [14]

A randomized study of glioblastoma patients who received brachytherapy (a form of radiotherapy involving placement of radioisotopes directly at the site of a tumor) with or without interstitial hyperthermia treatment showed an impressive doubling of 2-year survival rates from 15% to 31%. [15]

In another study of 36 patients with stage III and IV gliomas, low-radiofrequency deep hyperthermia produced partial remission or retardation of tumor growth. [16]

Irradiation alone produces a complete response in approximately 30% of cancer patients. Combining irradiation and hyperthermia increases the complete response rate to roughly 70%. [17]

Dr. James Bicher of the Bicher Cancer Institute in Los Angeles specializes in the use of hyperthermia. In one study, he used hyperthermia combined with fractionated low-dose radiotherapy to treat patients with early stage cancers, stage IIIA or less, of the breast (40 patients), head and neck (17), and prostate (15) who had refused conventional radiotherapy, surgery or chemotherapy.

Therapy was fractionated and hyperthermia to the tumor and areas of lymph node spread was given along with every radiation treatment, one hour each day, 5 days per week for 16-20 weeks. Progressively decreasing daily doses of radiation therapy were used, and the total radiation dose was 15-25% less than that of conventional radiotherapy

Dr. Bicher claimed complete response rates were 82% for cancer of the breast, 88% for head and neck, and 93% for prostate. Projected 5 year survival rates were 80% for breast patients, 88% for head and neck, and 87% for prostate patients. Side effects of the combination therapy were less than for radiotherapy alone.[18]

A 1986 study also by Dr. Bicher of 256 patients with various tumors also treated by multifraction hyperthermia and radiation therapy found an overall response rate of 94%, and a 62% complete response.[19]

Dr. Bicher has published a detailed description of the clinic's treatment program, along with numerous research papers.[20-27]

Hyperthermia (especially in combination with radiotherapy) has been used so extensively for decades, and is so well-documented in clinical settings, that it is more accurately described as a lesser-known conventional cancer treatment than as a form of alternative medicine.[28-45]

It has been used effectively to treat head and neck tumors, which are extremely difficult to treat surgically and are usually unresponsive to chemotherapy.[46-48]

It has been used to treat melanoma,[49] sarcoma,[50] cervical[51] and prostate cancer.[52,53,54]

In alternative medicine, whole-body hyperthermia or local hyperthermia has been combined with infusion therapies (Vitamin C, laetrile or oxygen) or insulin potentiation therapy and low-dose chemotherapy.[55]

Clinics

Hyperthermia clinics operating in the United States charge around $15,000 to $20,000 for a series of treatments. The Bicher Clinic is one of the oldest.

http://www.bichercancerinstitute.com/

The best hyperthermia clinics are in Germany, especially well known is the Issels Clinic. It is rumored that at least 2 presidents, including Ronald Reagan, were cured of cancer in Germany using hyperthermia.

Home Treatments

The Biomat is a hyperthermia vest for home use, priced at $550 to $2300.
It produces deeply-penetrating far infrared ray therapy.

http://www.biomat.com

References

(1) Gian F. Baronzio (2006). "Introduction". Hyperthermia In Cancer Treatment: A Primer (Medical Intelligence Unit). Berlin: Springer.

(2) Freeman Carolyn, Halperin Edward C, Brady, Luther W, Wazer David E., Perez and Brady's Principles and Practice of Radiation Oncology. 2008 Philadelphia: Wolters Kluwer Health/Lippincott Williams & Wilkins. pp. 637–644

(3) Gerweck LE. "Modifiers of thermal effects: Environmental factors." In Urano M. Douple E, eds: Hyperthermia and Oncology, p 83 The Netherlands, VSP BV Publishers, 1988.

(4) Punit Kaur, et al., "Combined Hyperthermia and Radiotherapy for the Treatment of Cancer." Cancers 2011, 3(4), 3799-3823

(5) Dollinger, Malin (2008). Everyone's Guide to Cancer Therapy; Revised 5th Edition: How Cancer Is Diagnosed, Treated, and Managed Day to Day. Kansas City, MO: Andrews McMeel Publishing. pp. 98–100.

(6) Mark Converse, , Essex J. Bond, Susan C. Hagness, Barry D. Van Veen, "Ultrawide-Band Microwave Space–Time Beamforming for Hyperthermia Treatment of Breast Cancer: A Computational Feasibility Study," IEEE

(7) Vernon CC et al. "Radiotherapy with or without hyperthermia in the treatment of superficial localized breast cancer: results from five randomized controlled trials." International Collaborative Hyperthermia Group. Int J Radiat Oncol Biol Phys 1996 Jul 1;35(4):731-44.

(8) Welzm S, Hehr T, Lamprecht v, Schesthauer H, Budach W, Bamburg M. "Thermoradiotherapy of the chest wall in locally advanced or recurrent breast cancer with marginal resection." Int. J. Hyperthermia, 2005; 21:159-167.

(9) Welz S, Hehr T, Lamprecht V, Scheithauer H, Budach W, Bamberg M. "Thermoradiotherapy of the chest wall in locally advanced or recurrent breast cancer with marginal resection." Int J Hyperthermia 2005; 21 (2): 159-167

(10) Perez CA, Kuske RR, Emerni B. "Irradiation alone or combined with hyperthermia in the treatment of recurrent carcinoma of the breast in the chest wall." Int J Hyperthermia 1985; 2:179-185.

(11) Sherer M et al. "Relationship between thermal dose and outcome in thermoradiotherapy treatments for superficial recurrences of breast cancer: data from a phase III trial." Int J Radiat Oncol Biol Phys 1997 Sep 1;39(2):371-80.

(12) Van der Zee J et al., "Comparison of radiotherapy alone with radiotherapy plus hyperthermia in locally advanced pelvic tumours: a prospective, randomised, multicentre trial." Dutch Deep Hyperthermia Group. Lancet 2000 Apr 1;355(9210):1119-25.

(13) Van der Zee J, Gonzalez GD, "The Dutch Deep Hyperthermia Trial: results in cervical cancer." Int J Hyperthermia 2002 Jan-Feb;18(1):1-12.

(14) Franckena Martine et al., "Long-Term Improvement in Treatment Outcome After Radiotherapy and Hyperthermia in Locoregionally Advanced Cervix Cancer: An Update of the Dutch Deep Hyperthermia Trial." International Journal of Radiation Biology Oncology Physics Volume 70 (4) Elsevier – Mar 15, 2008

(15) Sneed PK, Stauffer PR, McDermott MW, Diederich CJ, Lamborn KR, Prados MD, Chang S, Weaver KA, Spry L, Malec MK, Lamb SA, Voss B, Davis RL, Wara WM, Larson DA, Phillips TL, Gutin PH. "Survival benefit of hyperthermia in a prospective randomized trial of brachytherapy boost +/- hyperthermia for glioblastoma multiforme." Int J Radiat Oncol Biol Phys. 1998 Jan 15;40(2):287-95

(16) Hager ED, Dziambor H, App EM, Popa C, Popa O, Hertlein M. "The treatment of patients with high-grade malignant gliomas with RF hyperthermia." Proc ASCO 2003; 22:118, #470, Proc Am Soc Clin Oncol 22: 2003

(17) Perez, C.A.; Emami, B.N.; Nussbaum, G.; Sapareto, S. "Hyperthermia". In Perez, C.A.; Brady, L.W.. Principles and practice of radiation oncology. 15. p. 342.

(18) Bicher HI, Al-Bussam N. "Thermoradiotherapy with curative intent — Breast, head, neck and prostate tumors". Deutsche Zeitschrift für Onkologie 2006 38 (3): 116–122

(19) Bicher HI, Wolfstein RS, Lewinsky BS. "Microwave hyperthermia as an adjunct to radiation therapy: Summary experience of 256 multifraction treatment cases." Int J. Radiat Oncol Biol Phys 1986;12:1667-1671.

(20) Bicher HI, Sandhu TS, Hetzel FW. "Hyperthermia and radiation in combination: A clinical fractionation regimen." Int J. Radiat Oncol Bio: Phys 1980; 6:867-870.

(21) Bicher HI, Mitagvaria N. "Circulatory responses of malignant tumors during hyperthermia." Microvascular Research 1981; 21:19-26.

(22) Bicher HI, Hetzel FW, Vaupel P, Sandhu TS. "Microcirculation modification by localized microwave hyperthermia and hematoporhyrin phototherapy." Bibl Anat 1981:20:628-632.

(23) Bicher HI, Mitagvaria NP. "Changes in tumor tissue oxygenation during microwave hyperthermia clinical relevance." Advances in Experimental Medicine and Biology, 1985 180: 190-905.

(24) Bicher HI, Wolfstein RS, Chatham PL. "Hyperthermic adjunct treatment for specific sites: nasopharynx, pancreas, liver, chest and pelvis. Preliminary experience." Int J. Hyperthermia 1987; 3:551 (Abstract).

(25) Bicher HI, Wolfstein RS. "Clinical use of regional hyperthermia." Adv in Exp Med and Biol. 1990; 267: 1- 20.

(26) Bicher HI, Wolfstein RS. "Local hyperthermia for superficial and moderately deep tumors. Factors affecting response." Adv in Exp Med and Biol 1990; 267: 353-367.

(27) Bicher HI. "Thermoradiotherapy treatment of malignant tumors. Fractionation regimen and objective and points. An update." Proceedings of the XXVI

490

ICHS (International Clinical Hyperthermia Society) Meeting, Shenzhen, China, September 10th-12th, 2004.

(28) Warren SL (1935). "Preliminary study of the effect of artificial fever upon hopeless tumor cases". Am J Roentgenol 33: 75.

(29) Dewey WC, Hopwood LE, Sappareti S. "Cellular responses to combinations of hyperthermia and radiation." Radiology 1977;123:463-475.

(30) Dewey WC, Highfield D. Freeman M.L. "Cell biology of hyperthermia and radiation." In Okada S: 6th International Congress Radiat. Research, Tokyo, 1979, 832-841.

(31) Field SB, Bleechen NM. "Hyperthermia in the treatment of cancer." Cancer Treatment Rev 1979;6:63-78.

(32) Field SB. "Cancer therapy by hyperthermia drugs and radiation." The Third International symposium, Fort Collins, CO June 22-26, 1980 p 83 (abstract).

(33) Vaupel P, Ostheimer K, Muller Klieser W. "Circulatory and metabolic responses of malignant tumors during localized hyperthermia." J Cancer Res Clin Oncol 1980; 98:15-26.

(34) Goldin EM, Leeper DB. "The effect of reduced pH on the induction of thermotolerance." Radiology 1981;141: 505-508.Bicher Cancer Institute, Los Angeles, California, U.S.A.

(35) Gerweck LE. "Effects of microenvironmental factors on the response of cells to single and fractionated heat treatments." Natl Cancer Inst Monogr 1982;61:19-26.

(36) Arcangeli G, Cividalli A, Nervi C. "Tumor control and therapeutic gain with different schedules of combined radiotherapy and local external hyperthermia in human cancer." Int J Radiat Oncol BiolPhys 1983; 9:1125-1136.

(37) Scott RS, Johnson RJR, Kowal H, Bicher HI. "Hyperthermia in combination with radiotherapy: A review of five years experience in the treatment of superficial tumors." Int J Radiat Oncol Biol Phys 1983; 9:1327-1334.

(38) Marchosky JA, Morza C, Fearnot N In: 36th Annual Meeting of the Radiation Research Society(Abstract Ch. 7), 1983.

(39) Arcangeli G, Civadalli A, Lovisolo G. "The clinical use of experimental parameters to evaluate the response to combined heat and radiation." In Overgaard J (ed): Proceedings of 4th International Symposium on Hyperthermic Oncology, Vol 1 London. Taylor & Francis, 1984, 329-335.

(40) Scott RS, Johnson RJR, Story KV. "Local hyperthermia in combination with definitive radiotherapy: Increased tumor clearance, reduced recurrence rate in extended followup." Int J Radiat Oncol Biol Phys 1984; 10:19-24.

(41) Vaupel P, Kallinowski F. "Physiological effects of hyperthermia." Recent Results Cancer Res. 1987;104: 71-109.

(42) Valdagni R, Liu FF, Kapp DS. "Important prognostic factors influencing outcome of combined radiation and hyperthermia." Int J Radiat Oncol Bio Phys 1988;15:959-972.

(43) Marchosky JA, Babbs FC, Moran CJ, Fearnot NE, De Ford JA, Welsh DM. "Conductive Interstitial Hyperthermia, a new modality for treatment of intra cranial and tumors in consensus of hyperthermia for the 1990's." Ed. H. I. Bicher et al. Plenum Press N. Y., 1990.

(44) Marchovsky SA, Moran CJ, Fearnot NE. "Hyperthermia catheter implantation and therapy in the brain," J. Neurosurgery. 1990;72:975-980.

(45) Steward FA, Denekamp J. "Fractionation studies with combined x-rays and hyperthermia in vivo." British J of Radiology 1998;56 346-356.

(46) Arcangeli G, Barni E, Cividalli A. "Effectiveness of microwave hyperthermia combined with ionizing radiation: Clinical results on neck node metastases." Int J Radiat Oncol Biol Phys 1980; 6:143.2.

(47) Valdagni R, Amichette M. "Report of long-term follow up in a randomized trial comparing radiation therapy and radiation therapy plus hyperthermia to metastatic lymph nodes in head and neck patients." Int. J. Radiat Oncol, Biol Phys. 1994; 28:163-169.

(48) Datta NR, Rose AK, Kapoor HK. "Head and neck cancers: Results of thermoradiotherapy versus radiotherapy." Int J Hyperthermia 1990; 6:479-485.

(49) Overgaard J, Gonzales GD, Hushof MC, Arcangeli G, Dani O, Mella O, Van der Zee J. "Hyperthermia as an adjuvant to radiation therapy of recurrent or metastatic malignant melanoma. A multicentre randomized trial by the European Society for Hyperthermia Oncology." Int J yperthermia 1996; 12:3-20.

(50) Leopold KA, Dewhirst M, Samuiski T, Harrelson J, Tucker TA, George SL. "Relationships among tumor temperature, treatment time and histopathological outcome using preoperative hyperthermia with radiation in soft tissue sarcomas." Int J Radiat Oncol Biol Phys 1992; 22:989-998.

(51) Hornback R, Shupe RE, Shidnia H. "Advanced stage IIIB cancer of the cervix treatment by hyperthermia and radiation." Gyne Oncol vol 23 Issue 2 February 1986, Pages 160–167

(52) Algan D, Fosmire H, Hynynen K, Dalkin D, Cui H, Drack A, Balddasare S, Cassady JR. "External beam radiotherapy and hyperthermia in the treatment of patients with locally advanced prostate carcinoma. Results of long term follow up." Cancer 2000;89: 399-403.

(53) Kaplan I, Kapp DS, Bagshaw MA. "Secondary external beam radiotherapy and hyperthermia for local resurrence after 125-iodine explanation in adenocarcinoma of the prostate." Int J Radiat Oncol Biol Phys 1991; 20:551-554.

(54) Anscher MS, Sarolski IV, Dodge R, Prosnitz LR, Dewhirts MW. "Combined external beam irradiation and external regional hyperthermia for locally advanced adenocarcinoma of the prostate." Int J Radiat Oncol Biol Phys 1997; 37:1059-1065.

(55) Dr. Peter Wolf, Innovations in biological cancer therapy, a guide for patients and their relatives, Naturasanitas 2008 page 31-33

15. Alternative Cancer Clinics

American Clinics

Medical practitioners within the United States face restrictions from the FDA in the treatment methods they can employ. However, this does not mean that all alternative methods are completely unavailable within American borders. For example, An Oasis Of Healing, and Envita Medical Center, both in Arizona, offer intravenous vitamin C as well as other modalities.

American clinics are usually more expensive than foreign clinics; however, they are clean, well-regulated, and staffed by well-trained professionals.

http://www.anoasisofhealing.com/

http://www.envita.com/

German Clinics

Many cancer patients have heard about German clinics offering alternative cancer treatments. German clinics claim to have high cure rates for many forms of cancer. This is why many American celebrities and politicians, including supposedly President Reagan, have undergone medical treatment in Germany.

German clinics for alternative cancer treatment offer a variety of options including the following:

Acupuncture
Colon Hydrotherapy
Detoxification
Hyperthermia
Oxygen therapy
Ozone therapy Magnetic field therapy
Mistletoe therapy
Naturopathic programs
Neural therapy
Nutritional counseling
Photo dynamic therapy
Thermotherapy
Vitamin C intravenous

Colonic hydrotherapy – may be used for treatment of the colon area and help with general detoxification.

Hyperthermia – high temperatures are used to kill cancer cells in one or more areas of the body. There are different versions of this treatment including whole body hyperthermia and localized hyperthermia.

Fever therapy – similar to hyperthermia but performed by injection. Sometimes the term isn't used as often but gives effects like hyperthermia.

Mistletoe treatment – used to build up the immune system to help fight cancer cells.

Magnetic field therapy – this may not be known by many people but this like mistletoe is used to build up the immune system.

Many of these forms of treatment are not available in the United States. On average, German alternative treatments cost around $25,000, much less than conventional cancer treatment in America.

A German treatment package may, in some cases, include travel and accommodation, and medication costs. Some even provide another bed in the room of the patient to allow them to have a friend or loved one stay during treatment. There are clinics that offer organic foods as part of the diet plan for cancer patients. Many of the clinics are in a private setting, which can be relaxing for patients, with easy access to local airports, shops, and natural scenery.

Many of the German clinics also perform extensive testing including x-rays, ultrasounds, MRIs, and biopsies. Some of the clinics may combine the conventional treatment with the alternative therapy to improve results.

Not only do German clinics have alternative treatment options for cancer, but some also treat other health conditions including spinal disorders, arthritis, weakened immune systems, skin disorders, chronic fatigue, depression, and sleep disorders, to name a few.

Depending on the form of cancer and the treatment option chosen, the duration of the treatment may vary, usually from 4-6 weeks, with additional follow-up in 1 or 2 years after the initial procedure.

Even though some of the clinics offer testing onsite, you may need a physician's referral before being admitted.

Buyer beware: it is important to inquire exactly what is offered at each clinic, since these facilities are independently operated and not as standardized as American cancer treatment clinics, which offer the same three treatments (surgery, chemotherapy and radiotherapy) throughout the nation. **Hyperthermia**, for example, is not offered at all clinics, and it is a very successful treatment. Some German private clinics are not particularly alternative in their approach, and basically offer the same conventional techniques found in North America, along with some holistic side features.

The Issels clinic is probably the most reputable.

Clinics elsewhere in Europe do not have the high reputation of those in Germany. This does not always mean that they are bad, just that little is known about their success rate.

Mexican Clinics

Mexico has various clinics that offer a wide variety of treatments. There are several dozen alternative cancer clinics in Mexico, many of them conveniently located in Tijuana.

Some are run by American alternative practitioners who were harassed by the FDA and subsequently moved their clinics across the border. One example is Hulda Clark, who moved her practice to Tijuana.

Compared to the United States, Mexican regulatory authorities offer much more latitude in regards to allowable treatment options for patients.

Laetrile is still available at many Mexican clinics, though it is illegal in the United States. The Bio-Medical Center (Hoxsey Clinic) in Tijuana, established in 1963, uses Hoxsey herbal extracts and salves.

It supposedly has very good results on skin cancer, including melanoma, and breast cancer.

One large facility is CHIPSA, the base for the Center for Integrative Medicine, a 6 story, 70 bed, full-service hospital located in the beach area of Tijuana, Mexico. They offer lab and x-ray facilities, a pharmacy, physical therapy, and a pediatric ward. Comprehensive care is provided by fully licensed doctors, nurses and consultant medical specialists. This medical center is fully licensed by the city, state and the federal Mexican government authorities. It treats all forms of cancer and as well as other diseases.

The CHIPSA clinic offers the Coley's Toxins modalities, a modified Gerson Diet, enzymes and supplements, vaccine therapy, ozone therapy, hyperthermia, Laetrile, DMSO, chelation and biological dentistry.

A large number of patients who seek treatment through Mexico have already received conventional cancer treatment with unsuccessful results, and because of this, Mexican clinics are accustomed to treating patients with advanced illness. This creates an additional challenge for the clinics, as they must work to undo damage done through conventional treatment, as well as treat the cancer.

An online search for Mexican cancer clinics will pull up multiple listings, often with a list of services offered, along with phone numbers and addresses. Unfortunately, no guarantees are offered about the accuracy of the information, and it is the responsibility of the patient to check out each facility.

Because Mexico is a developing nation, and Americans often do not speak Spanish, extra care and caution is advised when seeking treatment options.

Some areas of Mexico are not kept up as well as others, and some hospitals and clinics may be in run-down areas. It helps to learn the location of the clinic or hospital in question. Patients may be able to tour the facility with staff members during the decision making process.

Because of their high percentage of American clients, most of these clinics have English-speaking staff, but be sure that you can communicate with them to your satisfaction.

There is a possibility of insurance being able to cover some of the costs, but you will have to check with your insurance carrier to see what their policy is regarding foreign coverage.

In many cases patients are required to provide upfront payment at Mexican clinics, since many insurance companies deny claims for Mexican treatment.

Buyer Beware: Mexican clinics have a reputation for inconsistent standards. Many people feel they cannot perform basic tasks well enough to do business, and are just out to part sick patients from their money. Service varies widely from clinic to clinic, so good references are important.

Even though there have been positive testimonials by patients who have gone through treatment, official advice from Canadian and American authorities is to steer clear of Mexican clinics. Statistics regarding success rates are unavailable and mostly unverified.

16. About the authors

This book was written by Johanna Schipper and Frank van der Lugt.

Johanna Schipper spent 5 years training in Medicine and years researching cancer.

Frank van der Lugt is a Chartered Accountant with a Bachelor of Science in Biology. Most members of his immediate family died of cancer. He has spent years researching cancer.

www.ingramcontent.com/pod-product-compliance
Lightning Source LLC
Chambersburg PA
CBHW072031190526
45165CB00017B/16